CW01486675

BRITISH MEDICAL BULLETIN   1995   VOL. 51   No. 3

BRITISH MEDICAL BULLETIN

British Medical Bulletin is published four times each year, in January, April, July and October.

Subscriptions and single-copy orders should be sent to: Pearson Professional Ltd, PO Box 77, Harlow, Essex CM19 5BQ. Tel: 01279 623760. Subscription rates for 1995 are: £134 (Europe), $222 (USA) or £137 (RoW). Single copies will be available at £49.95 (UK)

NEXT ISSUE

BRITISH
MEDICAL BULLETIN

VOLUME FIFTY-ONE
1995

CHURCHILL LIVINGSTONE
EDINBURGH, LONDON, MADRID, MELBOURNE,
NEW YORK, TOKYO AND HONG KONG

CHURCHILL LIVINGSTONE
Medical Division of Pearson Professional Ltd

Distributed in the United States of America by Churchill
Livingstone Inc., 650 Avenue of the Americas, New York,
NY10011, and by associated companies, branches and
representatives throughout the world.

© The British Council 1995

All rights reserved. No part of this publication may be
reproduced, stored in a retrieval system, or transmitted in any
form or by any means, electronic, mechanical, photocopying,
recording or otherwise, without the prior written
permission of the copyright owner, or a licence permitting
restricted copying in the United Kingdom issued by the
Copyright Licensing Agency Ltd, 90 Tottenham Court Road,
London W1P 9HE.

(Copyright in all materials published in *British Medical Bulletin*
prior to 1981 rests with the individual contributors and not with
the British Council.)

ISSN 0007-1420
ISBN 0-443-05335-9

Published by Pearson Professional Ltd
Printed in Great Britain by Bell and Bain Ltd., Glasgow

This journal is indexed, abstracted and/or published online in the following media:
Adonis, Biosis, BRS Colleague (full text), Chemical Abstracts, Colleague (Online),
Current Awareness in Biological Science, Current Contents/Clinical Medicine,
Current Contents/Life Science, Excerpta Medica/Embase, Index Medicus/Medline,
Medical Documentation Service, Reference Update, Research Alert, Science
Citation Index, Scisearch, SIIC-Database Argentina, UMI (Microfilms), USSR
Academy of Sciences

Notes to users in the USA: Authorisation to photocopy items for internal or personal use
is granted by Pearson Professional Ltd provided that the appropriate fees are paid directly to
Copyright Clearance Center, 222 Rosewood Drive, Danvers, Massachusetts 01923, USA. For
more information, please contact CCC. For territories outside North America, permission
should be sought direct from the copyright holder. This consent does not extend to other
kinds of copying, such as copying for general distribution, for advertising and promotional
purposes, for creating new collective works, or for resale.

British Medical Bulletin is published quarterly in January, April, July and October by
Churchill Livingstone c/o Mercury Airfreight International Inc Ltd, 2323 Randolph
Avenue, Avenel, New Jersey 07001. Subscription price is $222.00 per annum. Second Class
Postage paid at Rahway NJ (USPS No. 011-369). Postmaster: Send address corrections to
British Medical Bulletin c/o Mercury Airfreight International Inc Ltd, 2323 Randolph Avenue,
Avenel, New Jersey 07001.

Melanoma

Scientific Editor: *R. M. MacKie*

1995 Vol. 51 No. 3

Professor R M MacKie chaired the committee which included Professsor I Hart, Professor S B Kaye and Mr D Soutar which planned this number of the British Medical Bulletin. We are grateful to them for their help and particularly to Professor MacKie for her work as Scientific Editor.

British Medical Bulletin is published by Churchill Livingstone for The British Council, 10 Spring Gardens, London SW1A 2BN

British Medical Bulletin 1995, Vol 51, No. 3 pp. 523–547
©The British Council 1995

Epidemiology of malignant melanoma

P Boyle[1], **P Maisonneuve**[1], **J-F Doré**[1,2]

[1] *Division of Epidemiology and Biostatistics, European Institute of Oncology, Milan, Italy*

[2] *INSERM, Centre Leon Berard, Lyon, France*

Although cutaneous malignant melanoma is still a relatively rare neoplasm in many populations, incidence rates are increasing in Caucasian populations around the world. The incidence of skin cancer has increased dramatically this century particularly in Northern Europe: the most reliable statistics pertain to malignant melanoma which has doubled in incidence every 10 years in many countries. Indeed the rate of increase has exceeded that of any cancer except for lung cancer in women, although there is some evidence from the United States and Nordic countries that the rate of increase may be slowing in younger cohorts. The incidence of malignant melanoma in the United Kingdom and Germany is now approximately 10 per 100,000 per annum giving an approximate lifetime risk of 1 in 200.

The search for an understanding of the causes of these increases in malignant melanoma focuses on several areas. First of all, there is a strong tendency for melanoma to have a familial component to risk. This may be due to some basic genetic factor or it could be related to the tendency for melanoma risk factors to run in families. Those include red hair, blue eyes, light skin and atypical mole syndromes/dysplastic naevus syndromes and are also determined by genetic factors. The second major factor is that for individuals with no strong genetic susceptibility to malignant melanoma, there may be some environmental factor which is capable of altering the risk of melanoma and leading to the development of a clinical tumour.

A worrying aspect of the trends in melanoma and current understanding of risk factors is that these trends may be exacerbated by further increases in acute exposures to sunshine (sunbathing), and possibly the depletion of the stratospheric ozone layer. Thus, melanoma is identified as one form of cancer which will become very important in public health terms in coming decades in the absence of effective intervention. There are already an estimated 92,000 cases diagnosed world-wide in 1985 which represented 1.2% of the total cancer burden[1] and this burden seems set to increase for the fore-seeable future.

DESCRIPTIVE EPIDEMIOLOGY

Cutaneous malignant melanoma is generally classified into three major histological groups. In white-skinned populations of European origin, the majority are *superficial spreading* or *nodular* melanomas. *Lentigo maligna melanoma* (Hutchinson's melanotic freckle) generally has a peak occurrence later in life than the two major types of the disease. *Acral lentiginous melanoma* has not been studied epidemiologically due chiefly, to its relative rarity in white-skinned individuals: it comprises, however, a substantial proportion of melanomas in the Japanese population.[2] Unfortunately, the distinction between these histological types of melanoma is very rarely made in either descriptive or analytical epidemiological studies.

In many populations, malignant melanoma is as common in women as in men in contrast to non-melanoma skin cancer in which there is a marked male excess.[3] Although reliable population-based information is relatively rare, melanoma is proportionally commonest on the back and face in men and on the legs in women.[4] The incidence of melanoma per unit of body area is approximately similar on sites which are fully exposed to the sun, such as the face, and on partially exposed sites, such as the lower limbs in women and the back in men. The frequency on body sites that are usually covered is much lower.[5]

Geographic variation

Melanoma is essentially a disease of white-skinned individuals where the tumour occurs most frequently on the trunk in males and the lower limbs in females. In these populations the mortality rate has been increasing steadily. The incidence rate varies 100-fold internationally with the highest rates being reported in Australian populations, particularly Queensland, a population of northern European origin close to the Equator, where the rate is approaching 40 per 100,000 per annum. Where long time series are available, incidence rates have been found to be rising almost without exception and now cutaneous malignant melanoma is the leading cause of cancer incidence in white American males aged 35 to 44. Migrants from low-incidence areas (such as Europe) to high incidence areas (such as Australia) have been shown to acquire higher incidence rates than native-born males and females.[6] The incidence and mortality of melanoma are higher in higher socio-economic groups.

Six of the highest incidence rates of malignant melanoma of the skin recorded around the mid-1980s in men are recorded in States of Australia: Capital Territories (28.9 per 100,000), New South Wales (25.9), Western Australia (24.9), South Australia (17.8), Victoria (16.4) and Tasmania (13.6). In Australia, malignant melanoma is now the third or fourth most frequent malignancy in men and women in every State, and it comprises more than ten per cent of all tumours in Queensland and Western Australia. Around the world, there are low rates in black population groups and no cases were recorded during the five year period in Gambia, among Koreans in Los Angeles male blacks in Bermuda and female blacks in Gambia. The regions with the highest rates in women are similar to those with the highest rates in men (Table 1).

Unlike non-melanoma skin cancers, melanoma does not follow an anatomical distribution similar to that of sun exposure,[5] and

Table 1 Highest and lowest incidence rates of malignant melanoma in men and women (circa 1985)

Melanoma of skin, Male ICD9 172 Registry	Cases	Rate	Melanoma of skin, Female ICD9 172 Registry	Cases	Rate
Australian Cap. Terr.	174	28.9	Australian Cap. Terr.	165	25.3
Australia, N S W	4085	25.9	Australia, N S W	3810	23.8
Australia, Western	940	24.9	Australia, Western	911	23.4
US, Hawaii: White	181	22.2	New Zealand: Non-Maori	2053	23.0
New Zealand: Non-Maori	1571	18.6	Australia, South	890	20.3
Australia, South	747	17.9	Australia, Tasmania	242	18.8
Australia, Victoria	1905	16.4	Australia, Victoria	2254	18.0
US, Los Angeles: O. white	2028	14.6	US, Hawaii: White	114	14.9
US, Atlanta: White	490	14.0	Norway	1860	13.5
Australia, Tasmania	167	13.6	Switzerland, Zurich	504	12.1
India, Bangalore	11	0.2	US, Hawaii: Filipino	1	0.3
Japan, Osaka	55	0.2	Singapore: Chinese	12	0.3
US, Alameda: Black	1	0.2	Japan, Osaka	64	0.2
US, Bay Area: Black	2	0.2	India, Bombay	25	0.2
US, Detroit: Black	3	0.2	Kuwait: Kuwaitis	1	0.2
Kuwait: Kuwaitis	1	0.1	Japan, Yamagata	8	0.2
Thailand, Khon Kaen	1	0.1	China, Qidong	4	0.1
The Gambia	0	–	Kuwait: Non-Kuwaitis	2	0.1
US, Los Angeles: Korean	0	–	Algeria, Setif	1	0.1
Bermuda: Black	0	–	The Gambia	0	–

several studies have shown that indoor workers had an increased risk of melanoma.[7] A population-based survey in Australia in 1989 provides important data regarding sub-site distribution.[8] Over all Australia, the incidence rate was higher in men (30.2 per 100,000) than in women (23.9 per 100,000). The highest rates were observed for the male trunk (11.7 per 100,000) and the female lower limbs (8.8 per 100,000) and the most commonly specified morphology was superficial spreading melanoma. 52% of melanomas of **known** thickness were thinner than 0.76 mm with women having proportionately more thin melanoms than men and men having twice the rate of melanomas thicker than 3 mm. In an internal geographical comparison, incidence rates in northern latitudes were double those in the south.[8]

The risk for melanoma is related to latitude in Australia and in the United States, white populations living near the Equator being at higher risk than those living nearer the poles. The situation is less clear in Europe where rates in Scandinavia and Switzerland are higher than those in France or Italy, probably reflecting different skin pigmentation and the importance of intermittent or recreational sunlight exposure. There is a strong social class gradient in risk, non-manual workers being at greater risk of developing malignant melanoma than manual workers.[9]

The risk of melanomas increased for North European migrants to Australia and Israel. In both countries increasing incidence was related to duration of residence,[10,11] but for superficial spreading melanoma, migration to Australia after the age of 20 was not accompanied by an increased risk.

A high proportion of these tumours is found on the lower limbs in white females whereas trunk, head and neck are the most frequently affected sites in males. In African black populations, malignant melanoma tends to occur on the soles of the feet in relation to pre-existing pigmented lesions.[12] A subungual location is more frequent among American Blacks and Asians than among Whites. The high relative frequency of plantar melanoma may reflect a relative absence of malignant melanoma on other parts of the body surface, rather than a raised incidence.

An interesting phenomenon is the difference in the pattern of malignant melanoma in male and female adolescents (aged 10–19).[13] In the largest Cancer Registries of Canada, the SEER Programme of the United States and England and Wales, the incidence rate was found to be approximately two-fold in girls than in boys in the same communities. Further investigation of this, from histological confirmation of the diagnoses to detailed analytical studies of risk factors, could profitably shed some light on risk factors for this disease.

Temporal trends in incidence

A rapid increase has been observed in both sexes almost everywhere in the world (Table 2), even in countries where rates are low, as in Japan.[14,15] The greatest average annual increases are around 6% in the Nordic countries, 7% in New Zealand and as much as 11% in the Jewish population of Israel. Recent findings support the idea that the increase observed in cutaneous malignant melanoma over the past 60 years is real and not due to changes in diagnostic criteria.[16] In Afro-American men in the United States, although there has been an increase of around 3% per annum, the absolute level of incidence remains low; incidence has fallen in Afro-American women.

The consistency of the rapid increase in the incidence rate of malignant melanoma is notable, particularly in those member states of the European Union. Here, the increase averages around 30% every 5 years in both sexes. The highest estimates of the cumulative risk of developing melanoma in the age range 30–74 years are seen for the 1940 birth cohort in the Nordic countries (between 1 and 3%) with rates increasing between 20 and 30% every 5 years while the corresponding risks of dying from malignant melanoma are between 0.2 and 0.6% with rates increasing at around 105 every 5 years. The rates of increase decelerated during the 1980s and this was particularly evident for mortality.[17]

Melanoma incidence among Indian, Chinese and Japanese populations of Asia and Oceania is up to one order of magnitude lower than in Caucasian populations: interestingly there is little evidence of systematic changes in melanoma risk in these populations.[17]

Melanoma incidence has been increasing rapidly since the 1960s in the 5 Provinces of Canada with long term data available. There is still a three-fold difference in cumulative incidence between British Colombia and Quebec. The large differences in melanoma risk between the different racial groups in the United States are widening further. Incidence among Caucasian populations is between 10 and 25 per 100,000 per annum and increasing by 20–40% every five years. The lifetime risk of the 1940 birth cohort is approximately 2–3% in men and 1–2% in women. Incidence rates in Afro-American population groups is typically 10–20 times lower and the rates appear to be stable.[17] In South America, mortality is 3–5 times lower than in North America and no clear pattern of change is evident.

When examination has been made of temporal trends in the inci-

Table 2 Malignant melanoma (ICD-9 172) – Age standardized (world) rates per 100,000 for different time periods in countries or regions covered by a cancer registry

REGISTRY	Vol.1 60–62 M	Vol.2 63–66 M	Vol.3 69–72 M	Vol.4 73–77 M	Vol.5 78–82 M	Vol.6 83–87 M	Vol.1 60–62 F	Vol.2 63–66 F	Vol.3 69–72 F	Vol.4 73–77 F	Vol.5 78–82 F	Vol.6 83–87 F
CANADA, MARITIMES PROVINCES			2.03	3.05	3.95	5.88			2.71	4.18	4.95	6.83
CANADA, NEWFOUNDLAND	1.60	1.13	1.60	2.14	2.88	3.07	2.51	1.41	1.90	1.92	3.07	3.95
CANADA, MANITOBA	1.50	2.13	2.56	2.74	5.29	5.07	1.98	2.58	3.40	4.41	6.51	6.13
CANADA, BRITISH COLUMBIA			3.60	4.98	6.57	9.73			4.76	5.24	8.14	10.74
CANADA, QUEBEC	1.78	1.15	1.39	1.68	2.66	3.00	1.47	1.39	1.76	1.67	2.64	3.17
CANADA, NEW BRUNSWICK	2.25	1.51					2.70	2.83				
CANADA, ALBERTA	2.35	2.21	2.23	3.29	4.08	3.93	1.91	2.62	2.67	4.58	5.11	5.75
CANADA, SASKATCHEWAN	3.04	2.93	2.76	3.11	4.33	6.28	2.05	3.69	3.41	4.89	5.66	6.74
USA, HAWAII, CAUCASIAN	0.80	4.53	6.78	11.80	4.50	6.16	0.00	3.52	5.65	7.48	5.97	7.83
USA, HAWAII, JAPANESE		1.01	0.29	0.09	1.69	0.94		0.23	0.34	0.28	1.17	0.81
USA, HAWAII, CHINESE		3.03	0.00	0.00	0.49	0.79		0.00	0.00	0.00	2.24	0.70
USA, HAWAII, HAWAIIAN	0.32	0.26	0.92	3.42	1.24	0.89	0.00	0.00	1.02	1.32	1.17	0.47
USA, HAWAII, FILIPINO		0.87	0.29	1.58	1.13	0.89		1.15	0.00	0.63	0.85	0.29
USA, UTAH			5.47	6.98	9.84	12.62			5.05	8.03	8.82	11.67
USA, CALIFORNIA, SF BAY AREA, WHITE			6.28	8.42	10.32	13.30			6.55	8.36	9.02	10.95
USA, CALIFORNIA, SF BAY AREA, BLACK			0.90	0.70	0.70	0.18			0.65	0.87	0.70	0.67
USA, CALIFORNIA, ALAMEDA COUNTY, WHITE		3.79	5.35	7.46	9.56	12.29		3.89	5.95	8.18	8.90	10.83

Population										
USA, CALIFORNIA, ALAMEDA COUNTY, BLACK	0.48	0.94	0.77	0.48	1.18	0.19	0.38	0.48	0.67	0.70
USA, IOWA	7.22	6.57	4.65	2.72		8.04	6.33	4.77	3.21	
USA, MICHIGAN, DETROIT, WHITE	7.20	6.36	3.59	3.06		9.03	7.43	4.31	2.75	
USA, MICHIGAN, DETROIT, BLACK	0.40	0.64	0.56	0.60		0.16	0.72	0.55	0.52	
USA, CONNECTICUT			5.41	4.31	3.41			6.69	4.54	3.51
USA, NEW YORK STATE (LESS N-Y CITY)	5.96	5.49	4.40	3.03	3.16	7.79	6.63	5.35	3.38	2.30
USA, WASHINGTON, SEATTLE			0.81	0.77	0.94			0.80	0.72	0.89
COLUMBIA, CALI	2.28	3.00	1.37	1.99	2.65	2.36	3.35	2.40	2.08	3.78
JAMAICA, KINGSTON & ST. ANDREW			1.32	1.06	1.19			0.71	1.42	1.25
JAPAN, MIYAGI PREFECTURE			0.45	0.15	0.20			0.43	0.35	0.31
INDIA, BOMBAY	0.22	0.17	0.20	0.18	0.48	0.25	0.23	0.21	0.17	
SINGAPORE, CHINESE	0.26	0.40	0.45	0.31	0.42	0.40	0.75	0.69	0.60	0.57
SINGAPORE, MALAY	0.51	0.19	0.00	0.00		0.46	1.52	0.68	0.35	
SINGAPORE, INDIAN	0.55	0.36	0.58	0.88		0.34	1.30	0.00	0.35	
ISRAEL, ALL JEWS	8.00	7.41	5.79	4.47	1.68	6.79	5.81	4.50	3.38	1.35
ISRAEL, JEWS BORN IN ISRAEL	11.89	14.48	6.81	6.96	3.06	10.59	8.95	6.01	4.74	2.49
ISRAEL, JEWS BORN IN EUROPE OR AMERICA	9.88	9.33	5.57	4.82	2.11	8.46	7.30	4.73	3.38	1.45
ISRAEL, JEWS BORN IN AFRICA OR ASIA	2.09	1.61	1.28	0.60	0.23	1.61	1.27	1.49	0.94	0.66
ISRAEL, NON-JEWS	0.45	0.43	0.48	0.13	0.18	0.97	0.28	0.81	0.67	0.33
GERMANY (FEDERAL REPUBLIC OF), SAARLAND	4.83	4.25	2.56	2.31		4.77	3.66	2.04	2.28	

Table 2 (continued)

REGISTRY	Vol.1 60–62 M	Vol.2 63–66 M	Vol.3 69–72 M	Vol.4 73–77 M	Vol.5 78–82 M	Vol.6 83–87 M	Vol.1 60–62 F	Vol.2 63–66 F	Vol.3 69–72 F	Vol.4 73–77 F	Vol.5 78–82 F	Vol.6 83–87 F
GERMANY (FEDERAL REPUBLIC OF), HAMBURG	0.00	0.00	2.43	2.44	3.95		0.00	0.00	1.83	1.49	4.61	
SWITZERLAND, GENEVA			3.87	7.55	8.88	8.70			1.80	6.29	9.58	8.59
SPAIN, ZARAGOZA		1.52	0.33	1.04	2.18	2.32		2.17	0.28	0.52	1.38	1.98
YUGOSLAVIA, SLOVENIA	1.26	1.82	1.82	1.94	2.36		1.43	2.16	2.88	2.04	2.73	
GERMAN DEMOCRATIC REPUBLIC		1.98	2.14	2.30	2.89	3.78		2.35	2.28	2.72	3.57	4.42
HUNGARY, VAS		1.38	1.76	3.71	3.45	4.73		1.25	2.07	2.87	3.68	4.64
POLAND, WARSAW CITY			2.32	2.54	2.19	3.30			2.08	2.25	2.12	2.75
DENMARK	1.56	2.34	2.88	4.59	5.92	7.68	2.21	3.15	4.89	6.22	8.43	9.83
FINLAND	1.89	2.43	2.85	3.85	4.70	6.60	2.07	2.04	2.84	3.80	4.90	5.97
ICELAND	0.68		1.57		2.70	3.45	1.77		3.57		5.04	5.75
NORWAY	2.73	3.59	5.37	7.51	8.89	10.47	2.56	4.04	5.73	9.10	10.54	13.51
SWEDEN	2.37	3.02	4.10	5.20	7.23	9.54	2.77	3.37	4.93	5.66	8.23	9.60
UK, ENGLAND, TRENT REGION (SHEFFIELD)		1.02	1.07	1.60	2.35	2.54		1.53	1.51	2.29	3.19	4.61
UK, ENGLAND, OXFORD REGION	1.09	1.22	2.16	2.20	2.67	3.55	2.07	2.61	3.11	3.61	4.79	6.45
UK, ENGLAND, SOUTH THAMES REGION			1.65	2.11	2.55	3.48			2.84	3.93	4.33	5.79
UK, ENGLAND, SOUTH WESTERN	1.17	1.41	1.62		3.23	5.34	2.27	3.31	4.02		6.53	9.33
UK, ENGLAND, BIRMINGHAM	0.93	1.10	1.29	1.35	1.56	2.78	1.56	1.83	2.21	2.48	3.35	5.35
NEW ZEALAND, NON-MAORI		6.22	7.36	12.33	15.58	18.58		9.06	11.66	18.83	21.45	23.03
NEW ZEALAND, MAORI		0.82	1.50	3.01	3.74	1.96		3.50	1.54	1.59	1.30	3.86

Source: *Cancer Incidence in Five Continents Volumes I, II, III, IV, V and VI.*

dence of melanoma by sub-site of the body among birth-cohorts there have been several notable observations. There have been marked increases in melanoma of the skin of the trunk, particularly in men, and increases of melanoma of the leg and arm, particularly in women.[18-25] Examination of the data from Connecticut showed a 12–16 fold increase in melanoma of the skin of the upper arm and forearm in both sexes but much smaller increases in melanoma of the hand.[25] These different effects for different sub-sites in men and women are consistent with the influence of local effects of some environmental exposure which differs between the sexes.

Temporal trends in mortality

Not all available data regarding the international distribution of mortality rates from malignant melanoma can be presented, but data from 9 countries have been chosen to be representative of the international trends in mortality from malignant melanoma.

In **Canada**, both the truncated and overall age-adjusted mortality rates from malignant melanoma of the skin have been increasing since 1955 and in both males and females. Examination by birth cohorts shows an increase in rates in successive birth cohorts for almost all age groups examined in both males and females.

In **Japan**, although the mortality rates of malignant melanoma are very low, a consistent increasing trend has been observed for the truncated and overall age-adjusted mortality rates in both the males and females during the past decades. Examination by birth cohorts suggests an increase in rates in successive birth cohorts for almost all age groups examined in both males and females.

In **Czechoslovakia**, both the truncated and overall age-adjusted mortality rates have been increasing rapidly since 1955 and in both males and females. Examination by birth cohorts shows a sizeable and regular increase in rates in successive birth cohorts for all the age groups examined in both males and females.

In **Poland**, both the truncated and overall age-adjusted mortality rates show an increasing, if unchanged, trend since 1961 in both males and females. Birth cohort examination suggests an increase in rates in successive birth cohorts for most of the ages in males and females.

In **Germany**, both the truncated and overall age-adjusted mortality rates have been increasing since 1955 although the increase is more rapid in males than in females. Examination by birth cohorts shows a rapid increase in rates in successive birth cohorts for all the age groups examined in both males and females.

In **Denmark**, although the mortality rates showed a relatively large year to year variation (particularly for female age truncated mortality rates), a general increasing trend in rates is clear for both males and females since 1955. Birth cohort examination indicates an increase in rates in successive birth cohorts for most of the age groups examined in both males and females.

In **Italy**, both the truncated and overall age-adjusted mortality rates increased after 1955 in both males and females. However, the rates seem to have stabilised since 1981 (especially the overall age-adjusted mortality rates). Examination by birth cohorts shows a rapid increase in rates in successive birth cohorts for all the age groups examined and in both sexes.

In **Australia**, both the truncated and overall age-adjusted mortality rates increased after 1955 in both males and females. However, the increase in rates is much more dramatic in males. Birth cohort examination shows that in males a consistent increase in rates in successive birth cohorts for ages over 50. For ages below 50, the increase from recent birth cohorts seem to have slowed down. A similar birth cohort pattern was observed in females.

Discrepancy between incidence and mortality

In many countries there are large increases taking place in the incidence rates of malignant melanoma but more modest increases apparent in the mortality rates. For example, a five-fold increase in incidence in Sweden since 1960 has been accompanied by a much lower increase in mortality rate. This immediately leads to questions being raised about changes in survival[27] and the possible role of changes in prognostic factors through time being responsible for this phenomenon. A multivariate analysis of a random sample of patients in the Swedish Cancer Registry has recently revealed that there are a number of variables which are of prognostic significance. For example, women had a reduction of one-third in their mortality rate than men after every other prognostic factor had been taken into account. There was an increased mortality rate for melanomas of the external ear, scalp and neck and trunk-located melanomas. Regional metastases and tumour thickness remained independent prognostic indicators.[28]

In an attempt to investigate possible explanations for the discrepancy in incidence and mortality trends described above, temporal changes in the most important histological prognostic factor (tumour thickness) have been investigated recently. Comparing 574 cases of malignant melanoma recorded in the South Swedish Health

Care Region in 1965, 1976 and 1985, review of the histopathology revealed that in 71 instances a diagnosis of invasive cutaneous malignant melanoma could be rejected: this represents 13% of the evaluable material in this population-based study (26 cases were excluded because the sample collection or evaluation was not possible). Among the remainder, there was no significant decrease of tumour thickness of the invasive cutaneous malignant melanoma nor any changes in the level of invasion.[29] From these data, the discrepancy between the rates of increase of incidence and mortality from malignant melanoma could not be explained by the removal of melanoma of lesser thickness.[29]

Migration studies

Native residents of Australia[30,31] and New Zealand,[32] who themselves are mainly of British origins, experience incidence and mortality rates of malignant melanoma roughly twice those of recent British immigrants. Native Israelis have been shown to have a risk at least twice that of immigrants to Israel from Europe for at least three decades following immigration.[33] Differences in skin colour are attributed as being the reason underlying the higher incidence of melanoma found in white immigrants to Hawaii from the United States mainland.[34] Non-Hispanic migrants to Los Angeles County (California) from higher latitudes in the United States appear to be substantially protected against melanoma for decades following migration.[35]

Socio-economic status and occupation

Malignant melanoma is substantially more common in higher socioeconomic groups. In the United Kingdom, the distribution of melanoma in married women by social class is similar to that of men indicating that this may be a social rather than an occupational effect (the social class of a married women is determined by her husband's occupation).[36] Assessment of outdoor exposure on the basis of routine data on job descriptions showed that melanoma is commoner in indoor than in outdoor workers, even within the same socioeconomic group.[9] Cutaneous melanoma incidence rates during 1972–1976 in New Zealand revealed no pattern according to outdoor workplace[37] whereas analyses from England and Wales and Sweden suggested an elevated incidence among professional occupations.[38] Garland et al.[39] performed an analysis of malignant melanoma among United States Navy personnel and noted that the rate for indoor occupation was higher than that for outdoor workers.

ANALYTICAL EPIDEMIOLOGY

Wide geographic variation and increasing trends in the incidence and mortality from malignant melanoma of the skin have been reported from many population groups around the world.[17] There is at least a component of the remarkable changes in risk which are apparently real.[15] A detailed review of thousands of histological slides from centres in nine countries around the world from 1930, 1955 and 1980 identified the tendency for increasing uniformity of diagnosis with the passage of time and strongly suggests that little (if any) of the observed increase in the incidence of malignant melanoma could be simply explicable by changes in the diagnostic criteria for the classification of malignancy of pigmented cell lesions.[16] The generality of the increase in incidence and mortality from malignant melanoma is so striking that the exceptions to this increase which are present in Asian populations are notable.

Genetic susceptibility and host factors

Melanoma is known to have a familial component and blue eyes, fair or red hair and a pale complexion have been demonstrated to increase risk. Furthermore, individuals who sunburn easily are at an increased risk, the association being particularly strong for sunburn in childhood. Freckles, either in childhood or as an adult, are also associated with increased risk. Because these traits also tend to run in families it is difficult to determine whether the familial tendency for melanoma is due to genetic characteristics or to the related risk factors.

Malignant melanoma may appear to cluster in families with family cancer syndromes where there is clearly a predisposition to a variety of different tumours. However, there are a number of families which seem vulnerable to malignant melanoma alone. In the majority of such families the tendency to melanoma is associated with the presence of abnormal melanocytic naevi, the atypical mole syndrome (AMS) phenotype.[40] The cumulative 10 year risk of developing malignant melanoma in cases of AMS has recently been estimated at 10.7%[41] and was greater than expected in a second recent study.[42] There are also a number of families whose members are susceptible to melanoma but have normal naevi. At the present time, segregation analysis does not support a predisposition by a single dominant gene as an explanation for the AMS/melanoma syndrome and there has not yet been a single gene for melanoma defined. Loss of heterozygosity studies have suggested that there may be a tumour suppressor gene important in familial melanoma on chromosome 9 although it is not yet clear what percentage of familial melanoma may be attributable to this gene.[40]

The number of naevi is an indication of malignant melanoma risk, and there is strong evidence that melanocytic naevi are strongly associated with melanoma risk and are possibly precursors of melanoma. White et al.[43] performed a case-control study involving 256 cases and 273 controls in Washington State (United States). Sun sensitivity was found to be the host factor most closely associated with the risk of malignant melanoma: this was measured as reaction to chronic exposure to sun (OR = 9.0, 95% C.I. (3.8,21) for no tan referred to deep tan) or reaction to acute exposure to sun (OR = 5.7, 95% C.I. (2.6,12.6) for severe burn referred to tan). The number of raised naevi counted on both arms by the subject was also associated with an increased risk of melanoma (OR = 5.7, 95% C.I. (2.2, 15) for 10 or more referred to none). Sun exposure in adulthood and occupational exposure were not found to be related to the risk of melanoma[43] while increased vitamin E intake decreased risk and risk appeared to increase with obesity.[44] The authors hypothesised that the ability to develop a tan during childhood could reduce the risk of melanoma by offering protection from the effects of sunlight exposure.[43]

Melanocytic naevi have been identified as the most important phenotypic risk factor for malignant melanoma and there has been recent activity directed at a better epidemiological understanding of this topic. A case-control study from Germany, involving 513 cases and 498 controls, revealed that the most important risk factor for melanoma was the presence of large numbers of melanocytic naevi: the odds ratio was 7.6 for more than 100 naevi compared to the referent group of 10 or less.[45] Elevated odds ratios were also found for atypical melanocytic naevi (OR = 6.1 for at least 5 melanocytic naevi versus none), the number of actinic lentigines (OR = 3.5 for many compared to none), hair colour, skin type and reported melanocytic naevus growth. Interestingly, this same study reported no significant association between the risk of malignant melanoma and a large number of sun exposure parameters.[45] Whole body examination and diagnosis of pigmented lesions was recommended as an effective strategy for the identification of individuals at a high risk of malignant melanoma.[42]

In a recent study, a total of 1123 school-children in 3 Australian cities (Melbourne, Sydney and Townsville) aged 6, 9, 12 and 15 years of age were surveyed by the same group of medical observers.[46] The towns were selected to cover a wide rage of latitudes. The prevalence of melanocytic naevi was found to increase with decreasing latitude particularly among the younger children aged 6 and 9. Although the numbers of naevi were higher among children with light skin and fair hair, blue eyes and freckling the latitude gradient remained after adjustment for these and other factors. The authors concluded that latitude of residence is strongly related to naevus prevalence in young Australian children although these differences appear to diminish with age: the association with latitude of residence is held to implicate ambient ultra-violet radiation in the aetiology of melanocytic naevi.

A comparative study of naevi in school children (between 13 and 15) in Glasgow (Scotland) and Brisbane (Australia) was undertaken to examine the distribution of naevi in sub-tropical and tropical environments on children of similar ethnicity.[47] Children in Brisbane had significantly more naevi than those in Glasgow after adjustment for complexion variables with a greater difference apparent among boys than girls. In view of the results obtained by Kelly et al.[46] it may be more fruitful to extend this comparison to younger subjects, where the differences could be expected to be greater, although the data from Fritischi et al.[47] provide some evidence in support of the theory that naevus development is related to the level of sun exposure in childhood and adolescence.

Even in individuals with AMS many cutaneous melanomas do not arise in an existing naevus. Thus the presence of melanocytic naevi may be a clear indicator of an individual at high risk of developing malignant melanoma and, at the same time, may be the best surrogate of sun exposure in childhood.

Host factors

A large number of studies generally conclude that individuals with blue eyes (compared to brown eyes), fair or red hair (compared to brown or black hair), freckles (compared to no freckles) and fair skin (compared to olive or dark skin) are associated with an increased risk of malignant melanoma.[11,20,48–52] It is essential that these factors be measured and used as a basis for adjustment when sun-related variables are being assessed.

Epidemiological studies of sunlight and malignant melanoma

The descriptive epidemiology of melanoma suggests that exposure to sunlight is a major cause of the disease in susceptible populations but it is apparent from analytical studies that the association between exposure to sunlight and risk of melanoma is complex.

Evidence has accumulated that the major aetiological factor for melanoma is excessive exposure to sunlight. The first major piece of evidence for this is that melanoma is essentially a disease of white skinned peoples (fair skin being more susceptible to the ill effects of sunlight): the incidence of melanoma for example in Japan being only 0.2 per 100,000 person years. Furthermore, although the incidence of melanoma has increased annually in white peoples in Europe, the United States, Canada, Australia etc. there has been very little increase in incidence amongst pigmented peoples of African or Asian origin.

Second, there is a relationship between latitude and incidence of melanoma in white populations. The incidence of melanoma for example is highest in countries like Australia (50 per 100,000 per annum) and in hotter regions of the United States such as Southern Arizona. Furthermore there is a relationship between the length of time that an individual has lived at lower latitudes and risk of melanoma, presumably representing lifetime accumulated excessive exposure to the sun.

Third, case control studies within Europe have identified intense intermittent exposure to the sun recreationally as a risk factor for melanoma. Several studies have for example identified high social class, indoor occupation, sunburn and sunbathing holidays as risk factors for melanoma reinforcing the view that at least in some populations the relationship between risk of melanoma and sun exposure is not a simple cumulative one.

The simplest form of classification of sun exposure should come from details of occupations which are performed essentially outdoors (e.g. farmers, fishermen, forestry, construction industry etc.). The indicators from these studies are that melanoma risk may be greater among professional workers and among those who work indoors. Analytical studies of malignant melanoma which have examined occupation generally reveal that the risk appears to be reduced once host factors, especially skin colour, is taken into account.

The large number of studies which have investigated the role of sunlight exposure to the risk of malignant melanoma have been excellently reviewed in detail in the recent International Agency for Research on Cancer (IARC) Working Party on the *Carcinogenicity of Solar and Ultraviolet Radiation*.[53] Results are generally consistent with positive associations with residence in sunny environments throughout life, in early life and even for short periods in early adult life. Positive associations are generally seen between measurements of cumulative sun damage expressed biologically as micro-topographical changes or history of keratoses or non-melanoma skin cancer (IARC, 1992).

In contrast to the results from migrant studies involving all age groups,[30] the risk of malignant melanoma among migrants to Australia who arrive before the age of ten is as high as for native-born Australians.[11] There appears to be a risk associated with having lived at a southerly latitude in the United States[50,54] and there appears to be an increased risk associated with living near the coast in Australia[55] and in Denmark.[21] In the latter two studies it is assumed that living near the coast will involve more exposure to the sun and different behavioural patterns vis-à-vis sun exposure among such residents.

A history of non-melanoma skin cancers, solar keratoses, actinic tumours or changes on cutaneous microtopography are all indicators of cumulative sun exposure. Positive associations have been observed with these variables in studies conducted in Australia[56] and the United States[57,58] although not in Denmark.[21]

Associations with the risk of malignant melanoma and total exposure to the sun over a lifetime or in recent years are inconsistent.[53] This inconsistency may well be due to differences in the effects of chronic sun exposure and intermittent sun exposure on melanoma risk. Chronic sun exposure, as assessed through occupational exposure, appears in the larger studies, with the most detailed exposure assessment, to reduce the risk of melanoma (although not in a consistent manner) especially in men[11,21,59,60] in a way similar to the descriptive epidemiology.

Unlike non-melanoma skin cancers, melanoma does not follow an anatomical distribution similar to that of sun exposure and several studies have shown that indoor workers had an increased risk of melanoma. The 'intermittent sun exposure hypothesis' has been put forward to explain this.[61] This postulates that the incidence of melanoma is determined as much (or more) by the pattern of sun exposure as by the total accumulated 'dose' of sun exposure and that infrequent (intermittent) exposure of untanned skin to high doses of sunlight is particularly effective in increasing the incidence of melanoma. It is very difficult to assess **intermittent sun exposure**: this exposure has generally been assessed by posing questions about specific activities that would be likely to represent relatively severe intermittent exposure such as sunbathing, holidays in sunny places, or to seek information about recreational or holiday exposures. Despite this difficulty, however, most studies agree in showing positive associations with melanoma risk and exposure patterns consistent with intermittent sun exposure.[53] In Canada, positive associations were found between melanoma risk and recreational and holiday sun exposures in activities involving intense sun exposure such as beach activities.[59,60] In Denmark, increased risks were associated with regular participation in activities such as sunbathing, boating, skiing, swimming and vacations in sunny places.[20,21] In a multicentric European study, recreational exposure to sunlight emerged as an independent risk factor.[62] Weaker and less consistent associations were apparent in the large Australian study.[63,64]

Most studies show positive associations between melanoma risk and a history of sunburn (IARC, 1992): a straightforward interpretation of this association is complicated since it may equally likely reflect the tendency of an individual to sunburn, if exposed, or general intermittent sun exposure as it could a true effect of sunburn *per se*. **Severe sunburn** has usually been defined as a burn which causes pain lasting for at least two days and/or accompanied by blistering. A history of sunburn indicates unusually intense sun exposure and skin sensitivity and therefore both questions must be assessed in any study to make the data meaningful. The large studies from Canada,[59] Australia[63,64] and Europe[62] could demonstrate that the association was primarily with tendency to burn rather than with the history of sunburn itself. In marked contrast, equally good-quality studies have demonstrated a strong association between melanoma risk and sunburn history which persisted after controlling for tendency to burn and other measures of skin sensitivity.[21,57,65] The positive association between an additional effect of sunburn in childhood and melanoma risk has been questioned by a recent meta-analysis.[66]

Artificial sources of ultraviolet radiation include sunlamps and sunbeds, which are being increasingly used to maintain a year-round tan in many countries. Positive associations have been demonstrated between duration of use of sunbeds and sunlamps and the risk of malignant melanoma from two studies which have collected detailed exposure assessment.[67,68] Studies with generally smaller sample sizes and less detailed exposure assessments have not produced consistent support for this association.[53] Several studies have reported positive associations between the risk of malignant melanoma and exposure to fluorescent lighting, another potential source of ultraviolet exposure. The quality of the studies which have produced these positive associations[59,60,69,70] differs little from those studies which produced null findings on this association.[71,21] It is difficult to reach a simple conclusion regarding this association from the available data.

Possible aetiological mechanisms of cutaneous melanomas

Epidemiological studies, both descriptive and analytical, tend to show that melanomas are more frequent in sun sensitive individuals, with poor ability to tan and sensitivity to sunburns, with numerous moles and who may develop freckling as a result of sun exposure. However, as indicated in the above, the relationship between sun exposure and melanoma risk is more complex than the simple accumulation of exposures and almost certainly involves intense and intermittent exposure in adulthood as well as acute exposure in childhood.

Mutagenic and oncogenic activities of solar ultraviolet radiation are well documented and their responsibility in skin ageing and the induction of squamous cell carcinomas of the skin in experimental animals and in humans is well established.[53] However, the precise mechanism(s) by which solar ultraviolet might influence melanoma in man as well as the active wavelengths (action spectrum) are far from being fully unravelled.

Epidemiological studies in man show a complex but almost certain influence of sun exposure and rarely suspect the role of chemical carcinogens in the development of melanoma. Inversely, in experimental conditions melanocytic naevi and melanomas are easily induced in rodents following exposure to the carcinogen dimethylbenz(a)anthracene but exceptionally following exposure to ultraviolet light.[72] The promotional effect of ultraviolet radiation was demonstrated in several animal models where rodents were submitted to DMBA treatment: see for review Doré et al.[73] However, three recently developed experimental models may prove of value in the study of the role played by ultraviolet light in melanoma induction.

Invasive melanomas were induced in a marsupial, the South American opossum (*Monodelphis domestica*), following **chronic** exposure to ultraviolet light. 10 weeks after termination of irradiation (3 times a week for 70 weeks, 250 J/m^2 UV-B) 70% of treated animals developed melanomas.[74]

Hybrid fishes from backcrosses of interspecies hybrids of the genus *Xiphophorus* are exquisitely sensitive to melanoma induction following UV irradiation. In this model, short range UVB (280–320 nm), but also longer range UVA (320–400 nm) and even visible light were able to induce melanoma.[75]

Mintz[76] previously showed that melanocytic naevi and melanomas spontaneously develop in transgenic mice harbouring an activated oncogene under the control of the tissue specific promoter of the tyrosinase gene. This group recently showed that brief UVB irradiation (323 mJ/cm^2 on 4 consecutive days) of 4 day-old mice from the melanoma susceptible transgenic strain TyrSV40E induces in most animals melanocytic naevi that subsequently transform into invasive melanomas.[77]

The ultraviolet spectrum is divided into three sections by wavelength: ultraviolet C (100–280 nm), ultraviolet B (280–315 nm) and ultraviolet A (315–400 nm). The biological effects of these three types of radiation are compared in Table 3. It is clear that in experimental animals, there is sufficient evidence that each one of UVA and UVB and UVC is carcinogenic to experimental animals.[53] Thus, it is difficult to conclude which of these types of irradiation is carcinogenic to humans in view of the lack of clear guidelines from animal experiments and the inability to measure the cumulative lifetime exposure (and the intermittent exposure etc., etc.) in individuals. This has important implications for health recommendations regarding sunscreen use (see below).

One of the most dramatic human syndromes associated with defects in DNA repair mechanisms is *Xeroderma Pigmentosum* which is associated with an ultra-sensivity to the effects of ultraviolet light. Among these patients (there are approximately 800 identified and followed world-wide) malignant skin neoplasms were present in 70% at a median age of 8 years: 57% had non-melanoma skin cancers and 22% had a malignant melanoma.[78] This median age was 50 years younger than the general population. These findings clearly demonstrate the importance of DNA repair mechanisms in the aetiology of malignant melanoma and should point to future priorities for laboratory studies.

Table 3 Biological effects of ultraviolet radiation

Biological Effect	UVC	UVB	UVA
Tanning: immediate and transient	–	–	+ +
Tanning: delayed and prolonged	+	+ + +	+ +
Sunburn	+ +	+ + +	+
Thickening of epidermis	+ + +	+ +	–
Dermal elastosis	–	+ +	+ +
Vitamin D3	–	+ + +	–
Mutations of cells in culture	+ + +	+ +	+
Squamous cell, carcinoma in mice	+ +	+ + +	+

Adapted from Dore et al (1990)[73]

Prospects for prevention

The recent IARC Working Party concluded that: (1) there is sufficient evidence in humans for the carcinogenicity of solar radiation which causes cutaneous malignant melanoma as well as non-melanoma skin cancer; (2) there is limited evidence for the carcinogenicity of exposure to ultraviolet radiation from sunlamps and sunbeds; and (3) there is inadequate evidence in humans for the carcinogenicity of fluorescent lighting. Solar radiation is carcinogenic to humans although the precise contributions of ultraviolet A, ultraviolet B and ultraviolet C are not yet defined.[53]

Although the incidence of melanoma is still not very high in comparison to the more common tumours, a major aetiological factor in its causation has, therefore, been identified. In Europe, the increase in incidence has been linked with the desire to be suntanned which has been fashionable since the 1930's. It would seem imperative that if the trend to increasing numbers of melanoma patients is to be reversed, then we have to reverse these fashion trends. Use of artificial sources of ultra-violet (UV) exposure such as sunbeds should therefore be similarly discouraged.

The question of precisely what pattern of sun exposure is most harmful is not fully answered. The observations that at least in Northern Europe indoor workers get melanoma rather than their outdoor working compatriots along with the case control data above suggest that intermittency is crucial, i.e. it is the cycle of being white in the winter, red in the spring and brown in the summer which is harmful. The immunological ill effects of sunburn may be crucial here. However, there is undoubtedly evidence, particularly from Australia that total cumulative overdosage of sunlight is also important. Sun induced non-melanomatous skin lesions such as basal cell carcinomas and actinic keratoses (which have a simple relationship with cumulative sun exposure) for example are significant risk factors for melanoma. It is likely then, that the health education messages should be *avoid sunburn* and *reduce your total cumulative dosage of sun exposure*: the latter is another way of saying 'don't tan'.

It is not clear either what exactly could be the benefit of sunscreen against the risk of melanoma: whereas it may be used to block certain types of ultra-violet light from reaching the skin, it may allow an increased exposure to other types which may be harmful. UVA, UVB and UVC are all considered as carcinogenic to experimental animals.[53] In some case-control studies use of sunscreens has been associated with and increased risk of malignant melanoma.[52,64,79] This latter study took steps to exclude the possible bias induced by individuals who use sunscreens because they get easily sunburned or expose themselves heavily. Wolf et al.[80] demonstrated that protection against sunburn does not necessarily imply protection against other possible ultraviolet radiation effects such as enhanced melanoma growth in C3H mice and concluded from their experiment that sunscreen protection against UV radiation-induced inflammation may encourage prolonged exposure to UV radiation and thus may lead to increases in the risk of melanoma development. It is obvious that further research on the ability of sunscreen to influence the risk of melanoma is required.

There is some evidence that excessive sun exposure is particularly deleterious in youth and childhood. Migration studies of immigrants to Australia and Israel have for example shown a significantly greater risk of melanoma for adults born there. Furthermore case control studies linking sunburn to risk of melanoma have (although not universally) identified sunburn under the age of 15 years as particularly significant. Finally there was some evidence from the only prospective study, the United States Nurses Health Study,[81] that early excessive sun exposure was more significant in terms of risk of melanoma than sun in adult life. It is therefore necessary that prevention messages should specially address the question of sun protection for children.

ACKNOWLEDGEMENTS

This work was conducted within the framework of support from the Associazione Italiana per la Ricerca sul Cancro (Italian Association for Cancer Research).

REFERENCES

1 Parkin DM, Pisani P, Ferlay J. Estimates of the world wide incidence of eighteen major cancers in 1985. Int J. Cancer 1993; 54: 594–606.
2 Elwood JM. Epidemiology and control of melanoma in white populations and in Japan. J Invest Dermatol 1989; 92: 214S–221S.
3 Parkin DM, Muir CS, Whelon SL, Gao YT, Ferlay J, Powell J. Cancer Incidence in Five Continents, Vol. VI. IARC Scientific Publication 120, Lyon: IARC 1992.
4 Crombie IK. Distribution of malignant melanoma on the body surface. Br J Cancer 1981; 43: 843–849.
5 Elwood JM, Gallagher RP. Site distribution of malignant melanoma. Can Med Assoc J; 1983; 128: 1400–1404.
6 Armstrong BK, Wooding TL, Stenhouse NS et al. Mortality from cancer in migrants to Australia 1962–1971. NH & MRSC Research Unit in Epidemiology and Preventive Medicine, University of Western Australia, Australia, 1983.
7 Beral V, Robinson N. The relationship of malignant melanoma, basal and squamous skin cancer to indoor and outdoor work. Br J Cancer 1981; 44: 886–891.
8 Jelfs PL, Giles G, Shugg D, et al. Cutaneous malignant melanoma in Australia, 1989. Med J Aust 1994; 161: 182–189.

9 Lee JAH, Strickland D. Malignant melanoma—social status and outdoor work. Br J Cancer 1980; 41: 757–763.

10 Morshovitz, M, Modan B. Role of sun exposure in the etiology of malignant melanoma—epidemiologic inferences. J Nat Cancer Inst 1973; 51: 777–779.

11 Holman CD, Armstrong BK. Pigmentary traits, ethnic origin, benign nevi, and family history as risk factors for cutaneous malignant melanoma. J Natl Cancer Inst 1984a; 72: 257–266.

12 Lewis MG. Malignant melanoma in Uganda. The relationship between pigmentation and malignant melanoma on the soles of the feet. Br. J Cancer 1967; 21: 483–495.

13 Boyle P, Maisonneuve P. Epidemiology of cancer in adolescents. In: Bailey F, Selby P. Cancer in adolescents. Oxford: Blackwell Scientific Press, (in press).

14 Muir CS, Nectoux J. Time-trends, malignant melanoma of the skin. In: k Magnus ed. Trends in cancer incidence. 1982 pp. 365–385.

15 Armstrong BK, Kricker A. Cutaneous melanoma In: Gallagher RP, Elwood JM, eds. Epidemiological aspects of cutaneous malignant melanoma. Boston: Kluwer Academic, 1994, pp 219–240.

16 Van der Esch EP, Muir CS, Nectoux J. et al. Temporal change in diagnostic criteria as a cause of the increase of malignant melanoma over time is unlikely. (submitted for publication).

17 Coleman MP, Esteve J, Damiecki P, Arslon A, Renard H. Trends in cancer incidence and mortality. IARC Scientific Publications 121, IARC, Lyon, 1993.

18 Boyle P, Day Ne, Magnus K. Mathematical modeling of malignant melanoma in Norway, 1953–1978. Am J Epidemiology 1983; 118: 887–896.

19 Osterlind A, Jensen OM. Increasing incidence of trunk melanoma in young Danish women. Br J Cancer 1987; 55: 467.

20 Osterlind A, Tucker MA, Hou-Jensen et al. The Danish case-control study of cutaneous malignant melanoma. I. Importance of host factors. Int J Cancer 1988a; 42: 200–206.

21 Osterlind A, Tucker MA, Stone BJ et al. The Danish case-control study of cutaneous malignant melanoma. II. Importance of UV-exposure. Int J Cancer 1988b; 42: 319–324.

22 Thorn M, Bergstrom R, Adami HO, Ringborg U. Trends in incidence of malignant melanoma in Sweden, by anatomic site. 1960–1984. Am J Epidemiol 1990; 132: 1066–1077.

23 Mackie R, Hunter JA, Aitchison TC et al. Cutaneous malignant melanoma, Scotland 1978–89. The Scottish Melanoma Group. Lancet 1992; 339: 971–975.

24 Gallagher RP, Ma B, McLean DI, et al. Trends in basal cell carcinoma, squamous cell carcinoma and melanoma of the skin from 1971 through 1987. J Am Acad Dermatol 1990; 23: 413–421.

25 Dubrow R, Flannery JT, Liu WL. Time trends in malignant melanoma of the upper limb in Connecticut. Cancer 1991; 68: 1854–1858.

26 Scotto J, Pitcher H, Lee JAH. Indications of future decreasing trends in skin melanoma mortality among white males in the United States. Int J Cancer 1991; 49: 490–497.

27 Thorn M, Adami HO, Bergstrom R, Ringborg U, Krusemo UB. Trends in survival for malignant melanoma: remarkable improvement in 23 years. J Natl Cancer Inst 1989; 81: 611–617.

28 Thorn M, Ponten F, Bergstrom R, Sparen P, Adami HO. Clinical and histopathologic predictors of survival in patients with malignant melanoma—A population-based study in Sweden J Natl Cancer Inst 1994; 86: 761–769.

29 Masback A, Westerdahl J, Ingvar C, Olsson H, Jonsson N. Cutaneous malignant melanoma in South Sweden 1965, 1975, and 1985 – A Histopathologic review. Cancer 1994; 73: 1625–1630.

30 McCredie M, Coates MS. Cancer incidence in Migrants to New South Wales, 1972 to 1984. New South Wales Central Cancer Registry, Woolloomooloo, NSW, New South Wales Cancer Council, 1989; pp. 22–23, 62–63.

31 Khlat M, Vail A, Parkin M, Green A. Mortality from melanoma in migrants to Australia: variation by age at arrival and duration of stay. Am J Epidemiol 1992; 135: 1103–1113.

32 Cooke KR, Fraser J. Migration and death for malignant melanoma. Int J Cancer 1985; 36: 175–178.

33 Steinmet R, Parkin DM, Young JL, Bieber CA, Katz L. Cancer Incidence in Jewish Migrants to Israel, 1961–1981. IARC Scientific Publications No. 98. Lyon: IARC 1989; pp. 114–115, 134–135.

34 Hinds MW, Kolonel LN. Malignant melanoma of the skin in Hawaii, 1960–1977. Cancer 1980; 45: 811–817.

35 Mack TM, Floredus B. Malignant melanoma risk by nativity, place of residence at diagnosis, and age at migration. Cancer Causes Control 1991; 2: 401–411.

36 Lee JAH. Melanoma and exposure to sunlight. Epidemiol Rev 1982; 4: 110–136.

37 Cooke KR, Skegg DCG, Fraser J. Socio-economics status, indoor and outdoor work, and malignant melanoma. Int J Cancer 1984; 34: 57–62.

38 Vagero S, Swerdlow A, Beral V. Occupation and melanoma: cancer registrations in England and Wales in England and Wales and in Sweden. Br J Indust Med 1990; 47: 317–324.

39 Garland FC, White MR, Garland CF, Shaw E, Gorham ED. Occupational sunlight exposure and melanoma in the US Navy. Arch environ Health 1990; 45: 261–267.

40 Newton JA. Genetics of melanoma. Br Med Bull 1994; 50: 677–687.

41 Marghoob AA, Salopek TG, Slade J, Kopf AW. Solar nevogenesis: A surrogate for predicting a rise in incidence of malignant melanoma because of ozone depletion. J Am Acad Dermatol 1994; 31: 134–135.

42 Kang Sw, Barnhill RL, Mihm MC, Fitzpatrick TB, Sober AJ. Melanoma risk in individuals with clinically atypical nevi Arch Dermatol 1994; 130: 999–1001.

43 White E, Kirkpatrick CS, Lee JAH. Case-control of malignant melanoma in Washington State. 1. Constitutional factors and sun exposure. Am J Epidemiol 1994; 139: 857–868.

44 Kirkpatrick CS, White E, Lee JAH. Case-control study of malignant melanoma in Washington State. 2. Diet, alcohol, and obesity. Am J Epidemiol 1994;139: 869–880.

45 Garbe C, Buttner C, Weiss J, et al. Risk factors for developing cutaneous melanoma and criteria for identifying persons at risk—multicenter case-control study of the central malignant melanoma registry of the German Dermatological Society. J Invest Dermatol 1994; 102: 695–699.

46 Kelly JW, Rivers JK, Maclennan R, Harrison S, Lewis AE, Tate BJ. Sunlight— A major factor associated with the development of melanocytic nevi in Australian schoolchildren. J Am Acad Dermatol 1994; 30: 40–48.

47 Fritischi L, Mchenry P, Green A, Mackie R, Green L, Siskind V. Naevi in schoolchildren in Scotland and Australia. Br J Dermatol 1994; 130: 599–603.

48 Lancaster HO, Nelson J. Sunlight as a cause of melanoma: a clinical survey. Med J Aust 1957; 1: 452–456.

49 Elwood JM, Gallagher RP, Hill SB, Spinelli JJ, Pearson, JCG, Threlfall. W. Pigmentation and skin reaction to sun as risk factors for cutaneous melanoma: Western Canada Melanoma Study. BMJ. 1984; 288: 99–102.

50 Graham S, Marshall J, Haughey B, et al. An inquiry into the epidemiology of melanoma. Am J Epidemiol 1985; 122: 606–619.

51 Dubin N, Moseson M, Pasternack BS. Sun exposure and malignant melanoma among susceptible individuals. Environ Health Perspectives 1989; 81: 139–151.

52 Beitner H, Norell SE, Ringborg U, Wennersten G, Mattson B. Malignant melanoma: aetiological importance of individual pigmentation and sun exposure. Br J Dermatol 1990; 122: 43–51.

53 International Agency for Research on Cancer (IARC) Monographs on the Evaluation of Carcinogens. Solar Radiation, vol. 55. Lyon: IARC, 1992.

54 Weinstock MA, Colditz GA, Willett WC, et al. Nonfamilial cutaneous melanoma

incidence in women associated with sun exposure before 20 years of age. Pediatrics 1989; 84: 199–204.
55 Green A, Siskind V. Geographical distribution of cutaneous melanoma in Queensland Med J Aust 1983; 1: 407–410.
56 Holman CD, Armstrong BK. Cutaneous malignant melanoma and indicators of total accumulated exposure to sun: An analysis separating histogenetic type. J Natl Cancer Inst 1984b; 73: 75–82.
57 Green A, O'Rourke MGE. Cutaneous malignant melanoma in association with other skin cancerns. J Natl Cancer Inst 1985; 74: 977–980.
58 Holly EA, Kelly JW, Shpall SN, Chiu SH. Number of melanocytic nevi as a major risk factor for malignant melanoma J Am Acad Dermatol 1987; 17: 459–468.
59 Elwood JM, Gallagher RP, Davidson J, Hill GB. Sunburn, suntan and the risk of cutaneous malignant melanoma: the Western Canada Melanoma Study. Br J Cancer 1985a; 51: 543–549.
60 Elwood JM, Gallagher RP, Hill GB, Pearson JCG. Cutaneous melanoma in relation to intermittent and constant sun exposure: the Western Canada Melanoma Study. Int J Cancer 1985b; 35: 427–433.
61 Armstrong BK. Epidemiology of malignant melanoma: intermittant or total accumulated exposure to the sun? J Dermatol Surg Oncol 1988; 14: 835–839.
62 Autier P, Doré JF, Lejeune F et al. EORTC Malignant Melanoma Cooperative Group. Recreational exposure to sunlight and lack of information as risk factors for cutaneous malignant melanoma. Results of an EORTC case-control study in Belgium, France and West Germany. Melanoma Res 1994; 4: 79–85.
63 Holman CD, Armstrong BK, Heenan PJ. Relationship of cutaneous malignant melanoma to individual sunlight-exposure habits J Natl Cancer Inst 1986a; 76: 403–414.
64 Holman CD, Armstrong BK, Heenan PJ, Blackwell JB, Cumming FJ et al. The causes of malignant melanoma: results from the West Australian Lions Melanoma Research Project. Recent Results Cancer Res 1986b; 102: 18–37.
65 MacKie Rm, Aitchison T. Severe sunburn and subsequent risk of primary cutaneous malignant melanoma in Scotland. Br J Cancer 1982; 40: 955–960.
66 Whiteman D, Green A. Sunburn and melanoma. Cancer Causes Control 1994; 5: 564–572.
67 MacKie RM. Freudenberger T, Aitchison TC. Personal risk-factor chart for cutaneous melanoma. Lancet 1989; ii: 487–490.
68 Walter SD, Marrett LD, From L, Hertzman C, Shannon HS, Roy P. The association of cutaneous malignant melanoma with the use of sunbeds and sunlamps. Am J Epidemiol 1990; 131: 232–243.
69 Beral V, Evans S, Shaw H, Milton G. Malignant melanoma and exposure to fluorescent lighting at work. Lancet 1982; ii: 290–293.
70 Swerdlow AJ, English JSC, MacKie RM, et al. Fluorescent lights, ultraviolet lamps, and risk of cutaneous melanoma BMJ 1988; 297: 647–650.
71 English DR, Rouse IL, Xu Z, et al. Cutaneous milagnant melanoma and fluorescent lighting. J Natl Cancer Inst 1985; 74: 1191–1197.
72 Kripke ML. Effects of UV radiations on tumor immunity. J Natl Cancer Inst 1990;82: 1392–1396.
73 Doré JF, Muir CS, Clerc F. Soleil et Mélanome. Analyse des risques de cancers cutanés. Moyens de prévention. Paris, INSERM/La Documentation Française, 1990.
74 Ley et al, 1989
75 Setlow RB, Woodhead AD. Temporal changes in the incidence of melanoma: explanation from action spectra. Mutat Res 1994; 307: 365–374.
76 Mititz (1992).
77 Kleinszanto AJP, Silvers WK, Mintz W. Ultraviolet radiation-induced malignant skin melanoma in melanoma-susceptible transgenic mice. Cancer Res 1994; 54: 4569–4572.
78 Kraemer KH, Lee MM, Andrews AD, Lambert WC. The role of sunlight and

DNA repair in melanoma and non-melanoma skin cancer – The xeroderma pigmentosum paradigm. Arch Dermatol 1994; 130: 1018–1021.

79 Autier P, Doré JF, Schifflers E et al. for the EORTC Malignant Melanoma Cooperative Group. Use of sunscreens and the risk of cutaneous malignant melanoma: an EORTC case-control study in Belgium, France and Germany. Melanoma Res (in press).

80 Wolf P, Donawho CK, Kripke ML. Effect of Sunscreens of UV Radiation-Induced Enhancement of Melanoma Growth in Mice. J Natl Cancer Inst 1994; 86: 99–105.

81 Weinstock MA, Colditz GA, Willett WC, et al. Melanoma and the sun: the effect of swimsuits and a 'healthy' tan on the risk of nonfamilial malignant melanoma in women. Am J Epidemiol 1991; 134: 462–470.

British Medical Bulletin 1995, Vol 51, No. 3 pp. 548–569
©The British Council 1995

Cutaneous melanoma: pathology, relevant prognostic indicators and progression

A Slominski, J Ross and M C Mihm

Department of Pathology and Laboratory Medicine, Albany Medical Center, Albany, New York, USA

Malignant melanoma, one of the most rapidly increasing malignancies in man, has recently received substantial attention in the world literature concerning application of traditional morphologic and newer immunologic and molecular biologic methods of predicting progression and ultimate clinical outcome. Although clinical features of patient sex, age and anatomic site of the lesion are important, classic morphologic variables defining prognosis remain the cornerstone of predicting disease outcome. Extent of radial growth phase and the two microstaging methods of measuring tumor thickness and determining level of invasion remain the critical disease progression predictors. Assessment of mitotic rate, number of tumor infiltrating lymphocytes, and determining the presence of regression, ulceration, and epithelioid cell component, microscopic satellites and vascular invasion are also important. More recently a variety of molecular and biochemical prognostic markers have been cited for prediction of disease recurrence and metastasis. Both overexpression and down regulation of a variety of cell adhesion molecules have been implicated in disease progression as has alterations in the plasminogen activation system. A series of growth factors, growth factor receptors, oncogenes and tumor suppressor genes have also been considered. Structural and numerical genomic DNA abnormalities, cell proliferation markers and DNA ploidy status have also been considered. Recently a variety of serum and blood markers indicating disease persistence or progression have been studied including melanin synthesis precursors and intermediate compounds of melanogenesis. Molecular detection by PCR of melanogenesis specific mRNA may become the most sensitive prognostic marker of the future. At present histopathologic and clinical criteria remain the cornerstones of predicting prognosis in malignant melanoma.

Over the last decade, cutaneous malignant melanoma has been one of the most rapidly increasing malignancies in humans[1] and its incidence is predicted to rise with the further depletion of the ozone layer.[2] Melanoma frequently affects young adults and is refractory to currently established methods of therapy once metastases have occurred.[1-6]

Melanocytes derive from the neural crest cells that during embryonal development differentiate toward melanoblasts along their migration to the skin in a pathway marked and modified by mesenchyme.[7] After reaching the dermis, they migrate to the epidermis or hair follicle and differentiate, respectively, towards epidermal or follicular melanocytes or remain within the dermis and differentiate into nevomelanocytes.[7] The traditionally recognized function of epidermal melanocytes has been production and transfer of melanin granules to surrounding keratinocytes within an 'epidermal melanin unit'.[8] However, recent evidence supports the concept that epidermal melanocytes act as sensory and regulatory cells, which detect external signals and disturbances in cutaneous homeostasis, and translate them into organized biological responses.[9] Unstimulated epidermal melanocytes in vivo are mitotically inactive or can proliferate briefly after selected external signals such as UV radiation.[7-9] The follicular melanocytes on the other hand, are characterized by cyclic proliferative and melanogenic activity that is strictly coupled to the growing phase of the hair follicle (anagen) and determine the color of the mature hair shaft.[10] The function of dermal nevomelanocytes is currently unknown. In addition to the migratory and proliferative activity, which normally occur as described above, melanocytes or melanocyte-derived cells form one of the most common benign tumors of the body, the melanocytic nevus.[5] It has been suggested that cutaneous melanomas derive in approximately 70% from epidermal melanocytes, 30% from nevomelanocytes[11] but not from follicular melanocytes.

Based on clinical, histopathologic, immunological and genetic properties 5 stages of progression in the melanocytic system have been defined:[3]

1. Benign melanocytic nevi, which are characterized only by an abnormal growth pattern without cytologic atypia and have low propensity toward malignant transformation with the exception of the congenital nevus;
2. Dysplastic nevi with architectural and cytological atypia that can be considered as potential precursors to melanoma;
3. Radial growth of primary malignant melanoma;
4. Vertical growth phase of primary malignant melanoma;
5. Metastatic melanoma.

In this paper we will discuss characteristics of melanoma in relation to their prognostic values.

EVOLUTION OF MELANOMA IN RELATION TO PROGNOSIS

General overview

Histopathologic and clinical criteria have been used for staging melanoma to determine prognosis and treatment. The traditional system recognizes 3 stages of melanoma. These are stage I, localized disease without evidence of lymph node involvement; stage II, in which melanoma is present in regional lymph nodes; and stage III, that is characterized by distant metastases.[3–6,11] The 5 year survival rate declines as the stage of melanoma increases with an approximate survival rate of 79%, 36% and 5% for stage I, II and III, respectively. Since approximately 80% of melanoma patients present with stage I disease, the American Joint Committee on Cancer (AJC) has recommended a 4 stage system in which stages I and II indicate localized growth according to tumor thickness, stage III, tumor thickness greater than 4 mm, presence of satellites within 2 cm or involvement of regional lymph nodes, while stage IV indicates distant metastases (Table 1). The similar TNM classification issued by the UICC in 1978 and 1987 has found general acceptance in German speaking countries.[12]

Within stage I and II the 5 year survival depends on the level of microinvasion according to Clark levels or the measured tumor

Table 1   AJC staging system for melanoma

Stage	Primary tumor	Metastases
I	pT1	N0, M0
	pT2	N0, M0
II	pT3	N0, M0
III	pT4	N0, M0
	every pT4	N1 or N2, M0
IV	every pT	every N, every M

pT1: tumor ≤0.75 mm thick and/or Clark's level II
pT2: tumor 0.76–1.5 mm thick and/or Clark's level III
pT3: tumor 1.51–4.0 mm thick and/or Clark's level IV
   (a) tumor 1.51–3.0 mm thick
   (b) tumor 3.01–4.0 mm thick
pT4: tumor >4.0 mm thick and/or Clark's level V
   (a) tumor >4.0 mm thick and/or invasion of subcutaneous tissue
   (b) satellites within 2 cm of primary tumor
N0: regional lymph node metastases undetectable
N1: regional lymph node metastases ≤3 cm
N2: regional lymph node metastases >3 cm and/or in transit metastases
   (a) regional lymph node metastases >3 cm
   (b) in transit metastases
   (c) a and b
M0: metastases undetectable
M1: distant metastases
   (a) in skin, subcutaneous tissue or lymph nodes beyond regional nodes
   (b) visceral metastases
Sources: Balch et al 1992.[6]

thickness defined by Breslow[cf. 13,14] (Table 2). In general, when tumor thickness or level of microinvasion increase the predicted 5 year survival decrease with a 100% curability for melanoma *in situ* and 47% 5 year survival for melanoma of >4 mm thickness.[3–6,11–13] Other histologic criteria for stage I and II melanoma are mitotic rate, presence of tumor infiltrating lymphocytes (TIL), tumor cell type, vascular invasion, microscopic satellites, ulceration and regression. Clinical criteria include age, sex, anatomic site and involvement of regional lymph nodes (Table 2). The histomorphometry of melanomas is limited by lack of standarized criteria and the heterogeneity of tumors, and the validity of vascular invasion as a prognostic feature is hampered by interpretive difficulties and the presence of tissue artifacts.[11]

LOCALIZED MELANOMA (stages I and II according to AJC)

Prognosis of malignant melanoma according to the traditional subtypes

The prognosis for stage I and II disease correlates with the traditional melanoma subtype with better prognosis (5 year survival time) for

lentigo maligna melanoma (LMM) and superficial spreading melanoma (SSM) (85% to 90%) than for nodular melanoma (NM)(65%)
and acral-lentiginous melanoma (ALM).[3, 11] These types of melanoma are distinctive processes and most likely have different etiol-
ogies.[3-6,11] LMM (Fig. 1A), which accounts for 5% of melanomas
in Caucasians, is limited to the markedly sun exposed skin.[3-6,11] It is
characterized by a prolonged period of intraepidermal or radial
growth phase (RGP). This RPG is comprised of pleomorphic
melanocytes that are confined to the basal region of a markedly
atrophic epidermis. There is usually marked solar elastosis in the
dermis and a chronic inflamatory infiltrate. SSM (Fig. 1B and C),
which constitutes 70% of melanomas in Caucasians, is characterized
by a proliferation of malignant melanocytes in the epidermis with
similar morphologic features.[3-6,11] The intraepidermal growth in
SSM is usually of considerably shorter duration than in LMM.
The characteristic cells of the intraepidermal growth phase have
prominent nuclei with variable cytoplasm filled with fine melanin
granules. The other type of malignant melanoma with a RGP is
ALM (Fig. 1D). ALM constitutes 2–8% of melanomas in Caucasians
and is the most common form of melanoma in dark-skinned persons
that involves palms, soles and nail beds.[3-6,11] The histology is similar
to LMM in that atypical melanocytes are confined to the dermal-
epidermal junction. However, in ALM the epidermis is usually hyperplastic. The melanocytes have large uniformly atypical appearance
with prominent dendrites; the large cytoplasms of the cells are usually

---

Fig. 1 Pathological subtypes of malignant melanoma.

A. *Lentigo maligna melanoma.* In this markedly sun damaged skin there is a striking
proliferation of predominantly spindle shaped nevomelanocytes that form large
intraepidermal nests. Multifocal superficial invasion is present at the sites of the
chronic inflammatory host response.

B. *Superficial spreading melanoma in situ.* Note the extent of uniformly atypical cells
throughout the entire epidermis reaching to the granular cell layer. The cells are
predominantly singly disposed, although small nests of cells are present.

C. *Invasive superficial spreading melanoma.* This large expansile nodule of mixed
epitheliod and spindle shaped cells extends to the dermis from the epidermis in which
pagetoid cells can be noted. Note the striking coalescence of the many nests forming
the vertical growth phase.

D. *Acrolentiginous melanoma.* Large cells containing markedly hyperchromatic nuclei
and large cytoplasmic masses as evidenced by clear spaces are present along the basal
region in this biopsy taken from the sole of the foot. Dendritic processes are strikingly
prominent extending upward to the mid spinous layer. Note scattered cells in pagetoid
array.

E. *Nodular melanoma.* This polypoid excrescent lesion shows multifocal intraepidermal origin sites overlying the dermal tumor nodule composed of malignant
melanocytes. There is no lateral spread away from the tumour component.

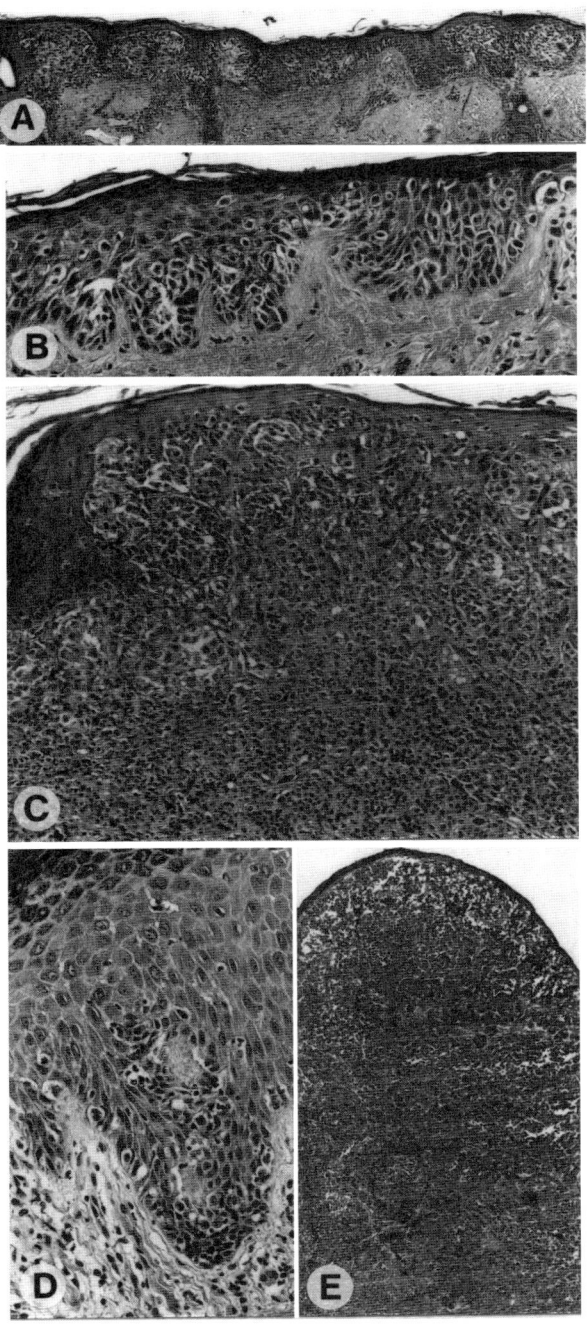

Table 2 Prognostic variable for localized melanoma (stage I and II according to AJC)

Variables	Categories	Effect on prognosis
HISTOLOGIC		
*Tumor thickness (mm):	<0.76	**93.2% of 8-yr survival
	0.76–1.69	**85.6% of 8-yr survival
	1.70–3.60	**59.8% of 8-yr survival
	>3.60	**33.3% of 8-yr survival
Levels of invasion:	I (intraepidermal)	**100% of 8-yr survival
	II (into papillary dermis)	**96.3% of 8-yr survival
	III (filling papillary dermis)	**76.1% of 8-yr survival
	IV (into reticular dermis)	**60.7% of 8-yr survival
	V (into subcutaneous fat)	**38.5% of 8-yr survival
RGP vs. VGP	–	Greater probability of metastases with VGP
*Mitotic rate (per mm^2)	0.0	**95.0% of 8-yr survival
	0.1–6.0	**79.4% of 8-yr survival
	>6.0	**38.2% of 8-yr survival
*TIL	brisk	**88.5% of 8-yr survival
	nonbrisk	**75.0% of 8-yr survival
	absent	**59.3% of 8-yr survival
*Regression	–	Increased risk for metastasis in tumors <1.0 mm with marked regression
*Ulceration	–	worse prognosis with ulceration >3.00 mm
Predominant cell type:	Spindle, small, other epithelioid	**86.4% of 8-yr survival **67.7% of 8-yr survival
Microscopic satellites	absent	**75.2% of 8-yr survival
	present	**40.0% of 8-yr survival
Vascular invasion	–	worse prognosis when present
Nodular growth	absent	**91.7% of 8-yr survival
	present	**65.2% of 8-yr survival
CLINICAL		
*Sex	–	women have better prognosis than man
*Anatomic site	–	better prognosis for lesions on extremities vs. head and neck area, palms, and soles
Age	–	morbidity and mortality with increasing age

*Independent values in some multivariate analyses
**Adapted from Clark et al. 1989[13]
Source: Barnhill, Mihm, Fitzpatrick, Sober 1993[3]; Balch et al. 1992[6]; Clark et al. 1989[13]; Mihm and Googe 1990[14a]

associated with prominent clear space surrounding them. This type of melanoma has more agressive behavior than LMM according to some authors.[3–6] The radial growth phase in LMM, SSM and ALM can be completely cured when surgically removed. It is only when a tumor enters the vertical growth phase (VGP), it acquires a significant potential for metastases. In fact, the survival time of VGP is inversely correlated with depth of invasion.[3–6,11,13] NM (Fig. 1E) has a frequency of 10–15% in Caucasians and is characterized by pure vertical growth phase disease.[3–6,11] It has no prolonged intraepidermal growth phase or RGP as an intraepidermal process before invasion occurs. Rather, as soon as the intraepidermal component appears, invasion takes place directly into the dermis with the formation of VGP. It should be emphasized that the classification of malignant melanoma into the above subtypes is a clinical-pathologic classification. While the histology is in most instances clearly identifiable for each type, clinical correlation is usually required for the most accuracy in subtyping. The prognosis depends on the type of growth and the type of invasion with good prognosis for RGP and poor prognosis for VGP that has a markedly deep measured depth of invasion.

Prognosis of malignant melanoma according to stage of evolution in radial and vertical growth phases

The simplified concept, favored by us, proposes that primary melanoma progresses through 3 steps: *in situ* RGP, invasive RGP and VGP or 'tumorigenic melanoma'.[13–15] The RGP of melanoma describes a step in the evolution of this malignant melanocytic process in which the malignant cells are confined almost exclusively to the intraepidermal component (*in situ* RGP, cf. Fig. 1B) and show single cell invasion or invasion by small nests of the papillary dermis (invasive RGP), thickness <0.76 mm in 97% or invasion at level II in 93%. The nests of cells in the epidermis and papillary dermis are similar in size and number (no more than 5–10 melanoma cells). They may be arranged either along the dermo-epidermal junction replacing the basilar region and/or may be present in pagetoid spread. Their cytology in the epidermis and the papillary dermis is similar. Mitoses are frequent in the epidermal but rare in the papillary dermal component. The nests do not form expansile aggregates. A host inflammatory response of lymphocytes is commonly present in the papillary dermis associated with the RGP. It is noteworthy that occasionally single cells may infiltrate into the upper reticular dermis. These cells are present only in the most superficial fibers of the RGP. This change does not confer VGP characteristics on the RGP. The RGP melanoma has metastasis-free survival for up to 13.7 years.[14,14a]

The VGP describes an expansile nodule of cells which distorts the papillary dermis (Fig. 1C). The cells in the nodule or nodules are in greater number than those in the intraepidermal component. The cytology of the cells is frequently different from those in the overlying epidermis. For example, the intraepidermal component may be composed of epithelioid cells with very fine melanin granularity, and the expansile nodule's VGP may show spindle cells or small epithelioid cells or a mixed pattern. Mitotic figures are variably present. Extension of the cells into the reticular dermis and even subcutaneous fat may be observed. The dermal nodules in the VGP are larger than the intraepidermal nests.

A pathological pattern has been suggested as the early VGP. Clinically, this lesion is different from the RGP, which is usually a flat or slightly elevated plaque and strikingly different from the fully evolved VGP, which is usually a prominent nodule. In the early VGP, a small papulonodule supervenes in the RGP. It is usually of a dark coloration and may even be blue/black in comparison to the admixture of brown/tan, pink/white observed in the RGP lesion. Histologically, there is a small expansile aggregate of cells in the papillary dermis. These cells are of different type than those in the RGP and their number (often 20–25) is larger than in epidermal nests. Mitotic figures may be observed.

The significance of these patterns of development of melanoma has direct relationship to prognosis. It appears clear that the RGP lesion, when excised with a margin of about 1 cm, is completely cured. The VGP lesions are excised with a margin up to 1.5 cm or greater, depending on the measured depth. The survival is directly related to the measured depth of invasion as well as other prognostic factors, including sex, age, anatomic site, and the presence of regression and a variable inflammatory infiltrate (tumor infiltrating lymphocytes: TILs). Melanoma cells in the VGP have the competence for metastatic spread.[13–14a]

In Clark's model,[13] the TILs are lymphocytes which infiltrate into the tumor nodule. Tumor cell lymphocyte satellitosis may be described as brisk, non-brisk and absent but further work is needed to establish the significance of this variable (See Fig. 2) (personal communications: Elder D, 1992; Clemente C, 1993).

Towards defining new prognostic markers

Melanoma at different stages of progression has not only different macroscopic and histological presentations but also is characterized by a distinctive antigenic profile.[15] For example, an antigenic profile in the RGP is similar to dysplastic nevi (DN), but changes in the VGP becoming closer to that of metastatic melanoma.[15] An effort

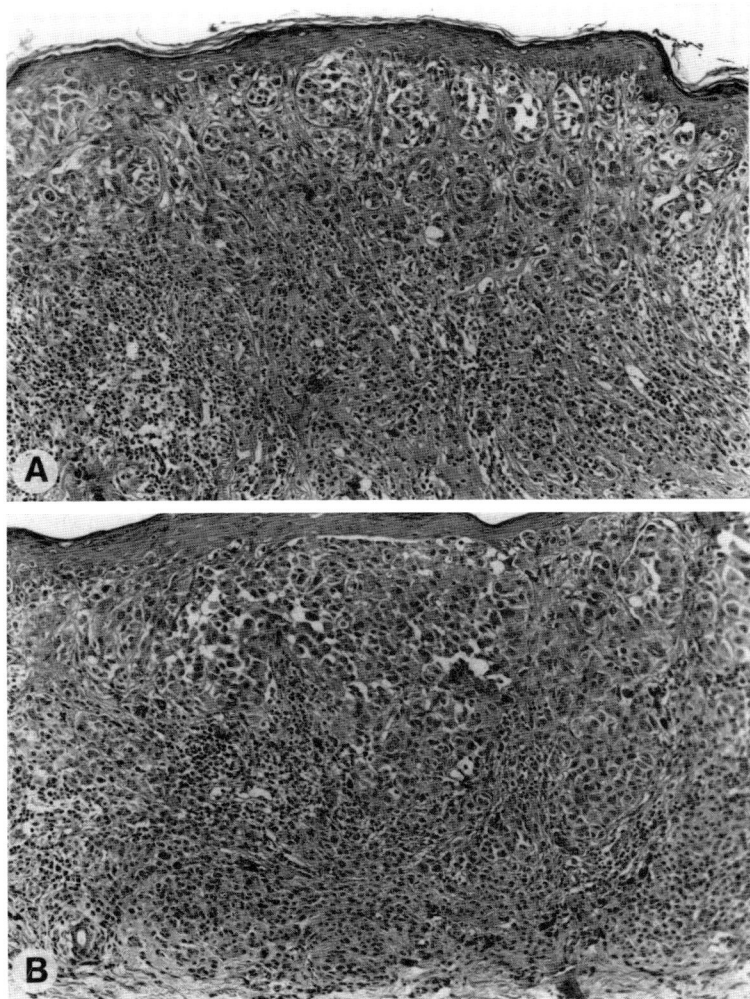

Fig. 2 Tumor infiltrating lymphocytes (TILs).
A. *Brisk response*. TILs are noted throughout the base of this vertical growth phase nodule.
B. *Non-brisk response*. Note the presence of TILs focally within the tumor nodule.
C. *Summary panel*. ABSENT: the lymphocytes are actually present but do not infiltrate the melanoma. Thus, they may be present along the base, in perivenular array but not extending into the tumor or stroma within the nodule. 'Absent' is also used for those cases where there are not lymphocytes in association with any part of the vertical growth phase. NON-BRISK: TILs are present in one or more foci of the vertical growth phase. BRISK: TILs are present throughout the substance of the vertical growth phase or present and infiltrating across the entire base of the vertical growth phase. Adapted from Clark et al. 1989.[13] and personal communications: Elder D, 1992; Clemente C, 1993. Large hollow ovals = melanoma cells; solid black dots = lymphocytes; grey circles = blood vessels.

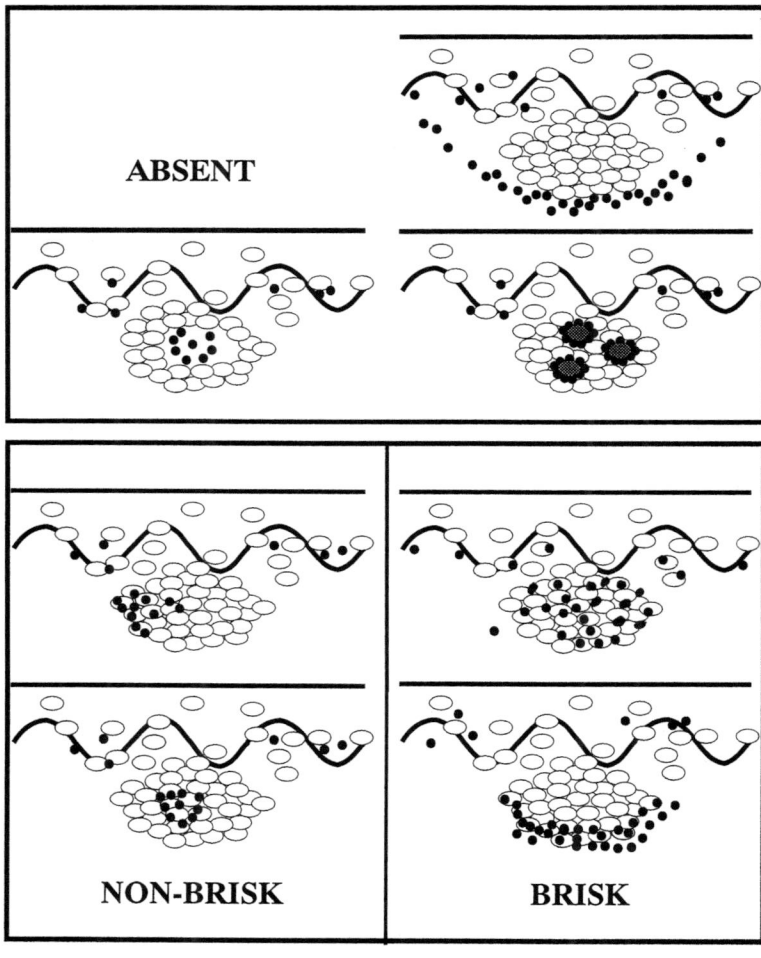

C

Fig. 2C (see previous page for details)

has, therefore, been undertaken to develop new molecular and bio-chemical prognostic markers of melanoma. Many of such markers have been proposed and include: cell adhesion molecules and related molecules, HLA antigens, melanoma and melanocyte differentiation markers, proteases, migration-associated molecules, angiogenesis related factors, glycosphingolipids, cytokines, growth factors, peptide hormones and their receptors, oncogenes and tumor suppressor genes, and metabolic factors.[15–33] Although these studies have been reviewed extensively,[3,5,11,16,22,28-30] no clear distinction has been made between phenomena specific to human disease and those operating only in animal or in vitro models. In this discussion we will analyse these observations briefly within the limits of human stage I and II disease with particular emphasis on those markers that have potential to act as prognostic variables in a particular clinicotherapeutic setting. The metastatic phenomenon is detailed in the following section.

One group of markers including HMB45 and tyrosinase, ultrastructural presence of melanosomes, expression of S100 protein, and other melanocyte specific proteins is already used in diagnosis of pigmented lesions.[3-6,16,27] Although there is no clear relationship between expression of melanocyte specific proteins and malignant behavior, recent findings that tyrosinase, gp100, MART 1/Aa, and Pmel17 can be classified as MHC class I-restricted tumor antigens[34-37] suggest that their expression in relation to specific human haplotype may be used as a guide for potential immunotherapy. The first possibly therapeutically useful model derives from the fact that specific peptides for these antigens are presented to CD8+ cytotoxic T cells (CTL) by HLA-A1 and HLA-A2 molecules.[34-37] The continuously growing family of MHC class I-restricted melanoma antigens include also MAGE proteins, which are expressed on melanoma cells but not melanocytes.[38]

HLA Class I and HLA Class II molecules, which present antigens and activate CD8+ and CD4+ lymphocytes, respectively, are expressed on melanoma cells.[5,16] It has been suggested that decrease in the HLA class I expression or changes in its specific subclasses may be associated with a progressive development of melanoma.[5,16] Specifically, a selective loss of HLA-A2 and/or A28 was described for 21% of the primary and 44% of metastatic melanoma.[21] Within HLA Class II molecules, it has been reported that the expression of HLA-DR and DP on melanoma cells increased with progression from the radial to vertical and metastatic growth phases.[5,16,17,29] It has been reported that the number of antigen presenting Langerhans cells (LC) increase around in situ and early invasive melanoma and decline around deeply invasive melanoma or cutaneous metastases.[39] Although these individual events may not neccessarily correlate with the degree of tumor progression, a pattern of their expression in a particular context may provide clinically useful information and be a guide for immunotherapy. For example HLA-A2 patients with melanoma presenting MHC class I restricted antigens to CD8+ lymphocytes should have a good prognosis, if we accept that their presence is an evidence of the intact loop necessary to recruit and expand CTL.

The stimulation of antibody production against cell surface antigens is the second immunotherapeutic approach tested intensively
in several laboratories. Gangliosides are promising candidates for
development of anti-melanoma vaccines.[5,16,22] The pattern of their
expression changes with tumour progression and includes increased
expression of GD3, GD2, GM2 and an appearance of GT3 and 9–
0–Ac-GD3.[5,16,22,40,41] Unfortunately, the expression of the particular
fraction of gangliosides in localized or metastatic lesions is
heterogenous and their proper identification requires additional
analyses such as high-performance thin-layer chromatography
(HPTLC).[42] Therefore, ganglioside pattern cannot be used as a diagnostic marker of melanoma progression. However, the analysis for
the presence of a particular fraction of gangliosides, e.g. GD2, GD3,
0–Ac-GD3 or GM2 should have a strong predictive value in the
context of immunotherapy using anti-ganglioside antibodies or
potential immunization with ganglioside containing anti-melanoma
vaccine.[22,30,40–44]

Additional potential diagnostic markers of melanoma
are high molecular weight melanoma-associated antigens
(HMWMAA),[16,23,24] such as calcyclin which shows stronger
expression in metastatic melanomas or melanomas with higher Clark
levels,[45] and neuroglandular antigen CD9 where expression appears
to be inversely related to metastatic potential of melanoma.[46] The
relationship between progression and a CD63 antigen seems to be
controversial.[46] The HMWMAA have been proposed as targets in
a specific antimelanoma therapy.[16,30]

Numerous groups have attempted to identify specific oncogenes
or tumor supressor genes potentially involved in melanoma
progression.[5,16,28] To date no clearly identifiable point mutation,
gene amplification, rearrangement nor expression that could serve
as a marker of melanoma progression has been detected.[16,28] On the
other hand, it has been found that non-random karyotypic abnormalities of chromosomes 1, 6, 7, 9 and 10 appear in parallel with
increasing agressiveness of melanoma.[4,6,47,48] However, primary cell
culture, necessary for karyotypic analysis, may not be possible for
small lesions, or may introduce an in vitro artifact. Therefore further
testing is required to determine whether specific numerical chro-
mosomal abnormalities could be used as markers of melanoma progression using the fluorescence *in situ* hybridization (FISH). This
technique employing centromere-specific probes has been successfully applied to detect numerical chromosome alterations in a
variety of solid tumors including uveal melanoma.[49] Similarly results
of the studies on relationship between melanoma progression and

DNA content or expression of proliferating cell nuclear antigens (PCNA) give varied results.[5,11,16,50] However, new findings support the concept that DNA ploidy may be an important prognostic variable for the course of malignant melanoma. Thus, melanocytic lesions with little or no cytologic atypia tend to be euploid, while those with high grade atypia are most likely aneuploid;[51] and metastases express significantly higher aneuploidy than primary tumors.[52] Since flow cytometry techniques used in many of previous studies can introduce artifacts and misinterpretation in the analysis of the data,[51,52] the existing controversy should be reconciled by careful *in situ* measurement of DNA content in melanoma cells with help of computer image analysis. This technique should eliminate potential artifacts connected with the preparation of heterogenous cell population and allow analysis of *in situ* fixed cells morphologically demonstrating aggressive behavior. Indeed, when measured by tissue section image analysis, DNA aneuploidy has correlated with disease progression in intermediate thickness level III melanomas, while diploid tumors have followed a benign course similar to thin, early stage cases.[53]

Results from cell culture systems have shown that cells from different stages of melanoma development have different growth potential, differ in an antigenic profile, expression of receptors, production and responsiveness to growth factors and cytokines.[5,16,28,54–55] However, since melanoma lines represent preselected, artificially obtained and maintained cell populations deprived of organ specific milieu characteristic for the human host, most of the findings in this experimental system may be specific only for the the in vitro condition and in fact are incompatible with the course of human disease. Therefore, for prognostic and clinical purposes such studies have to be de-emphasized, until their hypotheses have been otherwise proven. On the other hand, the *in situ* analyses of the expression and localization of receptors for NGF, transferrin, and epidermal growth factor (EGF),[15,17] and of growth factors such as transforming growth factor-β2 (TGF-β2)[31] and insulin growth factor-I (IGF-I)[32] suggest or have already showed some relationship with different stages of development of melanocytic lesion. An increased expression of TGF-β2, IGF-I and of receptor for EGF seems to correlate with depth of invasion and metastases in malignant melanoma.[15,31,32]

Recent findings of the POMC (proopiomelanocortin) expression in skin and localization of POMC products in melanomas[56–58] open potentially promising areas for melanoma diagnosis, e.g. cutaneous expression of the POMC gene, production of POMC neuropeptides and expression of corresponding receptors on skin cells in relation to progression of melanocytic lesions. Of particular interest are the findings that UV light ('melanocyte carcinogen',[3,5,11]) can stimulate POMC gene expression.[59,59a] Furthermore, POMC derived ACTH, MSH and β-endorphin can regulate functions of normal and malignant melanocytes and can act as immunomodulators.[56–60]

METASTATIC PHENOMENON (stage III and IV melanoma according to AJC)

Biology of melanoma development and progression

Since localized melanoma can be cured by surgical excision, the appearance of a new cell population with metastatic capability within VGP is a fundamental event in influencing the clinical course of disease. The process of melanoma metastasis is a dynamic one composed of several defined and interrelated steps that depend on both the intrinsic behavior of melanoma cells and host response. These steps according to Fidler[cf.11] include:

(1) extensive vascularization of a tumor mass which exceed 1 to 2 mm in diameter;
(2) local invasion of stroma including invasion of lymphatic and hematogenous capillaries;
(3) interactions with blood cell components and formation of small cell aggregates that allow survival in the circulation and arrest in target organs;
(4) adherence to capillary endothelial cells or subendothelial basement membrane;
(5) extravasation and further establishment of proper microenvironment for growth;
(6) proliferation in the parenchyma of the target organ, establishment of a tumor vascular network and continued evasion of the host immune system.

To produce clinically detectable metastases, melanoma cells must complete all of these processes.[11]

Prognostic factors and markers

The development of metastases causes a dramatic decrease in the survival of patients with stage III and IV melanomas.[3–6,11,13] When the regional lymph nodes are involved, the 5 year survival time decreases to approximately 30% to 40% with worse prognosis with increasing number of involved lymph nodes and presence of extra-nodal disease.[3-6,11,13] The prognosis has also been reported to be worse for primary tumors localized in the trunk versus extremities. Once distant metastases are formed, the disease is rarely curable and median survival time is approximately 6 months.[3,11] The prognosis worsens with increasing number of metastases, involvement of visceral sites and shorter duration of remission. Some authors suggest that sex can influence the course of the disease with worse prognosis for males than females.[3,11]

A group of possible prognostic markers is listed in Table 3. Since the first step in the metastatic cascade is dissemination of melanoma cells from the primary tumor mass, the expression of factors involved in cell adhesion, matrix degradation, migration and colonization is being investigated in relation to tumor development.[5,6,16,18-20,25,33,61-63] Most recent studies on the expression of plasminogen activators, their inhibitors and urokinase receptors suggest that plasminogen activation is an important step in malignant melanoma progression.[25,33] The expression of adhesion mol-

Table 3 Candidates for molecular and biochemical prognostic markers of metastatic melanoma

Source and Category	Marker	Citation
TUMOR		
Cell adhesion molecules:	ICAM-1	18, 29, 64
	MUC18	19, 29
	integrins	16, 20
	CD44	65
Plasminogen activation system:	uPA, PAI-1, PAI-2, uPAR	25, 33
Growth factors and receptors:	TGF-β2	31
	IGF-I	32
	EGF receptor	15, 17
	transferin receptor	15, 17
Genomic:	structural and numerical chromosomal abnormalities	4, 6, 47, 48
	DNA aneuploidy and polyploidy	51, 52, 53
BLOOD		
Whole blood:	tyrosinase mRNA	71
Serum or plasma:	intermediates of melanogenesis	27, 68–70
	enolase	67
	ICAM-1	64
	tyrosinase	66

EGF: epidermal growth factor; IGF-I: insulin growth factor-I; ICAM-1: intercellular adhesion molecule-1; PAI-1: plasminogen activator inhibitor type 1; PAI-2: plasminogen activator inhibitor type 2; TGF-β2: transforming growth fractor beta 2; uPA: urokinase-type plasminogen activator; uPAR: urokinase type plasminogen activator receptor.

ecules ICAM-1 and MUC18 on melanoma cells increase with increased tumor thickness and positively correlate with development of metastatic disease.[29,64] Increased serum levels of ICAM-1 is suggestive of poor prognosis.[64] Similarly increased or decreased expression of a particular class of integrins has been correlated positively with level of invasion in localized melanoma or development of metastases.[16,20] CD44, a lymphocyte homing, recirculating and cartilage attachement cell adhesion molecule, has been associated with increased cell motility and metastatic potential in malignant melanoma.[65]Thus, the expression of plasminogen activation components,[25,33] ICAM-1, MUC-18[18,19,29,64] or of selected integrins,[16,20] deserve further clinical testing for their usefulness as markers of melanoma progression.

It has been reported that serum activity of tyrosinase,[66] enolase[67] and serum and urine levels of precursors to melanin[27,68-70] correlate in certain degree with the progression of human melanoma. The measurement of serum tyrosinase activity has not been shown to be specific or sensitive enough to serve as a biochemical marker of melanoma.[66] However, the recent successful detection of mRNA for tyrosinase using RT/PCR technique in blood from melanoma patients promises that under certain conditions the expression of tyrosinase gene may act as specific and sensitive marker of melanoma progression.[71] Since transcription of tyrosinase gene appears to be restricted to cells of melanocytic origin,[7] the last finding may become an important step in establishing an assay to detect circulating metastatic melanoma cells before their presence can be assessed clinically.

The most promising markers of melanoma progression that can be detected in the serum of melanoma patients are intermediates of melanogenesis,[27,68-70] products of oxidation of tyrosine to DOPA and its multistep metabolism catalysed by tyrosinase and other enzymatic or nonenzymatic factors.[72, 73] In general it has been documented that patients with advanced stages of melanoma demonstrate an increased plasma or urine levels of melanin precursors including DOPA, 5-S-cysteinyldopa (5-S-CD), dihydroxyindole (DHI), its carboxylic form (DHICA) and O-methyl derivatives of DHI and DHICA.[27,68-70] Recent studies by the Jimbow group demonstrated that high plasma levels of 6-hydroxy-5-methoxyindole-2-carboxylic acid (6H5MI2C) are seen in all melanoma patients with tumor thickness > 3.0 mm independently of the presence or absence of metastasis, while in thinner melanomas this is seen only when metastases are present.[69] However, others have concluded that serum level of 5-S-CD is the best prognostic biochemical marker of melanoma progression.[70] Although it still remains to be clarified which of the two, 5-S-CD or 6H5MI2C, should be assayed to estimate melanoma progression, one can conclude that plasma levels of melanin precursors are good prognostic markers for malignant melanoma. In this context we emphasize that precursors to melanin can act as potent immunosuppressors,[74] and tyrosinase may be involved in the impairment of the immune system via oxidation of tyrosine and DOPA to lymphocytotoxic precursors of melanogenesis.[75] Thus, increased serum levels of intermediates of melanogenesis may also serve as indicators of a potential impairment of the host immune response against melanoma.

CONCLUSION

Development and progression of melanoma is a multistep process starting with malignant transformation of epidermal melanocytes or dermal nevocytes, followed by gradual or abrupt acquisition of one or more phenotypic and genotypic traits that increase melanocyte potential to proliferate, to invade surrounding tissues and to form local and distant metastases. The expression of these traits and their acquisition depends on multidirectional interactions between transformed pigment cells on the one hand, and local (skin) and systemic host factors, on the other, which may also be further modified by environmental stimuli. The malignancy of melanoma increases with growing autonomy of the tumor and is further accelerated with the aquisition by the tumor of an ability to regulate its own environment.

The complexity of this process makes the traditional histologic criteria (such as tumor thickness, depth of invasion, mitotic rate, presence of TIL, histologic regression and anatomic site) currently the best prognostic criteria for stage I-III (AJC) disease.[cf. 3–6,13–15] They are the visible reflection of multidirectional interactions between malignant melanocytes and other surrounding cells. In this context molecular factors expressed by melanoma cells should be defined as dependent variables of the above histologic criteria and serve only as additional guides in specific clinical settings. For example the expression of specific ganglioside fraction, of HMWMAA or the presence of MHC-I restricted CTL response via presentation of melanocyte specific peptides could determine type or outcome of therapy.

During the development of the metastatic phenomenon, one of the most important steps is detection of metastasizing cells before metastases become clinically evident. Detection of circulating melanoma cells by RT/PCR detection of melanogenesis-specific mRNA in blood of melanoma patients may serve as a potential prognostic marker.[71] Similar methodology using the tyrosine hydroxylase gene has been used to detect the metastasizing potential of neuroblastoma.[76] Additional serum markers that may be used in prognosis are levels of intermediates of melanogenesis[27,68-70] and perhaps levels of selected neuroectodermal antigens.[67] They could reflect increase in the total tumor mass in the host, recurrence of the disease or presence of occult melanoma. Presence of precursors to melanin deserve special attention because they can act as immunosuppressors,[74] and they reflect presence of melanogenesis related proteins in melanoma cells, which may be a potential future target in melanoma immunotherapy.[75]

In summary we currently favor the use of traditional histopathological and clinical criteria in assessment of the prognosis of melanoma and strongly recommend further clinical testing of the above listed potentially predictive serum markers of metastatic melanoma disease.

REFERENCES

1 Glass AG, Hoover RN. The emerging epidemic of melanoma and squamos cell skin cancer. JAMA 1989; 262: 2097–2100.
2 Marks R. Freckles, moles, melanoma and the ozone layer: a tale of the relationship between humans and their environment. Med J Australia 1989; 151: 611–613.
3 Barnhill RL, Mihm MC Jr, Fitzpatrick TB, Sober EJ. Neoplasms: malignant melanoma. In: Fitzpatrick TB, Eisen AZ, Wolff K, Freedberg IM, Austen KF, eds. Dermatology in general medicine. New York: McGraw-Hill 1993; 1: 1078–116.
4 Lejeune FJ, Chaudhuri PK, Das Gupta TK. Malignant melanoma. Medical and surgical management. New York: McGraw-Hill 1994.
5 Mihm MC, Murphy GF, Kaufman N. Pathobiology and recognition of malignant melanoma. Baltimore: Williams and Wilkins 1988.
6 Balch CM, Houghton AN, Milton GW, Sober AJ, Song S-J. Cutaneous melanoma. Philadelphia: JB Lippincott , 1992.
7 Levine N. Pigmentation and pigmentary disorders. Boca Raton: CRC Press, 1993.
8 Fitzpatrick TB, Breathnach AS: Das epidermale Melanineinheits-System. DerWoschenschr 1963; 147: 481–489.
9 Slominski A, Paus R, Schanderdorf D. Melanocytes as sensory and regulatory cells in the epidermis. J Theor Biol 1993; 164: 103–120.
10 Slominski A, Paus R. Melanogenesis is coupled to murine anagen: toward new concepts for the role of melanocytes and the regulation of melanogenesis in hair growth. J Invest Dermatol 1993; 101: 90S-907S.
11 Friedman RJ, Rigel DS, Kopf AW, Harris MN, Baker D. Cancer of the skin. Philadelphia: WB Saunders, 1991.
12 Haffner AC, Garbe C, Burg G et al. The prognosis of primary and metastasizing melanoma. An evaluation of the TNM classification in 2,495 patients. Br J Cancer 1992; 66: 856–861.
13 Clark WH Jr, Elder DE, Guerry IV DP et al. Model predicting survival in stage I melanoma based on tumor progression. J Natl Cancer Inst 1989; 81: 1893–1904.
13a Clark WH Jr, Elder DE, Guerry IV DP et al. A study of tumor progression: the

precursor lesions of superficial spreading and nodular melanoma. Hum Pathol 1984; 15: 1147–1165.

14 Guerry IV DP, Synneszvedt M, Elder DE, Schultz D. Lessons from tumor progression: the invasive radial growth phase of melanoma is common, incapable of metastasis, and indolent. J Invest Dermatol 1993; 100: 342S-345S.

14a Mihm MC, Googe PB. Problematic pigmented lesions. A case method approach. Philadelphia: Lea and Febiger, 1990.

15 Elder DE, Rodeck U, Thurin J et al. Antigenic profile of tumor progression stages in human melanocytic nevi and melanomas. Cancer Res 1989; 49: 5091–5096.

16 Weterman MAJ, Van Muije GNP, Bloemers HPJ, Ruiter D. Biology of disease.- Molecular markers of melanocytic tumor progression. Lab Invest 1994; 70: 593–608.

17 Carrel S, Dore JF, Ruiter DJ et al. The EORTC melanoma group exchange program: evaluation of a multicenter monoclonal antibody study. Int J Cancer 1991; 48: 836–847.

18 Johnson J, Stade BG, Holzmann B et al. De novo expression of intercellular-adhesion molecule 1 in melanoma correlates with increased risk of metastasis. Proc Natl Acad Sci USA 1989; 86: 641–644.

19 Lehmann JM, Riethmuller G, Pohnson JP. MUC18, a marker of tumor progression in human melanoma, shows sequence similarity to the neural cell adhesion molecules of the immunoglobulin superfamily. Proc Natl Acad Sci USA 1989; 86: 9891–9895.

20 Schadendorf D, Gawlik C, Haney U et al. Tumor progression and metastatic behaviour in vivo correlates with integrin expresion on melanocytic tumours. J Pathol 1993; 170: 429–434.

21 Kageshita T, Wang Z, Calorini L et al. Selective loss of human leukocyte class I allospecificities and staining of melanoma cells by monoclonal antibodies recognizing monomorphic determinants of class I human leukocyte antigens. Cancer Res 1993; 53: 3349–3354

22 Ravindranath MH, Irie RF. Gangliosides as antigens of human melanoma. In: Nathason L, ed. Malignant: biology, diagnosis, and therapy. Boston 1998: Kluwer Academic 1988; 17–43.

23 Kageshita T, Nakamura T, Yamada M et al. Differential expression of melanoma associated antigens in acral lentiginous melanoma and in nodular melanoma lesions. Cancer Res 1991. 51: 1726–1732.

24 Kageshita T, Kuriya N. Ono T et al. Association of high molecular weight melanoma-associated antigen expression in primary acral lentiginous melanoma lesions with poor prognosis. Cancer Res 1993; 53: 2830–2833.

25 De Vries TJ, Quax PHA, Denijn M et al. Plasminogen activators, their inhibitors, and urokinase receptor emerge in late stages of melanocytic tumor progression. Am J Pathol 1994; 144: 70–81.

26 Barnhill RL, Fandrey K, Levy MA et al. Angiogenesis and tumor progression of melanoma. Lab Invest 1992; 67: 331–337.

27 Jimbow K, Lee SK, King MG et al. Melanin pigments and melanosomal proteins as differentiation markers unique to normal and neoplastic melanocytes. J Invest Dermatol 1993; 100: 259S–268S.

28 Herlyn M. Molecular and cellular biology of melanoma. Austin: RG Landes,1993.

29 Johnson JP, Lehmann JM, Stade BG et al. Functional aspects of three molecules associated with metastasis development in human malignant melanoma. Invasion Met 1989; 9: 338–350.

30 Carrel S, Rimoldi D. Melanoma-associated antigens. Eur J Cancer 1993; 29A: 1903–1907.

31 Reed JA, McNutt NS, Prieto VG, Albino AP. Expression of transforming growth factor-$\beta 2$ in malignant melanoma correlates with the depth of tumor invasion. Am J Pathol 1994; 145: 97–104.

32 Fleming MG, Howe SF, Graf LH. Expression of insulin-like growth factor I (IGF-I) in nevi and melanomas. Am J Dermatopathol 1994; In press.

568   MELANOMA: CUTANEOUS AND OCULAR

33 Debaldo C, Masouye I, Saurat J-H, Vassalli J-D, Sappino A-P. Plasminogen
    activation in melanocytic neoplasia. Cancer Res 1994; 54: 4547–4552.
34 Brichard V, Van Pel A, Wolfel T et al. The tyrosinase gene codes for an antigen
    recognized by autologous cytolytic T lymphocytes on HLA-A2 melanoma. J Exp
    Med 1993; 178: 489–495.
35 Bakker ABH, Schreurs MWJ, DeBoer AJ et al. Melanocyte lineage-specific anti-
    gen gp100 is recognized by melanoma-derived tumor-infiltrating lymphocytes. J
    Exp Med 1994; 179: 1005–1009.
36 Cox AL, Skipper J, Chen Y et al. Identification of a peptide recognized by five
    melanoma-specific human cytotoxic T cell lines. Science 1994; 264: 716–719.
37 Kawakami Y, Eliyahu S, Sakaguchi K et al. Identification of the immunodominant
    peptides of the MART-1 human melanoma antigen recognized by the majority of
    HLA-A2–restricted tumor infiltrating lymphocytes. J Exp Med 1994; 180: 347–
    352.
38 Celis E, Tsai V, Crimi C et al. Induction of anti-tumor cytotoxic T lymphocytesin
    normal humans using primary cultures and synthetic peptide epitopes. Proc Natl
    Acad Sci USA 1994; 91: 2105–2109.
39 Stene MA, Babajanians M, Bhuta S, Cochran AJ. Quantitative alterations incu-
    taneous Langerhans cells during the evolution of malignant melanoma of the skin.
    J Invest Derm 1988; 91: 125–128.
40 Hamilton WB, Helling F, Llloyd KO, Livingston P. Ganglioside expression on
    human malignant melanoma assessed by quantitative immune thin-layer chro-
    matography. Int J Cancer 1993; 53: 566–573.
41 Ravidranath MH, Tsuchida T, Morton DL, Irie RF. Ganglioside GM3: GD3
    ratio as an index for the management of melanoma. Cancer 1991; 67: 3029–3035.
42 Tsuchida T, Saxton RE, Morton DL, RF Irie. Gangliosides of human melanoma.
    J Natl Cancer Inst 1987; 78: 45–54.
43 Portoukalian J, Carrel S, Dore JF, Rumke P, Humoral immune response indisease-
    free advanced melanoma patients after vaccination with melanoma-associated
    gangliosides. Int J Cancer 1991; 49: 893–899.
44 Livingston PO, Wong GYC, Adluri S et al. Improved survival in stage III-
    melanoma patients with GM2 antibodies: a randomized trial of adju-
    vantvaccination with GM2 ganglioside. J Clin Oncol 1994; 12: 1036–1044.
45 Weterman MA, Van Muijen GNP, Bloemers HP, Ruiter DJ. Expression of cal-
    cyclin in human melanocytic lesions. Cancer Res 1993; 53: 6061–6066.
46 Si Z, Hersey P. Expression of the neuroglandular antigen and analogues in mela-
    noma. CD9 expression appears inversely related to metastatic potential of mela-
    noma. Int J Cancer 1993; 54: 37–43.
47 Parmiter RH, Nowell PC. Cytogenetics of melanocytic tumors. J Invest Dermatol
    1993; 100: 254S–258S.
48 Holland EA, Beaton SC, Edwards BG et al. Loss of heterozygosity and homo-
    zygous deletions on 9q21–22 in melanoma. Oncogene 1994; 9: 1361–1365.
49 Gordon KB, Thompson CT, Char DH et al. Comparative genomic hybridization
    in the detection of DNA copy number abnormalities in uveal melanoma. Cancer
    Res 1994; 54: 4764–4768.
50 Evans ET, Blessing K, Orrel JM, Grant A. Mitotic indices, anti-PCNA immuno-
    staining, and AgNORs in thick cutaneous melanomas displaying paradoxical
    behaviour. J Pathol 1992; 168: 15–22.
51 Schmidt B, Weinberg DS, Hollister K et al. Analysis of melanocytic lesions by
    DNA image cytometry. Cancer 1994; 73: 2971–2977.
52 Karlsson M, Boeryd B, Carstensen J et al. DNA ploidy and S-phase fraction in
    primary melanomas and their regional metastases. Melanoma Res 1994; 4: 47–51.
53 Bjornhajen V, Auer G, Lagerlof B et al. DNA analysis in archival material from
    primary malignant melanoma. Anal Quant Histol Cytol 1991; 13: 335–342.
54 Krasagakis K, Garbe C, Orfanos CE. Cytokines in human melanoma cells:
    synthesis, autocrine stimulation and regulatory functions-an overview. Melanoma
    Res 1993; 3: 425–433.

55 Halaban R, Kwon BS, Ghosh S et al. bFGF as an autocrine growth factor for human melanomas. Oncogene Res 1988; 3: 177–186.
56 Slominski A, Paus R, Wortsman J. On the potential role of proopiomelanocortin in skin physiology and pathology. Mol Cell Endocrinol 1993; 93: C1–C6.
57 Slominski A, Wortsman J, Mazurkiewicz J, Matsuoka L, Lawrence K, Paus R. Detection of the proopiomelanocortin derived-antigens in normal and pathologic human skin. J Lab Clin Med 1993; 122: 658–656.
58 Slominski A. POMC gene expression in mouse and hamster melanoma cells. FEBS Lett 1991; 291: 165–168
59 Schauer E, Trautinger F, Kock A et al. Proopiomelanocortin-derived peptides are synthesized and released by human keratinocytes. J Clin Invest 1994; 93: 2258–2262.
59a Chakraborty A, Slominski A, Ermek G, Hwang Y, Pawelek J. UVB and MSH stimulate mRNA production of αMSH receptors and POMC-derived peptides in mouse melanoma cells and transformed keratinocytes. J Invest Dermatol. In press.
60 Pawelek J. Proopiomelanocortin in skin: new possibilities for regulation of skin physiology. J Lab Clin Med 1993; 122: 627–628.
61 Dekker SK, Vink J, Vermeer BJ et al. Differential effects of interleukin 1-α (IL-1α) or tumor necrosis factor-α (TNF-α) on motility of human melanoma cell lines and fibronectin. J Invest Dermatol 1994; 102: 898–905.
62 Bouffard D, Duncan LM, Howard CA et al. Actin-binding protein expression in benign and malignant melanocytic proliferation. Human Pathol 1994; 25: 709–714.
63 Etoh T, Thomas L, Pastel-Levy C et al. Role of integrin alpha-2/beta-1 (VLA-2) in the migration of human melanoma cells on laminin and type IV collagen. J Invest Dermatol 1993; 100: 640–647.
64 Kageshita T, Yoshii A, Kimura T et al. Clinical relevance of ICAM-1 expression in primary lesions and serum of patients with malignant melanoma. Cancer Res 1993; 53: 4927–4932.
65 Birch M, Mitchell S, Hart IR. Isolation and characterization of human melanoma cell variance expressing high and low levels of CD44. Cancer Res 1991; 51: 6660–6667.
66 Agrup P, Carstam R, Wittbjer A et al. Tyrosinase activity in serum from patients with malignant melanoma. Acta Derm Venereol (Stockh) 1989; 69: 120–124.
67 Wibe E, Hannisdal E, Paus E, Aamdal S. Neuron-specific enolase as a prognostic factor in metastatic melanoma. Eur J Cancer 1992; 28A: 1692–1695.
68 Rorsman H, Agrup G, Hansson C, Rosengren. Biochemical recorders of malignant melanoma. In: MacKie RM, ed. Pigment cell. Basel: Kargel, 1983; 6: 93–115.
69 Hara H, Walsh N, Yamada K, Jimbow K. High plasma levels of a eumelanin precursor, 6–hydroxy-5–methoxyindole-2–carboxylic acid as a prognostic marker for malignant melanoma. J Invest Dermatol 1994; 102: 501–505.
70 Horikoshi T, Ito S, Wakamatsu K et al. Evaluation of melanin-related metabolites as markers of melanoma progression. Cancer 1994; 73: 629–636.
71 Brossart P, Keilholz U, Willhauck M et al. Hematogenous spread of malignant melanoma cells in different stages of disease. J Invest Dermatol 1993; 101: 887–889.
72 Pawelek J, Korner A. The biosynthesis of mammalian melanin. Am Sci 1982; 70: 136–145.
73 Protta G. Melanins and melanogenesis. Orlando: Academic Press, 1992.
74 Slominski A, Goodman-Snitkoff G. DOPA inhibits induced proliferative activity of murine and human lymphocytes. Anticancer Res 1992; 12: 753–756.
75 Slominski A, Paus R. Inhibition of melanogenesis for melanoma therapy? J Invest Dermatol 1994; 103: 742.
76 Burchill SA, Bradbury FM, Smith B, Selby P. Neuroblastoma cell detection by reverse transcriptase-polymerase chain reaction (RT-PCR) for tyrosine hydroxylase mRNA. Int J Cancer 1994; 57: 671–675.

British Medical Bulletin 1995, Vol 51, No. 3 pp. 570–583
©The British Council 1995

Melanoma prevention and early detection

R M MacKie

Department of Dermatology, University of Glasgow, Glasgow, UK

In the absence of significant advances in non-surgical treatment of advanced malignant melanoma, efforts to reduce mortality must rely on earlier diagnosis of thinner lesions more likely to be cured by surgery, and also on primary prevention. early detection activities are in progress in many countries with varying levels of built-in audit of their efficacy. In general, however, it would appear that in most countries melanomas are currently detected and treated when they are thinner than was the case 10 years ago. Primary prevention activities are aimed mainly at encouraging sensible sun exposure. Measuring change in sun exposure habits of the public is difficult but surveys indicate that knowledge and attitude to sunburn and the desirability of a tanned skin has moderated over the past 10 years. There is as yet little evidence however that behaviour with regard to sun exposure has changed significantly.

In the field of cancer prevention and early detection it is important to clearly define the terms commonly used. Prevention of death from a malignancy, in this case malignant melanoma, can be brought about by either primary or secondary prevention. Primary prevention is the prevention of the development of the malignancy itself, and secondary prevention is the prevention of deaths from that malignancy, either by improved therapy or by earlier diagnosis. Thus in the case of melanoma primary prevention is usually centred around efforts to avoid excessive sun exposure, while secondary prevention concentrates on public education concerning features of early melanoma, and the encouragement of the public to self-examine their skin and attend for surgical treatment when any possible melanoma is at an early curable stage.

The terms **case finding**, **screening** and **surveillance** also require definition. Some of the current activities in the field of early detection, while described as screening are probably more appropriately termed opportunistic or invited case finding rather than screening.

Case finding is the dissemination of information either to the public or to the primary care team of the features of early malignant melanoma and inviting individuals to self-examine their skin and self-refer themselves to an appropriate referral centre if they feel they have a worrying skin lesion. Thus many of the skin cancer fairs held in the past, mainly in North America, are examples of case finding rather than true screening. At these case finding examinations, some centres offer a free total body skin examination, while others offer free examination of one specific lesion giving rise to concern. A problem with such exercises, discussed below, may be the lack of treatment available or offered and lack of any regular follow up to confirm that advice offered has been acted upon.

Screening for melanoma involves the systematic examination of a population. Population screening involves the systematic screening of a selected group coming from one geographic area. The individuals in this population to be screened may be selected on the basis of age, sex or other features. Screening may also be confined to those known to be at increased risk of melanoma, and thus could be confined to those who have a known family history of melanoma, who are known to have multiple naevi, or who have other risk factors.

Surveillance is the ongoing examination at regular intervals of individuals for development of new pigmented lesions which may be early malignant melanoma. The intervals at which surveillance examinations take place varies, but is usually between 3 and 6 monthly. This is clearly a labour intensive exercise and is currently confined to a small number of centres who have a research interest in this area examining individuals at known greatly increased risk of developing primary malignant melanoma. Examples of individuals subjected to surveillance in some centres include those who have already had one primary malignant melanoma and those individuals with both a family history of melanoma and large numbers of benign naevi.

There is as yet no statistically significant proven survival benefit in screening, case finding or surveillance activities other than in females in Scotland. While a number of centres have shown encouraging trends in reported diagnoses and removal of thinner presumed early melanomas in a population subjected to surveillance for example, no appropriate control group has been used. Well constructed controlled trials of the value of these activities are, therefore, urgently needed as there is a current trend to introduce screening programmes on the assumption that they must be of benefit. This does require to be proven.

In Europe at the present time activities are ongoing in several countries.[1] These mainly concern early detection and education exercises, but increasingly there is a movement towards primary prevention, with governments, public health departments, national dermatological associations and others mounting campaigns to encourage a cautious approach and advocate sensible sun exposure. In the UK, skin cancer has been targetted in the Health of the Nation Document, with the stated aim of reducing the year on year rise in the incidence of skin cancer by the year 2005.

Approaches to early detection of malignant melanoma depend on the hypothesis that if melanoma is detected and removed at an early stage, it will be a thinner tumour, and that this in turn will correlate with increased survival. It is well established from detailed clinicopathological studies correlating features of the primary tumour with prognosis that tumour thickness is in the great majority of such studies the most important determinant of survival. Thus 5 year survival for patients with tumours thinner than 1.5 mm is over 90%, while for those with tumours thicker than 3.5mm it falls to under 50%. However, studies on patients' history of pigmented lesion growth and tumour thickness suggest that the correlation of the stated duration of a new or growing lesion on the skin and tumour thickness is not absolute. This is clear, for example, in slowly growing melanomas of the lentigo maligna/lentigo maligna melanoma variants, in which the history of slow growth may extend over several years during which time the tumour has only invaded to 1 to 2mm. The other end of this spectrum is the rapidly growing nodular melanoma where the patient gives a clear history, sometimes supplemented by clinical photographs, of the absence of any lesion in the affected site 4 to 6 months prior to rapid development of a nodular melanoma which is already 3 to 4 mm thick at the time of excision.

However, for superficial spreading melanomas a reasonable correlation has been established by Temoshok, Clemente, Sweet, et al.[2] This shows that for superficial spreading malignant melanomas which comprise over 70% of all primary cutaneous melanomas there is a reasonable correlation between the patient's statement of duration of growth of the pigmented lesion in question and tumour thickness. Thus the early detection approach to malignant melanoma should be successful for superficial spreading lesions, but probably less so for nodular and lentigo maligna melanomas.

A further point to be considered is the question of lead time bias.

This has been investigated mainly in the field of breast cancer, and is the suggestion that the time from potential recognition of a tumour to death is constant, and that earlier recognition will not alter that point. Thus early diagnosis could lead to a longer period of follow-up during which time the patient is slowly developing progressive disease, but will not lead to a higher number of survivors at a distant point in time – perhaps 12 to 18 years after original diagnosis. The problem of lead time bias has not yet been addressed in the field of melanocytic lesions.

SECONDARY PREVENTION – PUBLIC EDUCATION ACTIVITIES

Early detection campaigns aimed at informing the public at large about the features of possible early malignant melanoma and advising them to seek medical advice require several important features (Table 1). The first of these is that there must be general agreement that early malignant melanoma is an entity which can be recognised or at least suspected by relatively untrained eyes. Studies assessing the pre-operative diagnostic accuracy of specialist dermatologists have suggested that around 70% of primary cutaneous malignant melanomas may be recognised pre-operatively by dermatologists[3] but no similar study has yet been carried out on family doctors and the general public. The accuracy of diagnosis by these groups is likely to be less than 70%, and could be very much less.

Given this fact, it is essential that the features advertised to the public as suggestive of malignant melanoma are relatively broad, and are sensitive but relatively non-specific. In other words, every effort must be made to identify all malignant melanomas and include these, although it has to be recognised that this will inevitably include a proportion of benign pigmented lesions. These may be either benign lesions arising from the melanocytic series or other pigmented lesions

Table 1 Requirements for public education campaigns in early detection of malignant melanoma

- Clear sensitive but relatively non specific description of **early** melanoma.
- Well publicised.
- Access to appropriate media for this.
- Primary care medical teams alerted to campaign and ready to handle resultant workload.
- Secondary referral facilities (e.g. pigmented lesion clinic available).
- Rapid diagnostic biopsy and pathology facilities.
- Rapid access to further definitive surgery as needed.

which do not arise from melanocytes, such as angiomas and occasionally pigmented basal cell carcinomas.

Once the clinical features suggestive but not diagnostic of malignant melanoma have been established and appropriately publicised, there must be an appropriate referral or self-referral centre available for members of the public who respond to these campaigns and require medical advice. Thus prior to any public education campaign, it is absolutely essential that the appropriate medical personnel in the area to be subjected to the campaign are primed about the aims and objectives of the campaign and are themselves up-to-date with regard to features of early malignant melanoma and its appropriate initial treatment. In many countries including the UK, this means preparing the primary care team to deal with pigmented lesions.

Because of the impossibility of entirely accurate pre-operative clinical diagnosis, a proportion of pigmented lesions self-referred by the public may require an excision biopsy to establish a histological diagnosis. This may be carried out either by the primary care physician, or at a specialised referral centre. Whichever is appropriate for the health care system in question, it is essential that members of these groups are acquainted with appropriate techniques and excision margins for excision biopsy of pigmented lesions about which there is any suspicion of early malignant change.

The next requirement is the availability of a rapid and accurate diagnostic pathology service. The accurate definition of early malignant melanoma and its separation on pathological grounds from reactive but benign melanocytic proliferations can be surprisingly difficult, and centres that plan a large melanoma recognition campaign do require to be sure that a specialist pathologist who has experience in this area is available. In addition, there must be adequate technical staff involved in pathological processing to provide high quality specimens relatively rapidly.

A proportion of melanomas diagnosed as a result of increased knowledge and thus self-awareness on the part of the patient and subsequent excision biopsy will require further surgery. Once again geographic areas planning early detection activities must be sure that the surgical services in their area have the manpower capacity to carry out any necessary definitive surgery rapidly and effectively.

From the above it will be seen that it is essential that the medical back-up service for early detection activities are in place. If any part of this necessary chain of medical activity is lacking, the result of an early detection campaign could be detrimental rather than beneficial, in that the system could become blocked by those alarmed by the publicity, but who do not have melanoma 'the worried well' thus preventing appropriate rapid management of those who do have true melanoma.

The public's attention can be drawn to malignant melanoma by a variety of media approaches. These can be transmitted by local or national newspapers, by television or radio, and also by purpose designed leaflets and posters. Research in many parts of the world has shown that television has the greatest power to reach the greatest number, certainly in those parts of Europe where the number of television channels available is relatively small.[4] However, in the US where there are a large number of television channels local newspapers have been found to be a more effective route. Audits of different approaches to public education have, however, demonstrated that all avenues of publicity do result in some response.

MELANOMA EARLY DETECTION ACTIVITIES

Europe

One of the first early detection exercises in Europe was that carried out by Cristofolini and colleagues in the province of Trento in Northern Italy.[5] Over the period 1977 to 1985 this group of trained dermatologists in the earlier recognition of malignant melanoma, informed general practitioners of these activities, and then explained to the public the necessary aspects of self-examination for early malignant melanoma using leaflets, conferences, television and radio. The control population for this study were the adjacent neighbouring areas of the Veneto, Alto Adige, and Lombardia. Cristofolini and colleagues in their publications do not indicate how they avoided these adjacent areas receiving television, newspaper or radio material.

Analysis of the effect of this campaign has been on the basis of expected and observed deaths in Trentino for the period 1977 to 1985. For men the expected deaths were 40 and the observed 26, while for women the expected deaths were 34 and the observed 26. Thus it has been calculated that 22 lives have been saved as a result of melanoma education. The cost of the campaign was $70,800, and the cost per year of life saved was calculated at $400.[6] It is of interest to note that this campaign appears to have been more effective in men than women, an observation in contrast to the early findings from the US and Scotland where it appears to have been easier to influence women than men.

In Scotland a similar campaign has taken place. In 1985 it was observed that a relatively high proportion of patients in Scotland had melanoma diagnosed when it was thicker than 1.5 mm.[4,7] A campaign was therefore launched, firstly to improve early detection of malignant melanoma by those working in the primary care sector, and thereafter to offer public information on the features of early malignant melanoma and encourage rapid self-referral.

This took place in the spring and early summer of 1985, and the results of these activities have already been published in detail.[8] Five audit measures were built in to the public education campaign (Table 2). These were a measure of increasing interest in malignant melanoma, increasing referrals of true malignant melanoma, an increase in the number of thin melanomas excised, an absolute fall in the number of thick melanomas excised, and a fall in melanoma mortality trends. From the early days of the campaign it was apparent that there was an increasing interest in melanoma with a sharp increase in the number of patients referred with histologically proven melanoma. Comparison of the Breslow thickness of melanomas excised in the whole of Scotland in the latter part of 1985/86 and 1987 by comparison with melanomas excised in the years 1980–1985 showed a significant increase in the proportion of thin tumours (less than 1.5 mm). Thereafter this was followed by a fall in the absolute number of thick tumours in women but not in men, and subsequently by a downward mortality trend in women but not in men. This campaign is one of the few which has been carefully audited from the outset, and has shown clear evidence that public education using television, radio, newspapers, leaflets, posters and other measures is an effective method of educating women with early malignant melanoma, but appears to have virtually no effect on men. The reasons for this sex difference are not immediately apparent. One feature, however, may be the extremely useful and informative wave of secondary education published in women's magazines. These may well be an underestimated avenue of health education.

Work carried out by Rampen and colleagues[9,10] in the Netherlands has also been published. This group offered screening in the town of Oss in 1989 and 1990, and 2564 individuals presented themselves for screening. Nine melanomas were suspected in this population, and the cost of the campaign was modest being estimated at only $6000.

Table 2 Appropriate audit measures to evaluate public education activities

- Is greater interest generated concerning melanoma?
- Are more melanomas diagnosed?
- After 2–3 years are those thinner melanomas than before?
- After 2–3 years does the absolute number of thicker melanomas fall?
- Longer term does melanoma mortality fall?

It is not clear from the publications whether or not all of these 9 were pathologically confirmed.

In Germany, Hoffman Dirschka Schatz et al[11] have reported on activities in the town of Bochum. There 1467 individuals attended a designated clinic after publicity was generated. Fourteen pathologically confirmed melanomas were diagnosed in this population giving a ratio of 1 melanoma diagnosed per 100 individuals examined.

In Austria campaigns carried out in 1988 and 1989 showed a sharp rise in number of melanomas diagnosed from 169 in 1988 to 213 in 1989.[12] The average thickness of these melanomas fell from 1.4 to 1.1 mm. However, in the years after 1989 a return to the 1988 pattern was seen, suggesting that regular reminder campaigns are necessary if the impetus begun by early detection activities is to be maintained.

Work carried out in Switzerland in the Canton of Basle has also been reported by Bulliard, Raymond, Levi et al.[13] This was carried out in 1986 with an augmentation campaign in 1989. These workers have reported a doubling in the number of newly diagnosed cases immediately after the 1986 campaign with a statistically significant drop in the age at diagnosis and a non-significant drop in tumour thickness. However, the recall campaign in 1989 did not appear to produce any significant changes.

Over the past decade similar exercises have been carried out in the USA, mainly under the guidance of the American Academy of Dermatology. These efforts have mainly related to offers of free skin cancer screening clinics, held at outdoor and social events such as county fairs, or at easy access sites such as shopping malls.[14-16] A major problem in the US studies to date is the fact that for ethical reasons, individuals thought to have melanoma have not been followed up, or offered treatment but only advised to contact their medical adviser. Attempts to review these individuals has indicated that by no means all so advised take this advice, and the published results of these activities suggest that they are labour intensive and expensive exercises for the yield of melanomas, although a reasonable number of non melanoma skin cancers are detected incidentally.

In Australia, early detection activities have been carried out for many years, mainly in Queensland.[17] Concomitant with this activity, there has been a fall in mean melanoma thickness at the time of excision, and it has been assumed that this is attributable to public education, although no specific review programme of the result of the educational activities has been published.

In summary, a large number of countries are currently carrying out early detection exercises. It is highly desirable that such activities are carefully audited to determine their true worth and to identify those areas of public education which are of greatest value. It is necessary, therefore, to know the number of melanomas and the distribution of tumour thickness in the population to be offered education for 3 or 4 years preceding any educational activity, and to follow these figures after the educational activity takes place. Over time it is also necessary to continue to observe tumour thickness. A fall in the absolute number of thick tumours would be an excellent marker of an effective campaign but a fall only in the **proportion** of these tumours would not be adequate as it is possible that the campaign had resulted in increased referral of only very early and possibly non progressor lesions. Mortality figures must of course be available. These activities are best carried out on a population basis, so the figures for the above measures must be available for the whole population, not just for one referral centre. This can give rise to problems in areas where there is an increasing trend for office based surgeons, dermatologists or plastic surgeons to excise thin melanomas in an office setting, as not all may be sent for adequate pathological reporting, leading to incomplete cancer registration.

Nevertheless the overall impression is that early detection and melanoma publicity campaigns do lead to presentation of thinner melanomas. If all thin melanomas are lesions that would have in time become thicker tumours, then these activities should lead to a fall in melanoma associated mortality. As yet this has only been demonstrated in Scotland.[8]

PRIMARY PREVENTION OF MALIGNANT MELANOMA

Primary prevention of malignant melanoma is a longer term exercise. From what is known about the growth kinetics of malignant melanoma, it is likely that trends in falling melanoma mortality and falling tumour thickness might be seen within 3 to 5 years of mounting a public education campaign aimed at secondary melanoma, but the latent interval between initiation of a tumour and development of melanoma may be longer than 20 years. Thus primary prevention activities need to be carried out on a very long-term basis. At the present time a large number of European countries are offering advice to their public on safe sun exposure,[1] on the assumption that excessive exposure to natural ultraviolet radiation is the most important aetiological agent in developing malignant melanoma. Epidemiological studies strongly support this hypothesis, and furthermore there is increasing evidence that sunlight exposure in early childhood is a significant risk factor for subsequent development of malignant melanoma as an adult some 20 to 30 years later. However the exact wavelength and action spectrum for the development of malignant melanoma is not yet established.

Activities currently in progress in the UK, Sweden and other European countries are aimed at encouraging a safe sun approach to exposure to natural ultraviolet radiation. Specific items in these safe sun approaches include avoidance of noonday sun, the use of shade such as trees or sun umbrellas, the use of protective clothing such as hats and T-shirts, and the use of a high SPF sunscreen at all times. These activities are inherently more difficult to monitor and audit than early detection activities, but there does appear on the basis of large surveys carried out by national magazines, to be greater awareness of the hazards of sun exposure both with regard to early ageing and to the development of cutaneous malignancy. However there is still considerable room for improvement and enhancement of knowledge on the part of the public. For example, in a large survey carried out on 22,000 individuals in the UK in 1993 conducted by a popular womans magazine, it was found that the most popular sunscreen had an SPF of only 4. In 1993 the UK Cancer Research Campaign mounted *Play Safe In The Sun* activity campaign similar to those promoted in Australia. The emphasis on these activities has been that it is possible to enjoy activities in European sunlight while taking appropriate precautions to prevent excessive sun exposure which could lead initially to sunburn and possibly later to cutaneous malignancy. The main points to be emphasised in the safe sun approach are avoidance of noonday sun, the use of natural shade (trees etc), the use of appropriate comfortable clothing (wide brimmed hats and cotton T shirts, and only then the sensible use of high SPF sunscreens (Table 3).

Because of the recently recognised importance of avoiding excessive sun exposure in early life, emphasis has switched to the education of young mothers and school age children. A wealth of educational material is now available for primary school children in a variety of European languages.

The field of assessment of primary melanoma prevention is a new

Table 3 Safe sun education points

- Avoid direct exposure to noonday sun.
- Seek natural shade (trees) or create it yourself (sun umbrellas).
- Use large brimmed hats and T-shirts as comfortable protective clothing.
- Use high SPF (> 15) broad spectrum sunscreens sensibly to reduce risk of damage.
- Apply thickly and reapply every 2–3 h.
- Protect the skin of children at all times.

one for many clinicians. This has been pioneered for many years in Australia,[18] and it is important to recognise that knowledge and attitude changes precede behavioural change. It is also essential to deliver primary prevention educational material in a way in which it is easily assimilated by the appropriate age range, and does not cause aversion due to alarm or fear. A recent publication by Boldeman and colleagues[19] from Sweden has illustrated that health education designed to encourage sensible sun exposure has been disseminated through Swedish pharmacies, schools, colleges of nursing science and pre-school teachers. Information diffusion has been good, and it remains to be seen whether or not there will be an associated change in behaviour.

Assessment of the efficacy of primary prevention campaigns is necessarily a long term goal. Clearly the desired end result is a fall in the incidence of malignant melanoma. With increasing availability of leisure time, and reports of a fall in ozone levels in the northern hemisphere, it would be expected that without any primary prevention activities that the incidence of malignant melanoma would continue to rise as has been the case in Europe for the past 20 years, and furthermore that this rate of rise might be rather steeper than had been observed to date. Thus is may be more realistic to expect some flattening of the increase in incidence curve following primary prevention campaigns rather than an absolute fall. There is not as yet any evidence of any reversing trend in the steadily rising incidence of malignant melanoma in all European countries for which data are available.

Primary prevention activities also refer to the avoidance of excessive exposure to artificial ultraviolet radiation as well as to natural sunlight. In northern European countries sunbeds and sun lamps have been popular mainly during the winter months, to promote the year round tan. There are now case control studies, from Canada, from the UK and from other European countries,[20-22] all of which show that excessive use of UV sunbeds is an additional risk factor for malignant melanoma. Primary prevention activities should, therefore, also advise against excessive exposure to artificial UV radiation.

One approach to primary prevention of melanoma is to target the section of the population at greatest risk of melanoma. In Europe this may be an appropriate strategy as the incidence of melanoma, although rising rapidly, is still relatively low. In contrast, policy decisions have been made in high incidence countries such as Australia that the whole population should be targeted.

An approach to defining the high risk sector of the population in the UK has been made by ourselves in carrying out a case control

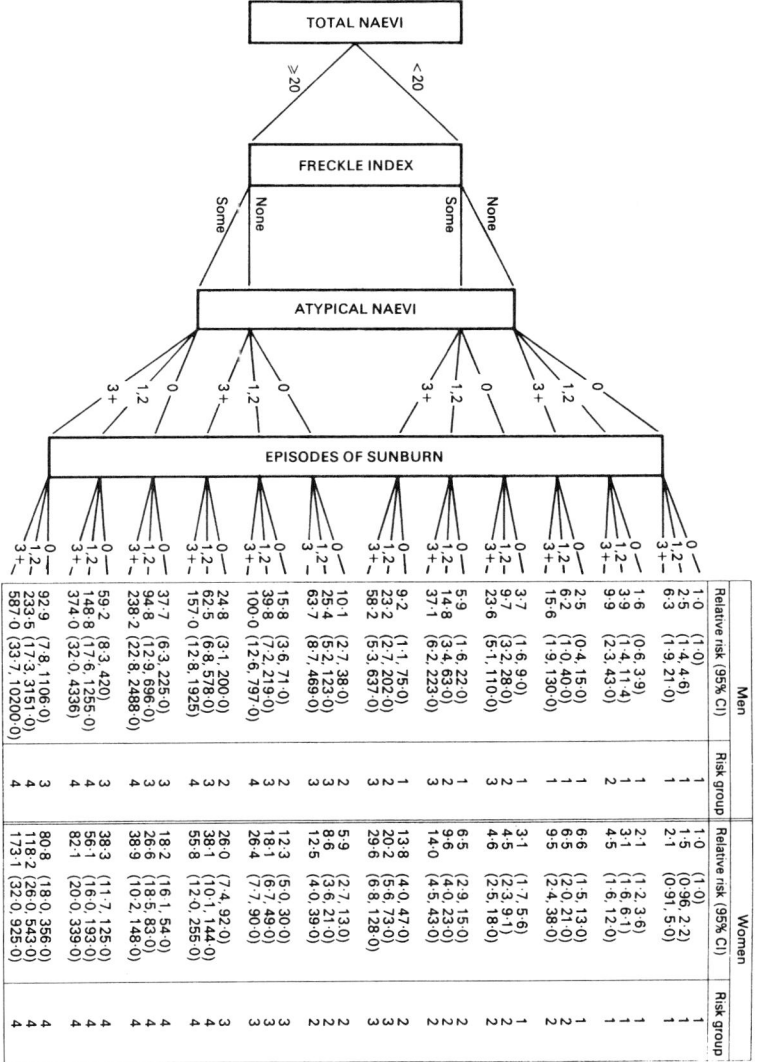

Fig. Flow-chart of risk factors for cutaneous malignant melanoma. Risk groups: 1 = marginally increased risk; 2 = increased risk; 3 = very increased risk; 4 = worryingly high risk. Relative risk coefficients used (for men/women, respectively): 10·1/5·9 for total naevi; 3·7/3·1 for freckles; 1·6/2·1 for atypical naevi; and 2·5/1·5 for episodes of sunburn.

study to determine the most important risk factors for melanoma. It was observed by appropriate statistical analysis that the 4 most important independent and statistically significant risk factors were total number of banal naevi, presence of freckling, presence of 3 or more clinically atypical or dysplastic naevi and a history of 3 or more episodes of severe sunburn. From this material a melanoma risk factor chart has been devised which is in regular use in a number of clinics. This categorises the population into 4 main groups, with group 4 being the group at significantly increased risk of developing melanoma who merit additional advice against excessive sun exposure, and possibly in some cases surveillance (Figure). The work carried out and published in 1989 in the UK[23] has recently been extended and confirmed in a German population.[24,25]

Sun avoidance and sensible sun exposure is the mainstay of advice on primary prevention. At the present time a number of manufacturers are encouraging the use of devices which give an indication when a certain measured level of UV has reached the device which is placed on the skin. These monitors which have a variety of trade names are suggested as being an appropriate way of offering 'safe' sun exposure.[26] However, it must be remembered that sun exposure has cumulative deleterious effect on the skin, and at the present time it is not possible to define any safe level of sun exposure. For this reason these sun exposure devices cannot be given any medical recommendation.

In conclusion, melanoma early detection and prevention in Europe is currently at a relatively early stage compared with that in Australia but appropriate educational activities for the incidence of melanoma and for the knowledge of the public are being identified.

It is essential that ongoing audit of the efficacy of these systems is carried out so that the more effective approaches can be widely disseminated and those which are less effective can be brought to an appropriate conclusion.

REFERENCES

1 MacKie RM, Osterlind A, Ruiter D et al. Report on consensus meeting of the EORTC Mealnoma Group on educational needs for primary and secondary prevention of melanoma in Europe. Eur J Cancer 1991: 27: 1317–1323.
2 Temoshok, L, Di Clement, RJ, Sweet DM et al. Factors relating to patient delay in seeking attention for cutaneous malignant melanoma. Cancer 1984; 54: 3048–3053.
3 Grin CM, Kopf AW, Welkovich B et al. Accuracy in the clinical diagnosis of malignant melanoma. Arch Dermatol 1990; 126: 763–766.
4 Doherty VR, MacKie RM. Experience of a public education programme on early detection of cutaneous malignant melanoma. BMJ 1988; 287: 388–391.
5 Cristofolini M, Zumiani M, Boi S, Piscioli F. Community detection of early melanoma. Lancet 1986; 1: 18.
6 Cristofolini M, Bianchi R, Sebastiana B, Decarli A, Hanau C, Micciolo R et al.

Analysis of the cost effectiveness ratio of the health campaign for the early diagnosis of cutaneous melanoma in Trentino, Italy. Cancer 1993; 71: 370–374.

7 Doherty VR & MacKie RM. Reasons for poor prognosis in British patients with cutaneous malignant melanoma. BMJ 1986; 292: 987–989.

8 MacKie RM & Hole D. Audit of public education campaign to encourage earlier detection of malignant melanoma. BMJ 1992; 304: 1012–1015.

9 Rampen FHJ, van Huystee BEWL & Kiemeney LALM. Melanoma/skin cancer screening clinics: Experiences in the Netherlands. J Am Acad Dermatol 1991; 25: 776–777.

10 Rampen FHJ, Berretty PJM, Van Huystee BEWL, Kiemeney LALM, Nijs CHHM. Lack of selective attendance of participants at skin cancer/melanoma screening clinics. J Am Acad Dermatol 1993; 29: 423–427.

11 Hoffmann K, Dirschka Th, Schatz H, Segerling M, Tiemann Th, Hoffmann A. A local education campaign on early diagnosis of malignant melanoma. Eur J Epidemiol 1993; 9: 591–598.

12 Pehamberger H, Binder M, Knollmayer S, Wolff K. Immediate effects of a public education campaign on prognostic feature of melanoma. J Am Acad Dermatol 1993; 29: 106–109.

13 Bulliard JL, Raymond L Levi, F Schuler, G Enderlin, F Pellaux J et al. Prevention of cutaneous melanoma: An epidemiological evaluation of the Swiss campaign. Rev Epidemiol Sante Publique 1992; 40: 431–438.

14 Koh HK, Lew RA, Prout MN. Screening for melanoma/skin cancer: theoretic and practical considerations. J Am Acad Dermatol 1989; 20: 159–172.

15 Kohl HK, Geller AC, Miller DR et al. Who is being screened for melanoma/skin cancer? J Am Acad Dermatol 1991; 24: 271–277.

16 Goldenhersh MA. Melanoma Screening: Critique and proposal. J Am Acad Dermatol 1993; 28: 642–644.

17 Mcleod GR. Control of melanoma in a high risk population. Pigment Cell 1988; 9: 131–140.

18 Marks R, Hill D. The Public Health approach to melanoma control: Prevention & Early Detection. Australian Cancer Society, 1992. ISBN 0 947283 23 4

19 Boldeman C, Ullen H. Mansson-Brahme E, Holm LE. Primary prevention of malignant melanoma in the Stockholm Cancer Prevention Programme. Eur J Cancer Prevent 1993; 2: 441–446.

20 Walter SD, Marrett LD, From L, Hertzman C, Shannon HS, Ray P. Association of cutaneous malignant melanoma with the use of sunbeds and sunlamps. Am J Epidemiol 1990; 131: 232–234.

21 Sverdlow AJ, English JSC, MacKie RM et al. Fluorescent lamps ultraviolet lamps and the risk of cutaneous melanoma. BMJ 1987; 297: 647–650.

22 Autier P, Dore J-F, Lejeune F et al. Cutaneous malignat melanoma and exposure to sunlamps or sunbeds: An EORTC multicenter case-control study in Belgium, France and Germany. Int J Cancer 1994; 58, 809–813.

23 MacKie RM, Freudenberger T, Aitchison TC. Personal risk factor chart for melanoma. Lancet 1989; II: 487–490.

24 Garbe C, Buttner P, Weiss J et al. Risk factors for developing cutaneous melanoma and criteria for identifying persons at risk: Multicenter case-control study of the central malignant melanoma. J Invest Dermatol 1994; 102: 695–699.

25 Garbe C, Buttner P, Weiss J et al. Associated factors in the prevalence of more than 50 common melanocytic nevi, atypical melanocytic nevi, and actini lentigines: Multicenter case-control study of the central malignant melanoma registry of the German Dermatological Society. J Invest Dermatol 1994; 102: 700–705.

26 Moseley H, MacKie RM, Ferguson J. The suitability of SunCheck patches and Tanscan cards for monitoring the sunburning effectiveness of sunlight. Br J Dermatol 1993; 128: 75–78.

British Medical Bulletin 1995, Vol 51, No. 3 pp. 584–608
©The British Council 1995

Surgical management of malignant melanoma

A S Ball and J Thomas

Academic Surgical Unit, The Royal Marsden Hospital, London, UK

Wide and mutilating surgical excision is contra-indicated for primary malignant melanoma. Tumours less than 1 mm thick require only 1 cm excision margins while those 1–4 mm thick need only 2 cm margins. Primary closure without skin grafting should always be attempted. Axillary and inguinal block dissection remain standard treatment for established lymphatic metastases but elective block dissection is still controversial and should only be performed in the context of a clinical trial. Selective lymphadenectomy based on intraoperative lymphatic mapping is being evaluated. Isolated limb perfusion plays an important role in palliation, and perfusion with a combination of cytotoxic agents and cytokines is an exciting therapeutic advance. Laser vapourization under local or general anaesthesia is an alternative way of treating multiple small cutaneous and subcutaneous lesions and is much better tolerated.

BIOPSY

Excision biopsy

Excision biopsy remains the standard way of diagnosing malignant melanoma, providing the histopathologist with a complete specimen for microstaging.[1] It can be accomplished without difficulty for lesions under 1.5 cm in diameter. A margin of 1–2 mm of normal skin is taken using an elliptical incision with its long axis in the line of the natural skin creases.

Incision biopsy

Evidence on the risk of incision biopsy is conflicting. Retrospective studies are hard to interpret because details of tumour thickness are absent or incomplete and aspects of treatment are not comparable. Worse survival figures after preliminary biopsy, as reported by Ironside et al.,[2] may simply reflect more advanced tumours. Epstein et al. compared the survival rate of 115 patients on the California Tumor Registry who had an incision biopsy or 'incomplete excision' before definitive treatment with that of 55 patients who did not and found no evidence of a detrimental effect from biopsy.[3] Biopsy included 'simple excision' in an unspecified number of cases and details of tumour thickness were not recorded, so the conclusions of the study have to remain suspect.

Bagley et al. compared the local recurrence and survival rates of 22 patients who underwent initial incision biopsy with 103 patients who did not and found no difference between the two groups, which were stratified according to tumour thickness.[4] On the other hand, in a study by Rampen et al. of 76 patients treated between 1961 to 1970, 14 of whom had undergone well-documented preliminary incision biopsy, univariate analysis demonstrated a worse prognosis after incision biopsy and multivariate analysis showed incision biopsy to have a strongly adverse prognostic effect.[5] The study can be criticized, however, for the small number of patients in the risk group and its data on tumour thickness which were sought retrospectively.

Apart from any effect on prognosis, incision biopsy has the major disadvantage that it may compromise accurate microstaging. Griffiths and Briggs reported that histological specimens were unassessable in over 30% of incision biopsies compared with only 5% of excision biopsies and 0.5% of primary wide excisions.[6] Incision biopsy is best reserved for patients with large or subungual lesions to confirm the diagnosis before further treatment. It can be accomplished either by taking a punch biopsy or by wedge resection.

SURGERY OF PRIMARY MALIGNANT MELANOMA

The tradition of taking a wide margin of normal skin around the primary tumour is attributed to William Sampson Handley whose advice was based on the prevailing principles of surgery for breast cancer at the turn of the century and on his observations from a single postmortem on a patient with metastatic disease from a primary lesion on the heel. As the primary had already been excised Handley admitted: 'No opportunity of investigating the spread of permeation around a primary focus of melanotic growth has fallen to me'.[7]

Handley never specified exact margins but in the second of his Hunterian Lectures in 1907 he recommended making an incision 'about an inch' from the edge of the tumour, raising skin flaps 'about two inches in all directions round the skin incision' and taking a similar margin of muscle down to and including the deep fascia.[8] A variety of other excision margins were recommended by different authorities over the next few decades: 5 cm by Raven,[9] 8 cm by Pack,[10] and even 15 cm in some cases by Peterssen,[11] but the results of radical sugery were universally disappointing, presumably due to the high proportion of thick tumours. Pack, for example, practicing wide and 'ruthless' (sic) excision, reported a definitive 5 year disease-free survival rate of 38% in 189 patients treated between 1948–1951.[12]

Taking broad margins of normal skin around malignant melanomas continued to be standard practice until recently. The chief reason for this was the description of an abnormal appearance and distribution of melanocytes in the vicinity of a malignant tumour.[13,14] According to Fallowfield and Cook, these changes are due to chronic sun exposure.[15]

A more conservative surgical approach gradually emerged with the advent of microstaging as it became apparent that thin melanomas had a better prognosis than thick ones.[16–18] Breslow reviewed 62 patients with melanomas <0.76 mm thick who had been followed up for 5 years or more.[19] None of them had developed distant recurrence, including (of especial note) 14 cases with excision margins of <0.5 cm.

Aitken et al. analysed survival data from 118 patients with localized melanoma and found that excision margins of <2 cm were associated with a worse prognosis than wider margins, if tumours were over 2 mm thick or 1 cm in diameter, but above 3 cm the width of excision margin had apparently no influence on survival.[20] Likewise, Schmoeckel et al. found no correlation between the rate of metastasis over 5 years and the width of excision margin in 577 patients who had undergone excision with a variety of excision margins.[21]

Unlike the risk of metastases, that of local relapse appears to be more closely related to the extent of local surgery. Local recurrence is usually defined as relapse within 5 cm of the perimeter of the primary closure or skin graft; relapse beyond 5 cm is defined as in-transit metastasis.[22] The incidence of local recurrence in most series is between 2 and 6%.[23]

Cascinelli et al reviewed data on 593 patients with clinical stage I (CS-I) tumours collected between 1967 to 1975 by the WHO Collaborating Centres for Evaluation of Methods of Diagnosis and Treatment of Melanoma.[24] The local relapse rate was 9% (9/96) for margins <2 cm wide and 3% (16/497) for margins >2 cm wide but this trend was not confirmed when relapse rates for tumours <2 mm and >2 mm thick were examined individually, suggesting that the effect of the excision margin may have reflected the distribution of tumour thickness. Rampen pointed out though that a threefold increase in the local recurrence rate with margins <2 cm was again evident when clinical stage II (CS-II) cases were included in the analysis and the study therefore demonstrated a strongly adverse effect from narrow margins.[25]

Bagley et al. reviewed the records of 147 patients treated at the Lahey Clinic between 1955–1979, two thirds of whom had 5 year follow-up.[4] There were 6 local relapses, 4 of them in patients whose excision margins had been <1 cm. The rate of local relapse in cases whose excision margins were <1 cm was 12% compared with only 2% in those whose margins were wider. All but one of the relapses occurred in patients with melanomas either >0.76 mm thick or Clark level III.

Similar results were reported by Kelly et al.[26] The local recurrence rate was 7.8% in 51 cases with excision margins of <1 cm but only 3 per cent in 295 cases with wider margins of excision. Schmoeckel et al. noted a local recurrence rate of 10% in patients with excision margins of <3 cm but of only 2.9% with margins of 3 cm or more.[21]

Equally good results with narrow excision margins were reported by others. Urist et al. reported that among 936 consecutive patients with tumours under 1 mm thick treated at the Sydney Melanoma Unit and 115 similar patients treated in Alabama there was only one local recurrence after a minimum of 5 years follow-up.[23] 62% of these patients had excision margins of 2 cm or less. Welvaart et al. reviewed the results of excision in 216 patients treated between 1960 and 1982 in the Netherlands. Local recurrence occurred in just a single patient although 47 had excision margins of <2 cm.[27]

The relationship between tumour thickness and excision margins has been demonstrated most clearly by Milton et al. who analysed the results of treatment in 1839 patients with 5 years follow-up.[28] The overall incidence of local recurrence was 7.6%. With narrow excision margins (<2 cm) the local recurrence rate ranged from 2% for thin tumours (0.1–0.7 mm) to 21% for thick tumours (>3 mm). With wider excision margins (>2 cm) it ranged from <1% to 9%. Patients with thick tumours treated with narrow resection margins had a local recurrence rate 2.5 times higher than that of patients treated by wide excision.

Taylor and Hughes reported the results of treating 163 patients over a 10 year period according to a simple practical plan in which the width of excision was based on palpation, which was reckoned to correlate roughly with tumour thickness.[29] Thus impalpable lesions (<0.76 mm) were excised with a 1 cm margin, macular lesions (0.76–1.49 mm) with 2 cm margin and nodular lesions (>1.5 mm) with 3–5 cm margins. Of the 163 patients, at least 34 had inadequate treatment based on the definitive tumour thickness and a similar number probably had wider excision margins than necessary, making the treatment plan unattractive. There were a total of 11 local recurrences. None occurred in patients with tumours <0.75 mm thick and only one in those with tumours 0.75–1.49 mm thick. Ten relapses occurred in patients with tumours >1.5 mm thick, 2 occurring in cases with less than 3 cm clearance, 3 in cases with 3 cm clearance, and 5 in cases with over 3 cm clearance.

All the studies suggest that there is a minimum safe margin of excision which depends on the depth of invasion of the tumour. Even so they are all subject to the usual deficiencies of retrospective reports. To rectify this, the World Health Organization Melanoma Group embarked on a prospective randomized trial in 1979 to compare excision margins of 1 and 3 cm for CS-I melanomas 2 mm thick or less.[30] By 1987 there were just over 300 patients in each group. Prognostic criteria, including tumour thickness, were comparable in both. Disease-free and overall survival rates after a mean follow-up period of 55 months were similar, and the incidence of distant, regional and in-transit metastases were similar for both margins (narrow margin – 7 distant, 14 regional, 2 in-transit; wide margin – 8 distant, 20 regional, 1 in-transit). Local recurrence developed in 6 patients (0.9%) but it was the only site of relapse in just 3 – in whom the tumours were all >1 mm thick and removed with a narrow margin.

The results were updated in 1991 with a mean follow up of 90 months.[31] There were no significant survival differences according to the margin of excision and the distribution of metastases was again similar (narrow margin – 17 distant, 21 regional, 2 in-transit; wide margin – 14 distant, 24 regional, 2 in-transit). Isolated local recurrence was now reported in 4 patients with a narrow excision margin, all of whom had melanomas of 1.01–2.00 mm thick, but in none of those with wide margins. The most recent update reports a single isolated local recurrence in the wide margin group and 5 local recurrences in the narrow margin group; all of them after excision of tumours >1 mm thick.[32]

The results of this trial did not make clear whether or not melanomas 1–2 mm thick should be treated with 1 cm or 3 cm margins to reduce the small risk of local recurrence.[33] Nonetheless, the results of the WHO study lent support to the conclusions of retrospective studies and it is now generally accepted that an excision margin of 1 cm is adequate for melanomas < 1 mm thick.

In 1993, the Intergroup Melanoma Committee (USA and Canada) reported the results of a prospective randomized trial to compare 2 and 4 cm margins for melanomas 1–4 mm thick.[34] This multicentre study involved 486 patients with melanoma of the trunk and proximal extremities and had a median follow-up time of 6 years. There were 244 patients in the 2 cm arm and 242 in the 4 cm arm and prognostic variables were closely matched. Distant and in-transit relapse rates were similar for both groups (2 cm – 10.9% distant, 2.5% in-transit; 4 cm – 8.5 per cent distant, 2.1% in transit). Local recurrence occurred in 2 patients with 2 cm excision margins and 4 patients with 4 cm excision margins ($P = NS$); 5 of these patients died of metastases. The overall 5 year survival rate was 79.5% for the 2 cm margin patients and 83.7% for the 4 cm margin patients ($P = NS$). Patients with narrower excision margins required less time in hospital because they did not need skin grafts. The trial design included randomization for elective regional lymph node dissection but follow-up was not sufficiently mature.

The use of 4 cm excision margins in this study for cases with a melanoma 1 mm thick has been criticized.[35] In the United Kingdom the Melanoma Study Group and British Association of Plastic Surgeons are currently conducting a trial comparing 1 and 3 cm margins for melanomas 2 mm or more in thickness on the limbs or trunk.

Deep fascia

Olsen examined the effect of excising fascia with the primary tumour.[36] From a series of 500 patients with melanoma he selected those with CS-I tumours located on the abdominal wall and extremities (where fascia is well-developed) and reviewed their outcome. Excision of fascia ceased after 1958 but was freely undertaken before that date. Of 67 patients treated before 1958 lymphatic metastases developed in 14/31 (45%) of those who underwent fascial excision but only 5/36 (14%) of those who did not. Of 51 patients treated after 1958 only 5 (10%) developed lymphatic metastases. Olsen argued that if the association of fascial excision with metastasis just reflected excision of more advanced tumours, a higher incidence of lymphatic metastasis would be expected among those treated after

1958. The low incidence of metastases in those treated after 1958 suggested that excision of fascia had a detrimental effect. A similar study was undertaken more recently by Kenady et al. at M D Anderson Hospital comparing the results of surgery in 107 patients treated before 1969, when excision of fascia was routine, with those in 95 patients treated subsequently, when fascia was preserved.[37] The distribution of tumours according to microstaging was similar. Survival and recurrence rates were not significantly different between the two groups.

Both these studies used historical controls and are thus subject to potential bias. Fascia is not routinely excised nowadays, but a definitive answer to the question of whether its excision is harmful or not still awaits the results of a controlled prospective study.

Skin closure and grafting

Pritchard et al. reviewed the type of wound closure employed in a series of 256 melanomas treated between 1972 and 1986.[38] Primary closure was used for only 30% of wounds between 1982–1986 but for 54% between 1982–1986. The change was explained partly by an increase in the number of thin melanomas treated in the latter period of study but also by the use of a multilayer closure technique whereby seroma formation is discouraged by using a continuous subcutaneous suture.

Aitken et al. included means of closure as a prognostic parameter in a retrospective analysis of 118 patients treated between 1952 to 1976.[20] No survival difference was found between those having a skin graft and those undergoing primary wound closure.

Traditionally, split skin grafts have been taken from the contralateral limb for fear that an ipsilateral donor site might be complicated by in-transit metastases. Flook et al. reviewed a series of 186 patients who underwent split skin grafts after melanoma excision.[39] In a quarter of the cases the graft was harvested from the ipsilateral limb proximal to the tumour. Only one patient had recurrence at a donor site and this occurred outside the lymphatic drainage of the limb. It is thus more sensible to harvest grafts from the same limb as the tumour so that any recurrence lies within the field of limb perfusion.

Subungual melanoma

The optimal treatment for these lesions is uncertain as they are not common, but the trend is away from proximal amputation.[40] When the tumour is confined to the nail bed alone it is often possible to amputate through the adjacent interphalangeal joint,[41] and to use a long volar skin flap. For more extensive tumours, amputation through the base of the proximal phalanx, distal to the insertion of flexor and extensor tendons may be possible.

Head and neck melanoma

In a study of 203 patients with CS-I melanoma of intermediate thickness (0.76–1.69 mm) Day noted that 11 of the 12 deaths occurred in patients whose primary lesion was on the upper back, posterior arm, posterior neck and posterior scalp (BANS).[42] He suggested that patients with lesions in the BANS area had a worse prognosis than those with lesions of equivalent thickness at other sites and that such patients might be suitable for elective lymph node dissection. However, when Cascinelli et al. examined the prognostic importance of BANS lesions in patients in the WHO Melanoma Group study, he found that survival was not significantly worse for those with BANS lesions, and that the BANS distribution did not emerge as a significant prognostic variable on multivariate analysis.[43]

Orr et al. reported the results of treatment in 91 cases of malignant melanoma of the head and neck.[44] Tumours were excised with margins of 1 cm or 2 cm depending on whether the lesion was impalpable or palpable, except when a poor cosmetic result was anticipated in which case a preliminary biopsy was taken. No patient had an inappropriately wide biopsy as a result of clinical overestimation of tumour thickness. Wounds were closed by direct suture in 27% of cases, by local flaps in 44% of cases and by skin grafting or distant flaps in 25% of cases. Local recurrence developed in 10 cases and regional recurrence in 13, all of whom had tumours >2 mm thick. A conservative policy with respect for cosmetic results appears to be acceptable.

REGIONAL LYMPH NODE DISSECTION

Elective regional lymph node dissection (ELND)

Controversy still surrounds the role of elective lymphadectomy, though in the United Kingdom there is a consensus that the evidence currently available does not warrent ELND for limb lesions.[45]

The rationale for ELND is based on the proposition that micrometastases disseminate sequentially from primary tumour to regional lymph nodes and then to distant sites. Theoretically, survival should be increased if nodal micrometastases are removed before they spread further. By the time lymph node metastases are clinically detectable 70 to 85% of patients have distant metastases and the 10 year survival is only 25%.[46]

The overall incidence of occult metastases in specimens obtained at ELND varies according to source from around 5% in some[47,48] to 20% and more in others.[49,50] Some authorities have proposed that ELND should be delayed for 14 days after excising the primary lesion but so far no studies have demonstrated any benefit from interval ELND.[45]

The counterarguments to ELND are that it represents over-treatment in patients without micrometastases, that morbidity is not insubstantial, and that the procedure is unlikely to confer any real survival benefit even when occult nodal metastases are present because lymphatic spread occurs in parallel with, rather than in series with, blood borne dissemination.[45,51] Moreover, in one study of 1164 patients treated without ELND, 516 of whom suffered relapse within 10 years, only 51% presented with a first recurrence in the regional nodes alone, the rest had either distant or simultaneous regional and distant disease.[52]

Most of the evidence in favour of ELND comes from retrospective studies conducted in the USA and Australia. Some are described as partly prospective but published results incorporate retrospective data as well, limiting their value.

Balch et al. reviewed results of surgery in 287 patients attending the Alabama Melanoma Registry from 1960 to 1977.[53] Patients with melanomas 0.77–3.99 mm thick who had wide excision and ELND had an actuarial 5 year survival rate of 86% compared with 58% among those having wide excision alone. The greatest advantage was seen in patients with tumours 1.50–3.99 mm thick but no benefit from ELND was apparent in those with lesions <0.76 mm or >4.00 mm thick. Balch et al. subsequently reported results of a retrospective study of 1786 patients attending melanoma clinics at the Universities of Alabama and Sydney, 491 of whom had undergone ELND.[54] Follow-up was over 2–25 years. Actuarial survival analysis again showed a marked survival benefit with ELND for tumours 1.50–3.99 mm thick and a further benefit for tumours 0.76–1.49 mm thick was noted in the Australian patients.

Milton et al. reviewed 1319 patients of whom 380 had ELND as well as wide local excision.[47] Patients were stratified according to sex, tumour thickness and location of lesion, which had been identified as independent prognostic factors on multivariate analysis. The distribution of these features was similar in those patients undergoing ELND and those undergoing wide excision alone. Follow-up was over 2–32 years. Survival analysis showed significantly improved survival rates after ELND in men with extremity lesions 1.6–3.0 mm thick. Improved survival was also noted in women with extremity lesions over 3.0 mm thick, but this was not significant.

McCarthy et al. undertook a non-randomized prospective study of 2347 patients with lesions confined to the trunk and limb, 628 of whom underwent ELND.[48] At 10 years a significant survival benefit was noted in men with lesions 1.6–3.0 mm thick on the trunk and extremities and in women with extremity lesions over 1.6 mm thick.

A recent study from 9 medical centres in Germany involving 3616 patients produced similar results.[55] A 20% improvement in 5 year survival was reported for male patients with axial and acral melanomas >1.5–4.5 mm thick who underwent ELND. In women only those with thick tumours appeared to benefit.

All these studies demonstrate a survival advantage from ELND for patients with tumours of intermediate thickness and a recent meta-analysis of ELND for CS-I cases has confirmed the apparent benefit in 5 year survival after ELND for melanomas of intermediate thickness.[56] Balch and Milton maintain that these are precisely the patients expected to benefit as they have a high risk of occult regional metastases but a low risk of systemic metastases.[46]

The most important evidence against ELND comes from two prospective randomized trials: an international cooperative study conducted by the WHO and another conducted by surgeons at the Mayo Clinic.

The WHO Melanoma Group study involved 530 patients with CS-I primary melanoma on the distal two-thirds of the limbs treated between September 1967 and January 1974.[57] Of these patients, 286 (52%) were randomized to receive wide exision of the primary lesion and node dissection if disease in regional nodes became clinically detectable later, 267 (48%) to receive wide local excision and ELND. Both groups were matched according to major prognostic criteria. After a mean follow-up period of over 10 years no difference in survival was found between the two groups. An updated report confirmed the conclusions.[49]

The Mayo Clinic Trial reported by Sim et al.[58,59] involved 171 CS-I melanoma patients with trunk and limb lesions randomized to one of three groups: (a) 62 had wide local excision alone, (b) 54 had wide local excision and simultaneous ELND and (c) 55 had wide local excision and ELND delayed 2 to 3 months. Patients with midline trunk and head and neck tumours were excluded. Median follow-up was 4.5 years Analysis of survival by the logrank test showed no significant differences in overall or disease free survival between the three groups.

The WHO trial has been criticized on a number of points. Multi-centre trials can be subject to wide variations in the standard of staging and treatment and the clinical diagnosis of node involvement is notoriously unreliable. In the WHO trial the proportion of patients with histologically positive but clinically negative regional nodes varied markedly among participating centres suggesting that the assiduity with which the pathologist sought lymphatic metastases may also have varied between centres.[46] Another potential source of difficulty is that the trial was confined to melanomas of the lower limb occurring chiefly in women (79%). It therefore only included patients with a relatively good prognosis, making survival differences more difficult to detect.[45]

As the trial was initiated before tumour thickness and ulceration were recognized as important prognostic factors, these factors were not included as stratification criteria.[60] Indeed, less than half of the patients entered into the original trial had full pathological and clinical data available. Balch undertook a multivariate analysis on the data from the WHO Melanoma Group study and confirmed that tumour thickness and ulceration were the dominant variables. He also found that although tumour thickness was equally divided between the two arms of the trial there were more patients with ulcerated lesions in the ELND group, possibly counteracting the benefit of ELND.[45] A reanalysis of the WHO data by Cascinelli, using data only from patients whose tumour thickness was known, showed a better survival rate among patients with intermediate thickness tumours who underwent ELND than in those who did not. The numbers in this group was small however.[61]

Currently awaited are the results of two international prospective randomized trials. In the NCI sponsored Intergroup Melanoma Committee protocol (USA and Canada), whose report on excision margins already has been discussed (*vide supra*), wide local excision is compared with wide local excision and ELND in patients with intermediate thickness melanomas (1 to 4 mm), and in the WHO Melanoma Group study (Europe), patients with trunk melanomas over 2 mm thick are randomized to wide local excision and thera-peutic lymph node dissection if required or wide local excision and ELND.

Intraoperative lymph node mapping and selective lymphadenectomy

Morton et al. have devised a method of identifying the 'sentinel node', the lymph node nearest the site of the primary tumour on the direct drainage pathway, making it possible to sample this lymph node and look for metastases.[62] The regional lymph node basin is identified by cutaneous lymphoscintigraphy (with technetium-labelled dextran) in patients whose melanoma has an ambiguous drainage route, a technique which has been verified in a number of studies.[63–65] At operation 0.5–1.0 ml of patent blue-V or isosulfan blue is injected intradermally at the site of the primary melanoma and the injection repeated every 20 minutes. Lymphatic channels can then be visualized during dissection and traced to the sentinel lymph node which is sent for frozen section. Morton et al. have reported that a sentinel lymph node (or nodes) was identified in 194/237 (82%) of lymphadenectomies, most successfully in cases with lesions draining to the groins. All cases underwent ELND and metastases were found in 20% of sentinel nodes. The positive predictive value of the technique for identifying involved regional nodes was 100%; the sensitivity, specificity and accuracy were 75%, 100% and 95% respectively.

Morton et al. believe that intraoperative mapping could avoid unecessary lymphadenectomy in 80% of CS-I cases and also in 20% of CS-II cases with palpable lymph nodes in the absence of metastases. The success of the technique is operator dependent, however, and most of the cases reported (128/237) had axillary surgery requiring less extensive dissection. Recent studies have reported successful lymphatic mapping using a gamma-probe after injection of technetium-labeled sulphur colloid and this approach may well have further application.[66,67]

Therapeutic regional lymph node dissection

There is no doubt about the benefit of therapeutic lymph node dissection (TLND) in controlling locoregional disease though its effect on survival is probably minimal.[68] Morbidity is greater after inguinal dissection than after axillary dissection. Wound complications can be reduced by trimming back skin flaps before the wound is finally closed, and transposing the sartorius muscle to cover the femoral vessels.[69] In a recent report of 168 patients undergoing inguinal dissections at M D Anderson Cancer Centre, wound problems occurred in around 20% of cases, and were related to age > 50 years and smoking.[70] In a series of patients treated by axillary dissection at Roswell Park Memorial Institute, wound complications occurred in 10% of patients and oedema of the arm in 4%.[71,72]

Besides anecdotal reports, there is no convincing evidence that survival is better after radical ilio-obdurator lymph node dissection

(RID) than after superficial femoral dissection (SFD). However, in a retrospective study of 133 patients at the Royal Marsden Hospital, groin recurrence was significantly more frequent after SFD (57.1%) than after RID (23.3%).[73] Multiple regression analysis also showed that the chief prognostic factors were the number of involved lymph nodes in the superficial femoral and ilio-obturator compartments. In a more recent study from the Memorial Sloane-Kettering Cancer Centre, favourable prognostic factors in patients with established regional node disease were found to include nontruncal primary site and absence of extranodal disease.[74]

The practice of ELND in patients with with melanoma of the head and neck is losing favour as the proportion of patients with occult disease does not justify such radical surgery.[44] In a recent study from Australia lymph node metastases were identified in only 7% of ELND specimens, and yet 13% of patients still developed regional recurrence after ELND. Improved survival after ELND, apparent on univariate analysis, was not demonstrated on multivariate analysis.[75,76]

Preauricular lymph nodes are a common site of metastasis from tumours of the head and neck and their excision usually requires parotidectomy with or without radical neck dissection (RND). Our policy in such cases is to get a frozen section of a jugulo-digastric lymph node during surgery and to proceed to RND only when a metastasis is demonstrated.[77] In a small series of patients with preauricular lymph node metastases, half of them had occult jugulo-digastric lymph node metastases and underwent RND.[78]

Minimal access techniques have been used to perform ilio-obturator node dissection[79] but there is insufficient data to draw any conclusions yet about their future application.

ISOLATED LIMB PERFUSION

Therapeutic perfusion

Isolated limb perfusion (ILP) was described by Creech et al. in 1958.[80] The principle is to deliver a cytotoxic agent at high concentration to a limb isolated from the systemic circulation by means of a tourniquet. The limb is perfused with cytotoxic via its main artery and vein. A concentration of cytotoxic 6–10 times that produced by systemic administration can be achieved without systemic side effects.

There have been abundant reports on the use of ILP for melanoma but assessing them is not easy. Until recently there has been no consistent staging system, and the M D Anderson system (Table 1), which is the most popular, is not ideal as it fails to take account of a variety of prognostic factors.[81] (In the present chapter an asterisk indicates the M D Anderson classification; the TMN system is not used.) There has also been no consistent method of reporting results. Overall survival rates are often the main emphasis of published reports but equally important are complete and partial response rates, disease-free intervals and times to progression of disease. Other difficulties include comparing dose schedules and the best way of calculating them.

Early reports demonstrated a clinical response to perfusion with melphalan.[80] Stehlin and Clark reported their experience with this drug in 221 cases with primary and recurrent malignant melanoma of the limbs. Overall survival of stage III* patients was better after ILP than after conventional treatment and loco-regional recurrence was much less.[82] In a subsequent report, McBride and Clark reported 5 year survival rates for stages II* and III* disease of 57 and 24% compared with rates of 38 and 18% in non-perfused cases. The local recurrence rate for lower limb lesions was only 4% compared with 20% after conventional surgery.[83]

Krementz and Ryan reviewed the results of ILP with melphalan, thiotepa or nitrogen mustard in 480 patients with melanoma treated between 1957 to 1971.[84] All tumours were Clark's level III or deeper. Of 39 patients with satellitosis, 11 were free of disease at 5 years and of 18 patients with unresectable primary tumours and regional

Table 1   Clinical staging systems

Standard System		
I	Localized primary melanoma	
II	Regional lymph node metastases	
III	Disseminated disease	

M D Anderson System		
I	Localized primary melanoma	
II	Local recurrence or satellites < 3 cm from primary	
IIIa	In-transit metastases	
IIIb	Regional lymph node metastases	
IV	Distant metastases	

TMN Classification		
I	< 1.5 mm	(Level I-III)
II	> 1.5–4 mm	(Level IV)
III	> 4 mm/satellites	(Level V)
	Regional lymph node metastases	
IV	Distant disease	

In the present chapter an asterisk indicates the M D Anderson classification. The TMN system is not used.

metastases, 5 were disease free at 5 years. Similarly, Koops et al. reported the results of ILP with melphalan in 17 patients with stages II* and III* disease of the extremities.[85] Only 3 patients had recurrence in an extremity. After two years 11 were still alive and after five 6 were still disease-free.

Cytotoxics other than melphalan have been examined, alone and in combination. Golomb observed impressive examples of tumour regression with intravenous actinomycin D after ILP with the same drug.[86] He also reported the results of perfusion with combinations of melphalan, actinomycin D, and thiotepa in patients with recurrent melanoma of the extremity: over 70% exhibited regression of the lesions and 22% had complete resolution lasting 7–124 months.[87] McBride reported the results of ILP in 50 patients with stage III* disease using a triple combination of melphalan, actinomycin D and nitrogen mustard. Half the patients were free of recurrence at 2 years but a quarter had local recurrence, though the local recurrence rate in patients without evidence of dissemination was only 9%.[88] Other cytotoxic agents have not been found to be superior to melphalan.[81] Imidazole carbamoxide (DTIC) which has been used for systemic treatment requires hepatic microsomal activation and is therefore not a rational choice for ILP.

Hyperthermic perfusion was introduced by Stehlin et al. in 1975 who reported its benefit in 165 patients with melanoma of the extremities, stages I–III*.[89] Limb temperatures were elevated to 38.8–40.0°C. The best results were achieved in patients with stage IIIa* disease who had a 5 year survival rate of over 70% compared with only 22% after normothermic ILP.

Recent studies have confirmed the value of hyperthermia.[90] In a review of the results of hyperthermic ILP perfomed in Italy using a variety of cytotoxic agents and combinations, tumour temperature proved to be the most important parameter for response, with complete response rates of 54–75% at tumour temperatures over 41°C.[91]

Ghussen et al. reported the results of a prospective randomized trial undertaken between 1980 and 1983 in patients with melanomas > 1.5 mm thick, stages I–III*, to compare wide local excision and regional lymph node dissection with wide local excision, regional lymph node dissection and hyperthermic ILP with melphalan.[92] Mean follow-up time was 6 years. There were 54 patients in the control arm and 53 in the perfused arm of the trial. Tumour thickness and clinical stage were similarly matched. Analysis of the results at the conclusion of entry into the trial already revealed a marked difference in relapse rate. Among the non-perfused controls there were 21 local recurrences while among the perfused cases there were only 4. By 1988, 26 of control patients had relapsed while only 6 of the perfused patients had relapsed.

Hafstrom et al. in Sweden also reported the results of a controlled trial of hyperthermic ILP with melphalan, wide excision and regional node dissection in patients with recurrent melanoma of the extremities.[93] There were 36 control patients and 33 perfused patients. Mean follow-up time was 39 months. Although disease-free survival was significantly better in perfused patients than controls, there was no significant difference in survival in this study.

Recent studies in the Netherlands have shown that a second perfusion 3–4 weeks after the first can result in significantly higher response rates although the effects are not long-lasting.[94,95] In a multivariate analysis of prognostic factors associated with a response to ILP with melphalan, a multiple perfusion schedule, uninvolved regional lymph nodes and origin on the lower limb were associated with complete remission while solitary lesions, complete remission and female sex were associated with a prolonged recurrence-free interval. There is no firm evidence at present that ILP is of particular benefit in cases with subungual melanoma.[96]

The majority of patients treated in our own unit have been referred with advanced local disease (Ia/IIIa*).[97] An overall response rate of 78% was obtained in 91 patients using hyperthermic perfusion with melphalan. Local progression occurred in 25% of all cases and in 30% of those with stage IIIa* disease. Among the latter group there was a higher recurrence rate and a shorter disease-free interval after femoral than after iliac perfusion. A recent study from the Netherlands, however, failed to demonstrate any significant reduction in inguinal node metastases after iliac perfusion.[98]

The most exciting new developments in ILP involve combination therapy with cytotoxics and cytokines. Tumour necrosis factor (TNF) was first discovered in the serum of animals treated with BCG (bacille Calmette-Guerin) or endotoxin and was found to produce haemorrhagic necrosis and tumour regression in animals. Subsequent developments led to the production of recombinant tumour necrosis factor (rTNF) in *Escherischia coli*. Phase I studies however showed that response to rTNF was limited by the maximum tolerated dose.[99]

Lejeune et al. undertook a pilot study of hyperthermic ILP with rTNF in three patients with extensive in-transit disease of the lower limb.[100] All patients developed fevers and two became temporarily shocked when cytokine entered the systemic circulation. All of them however exhibited some degree of tumour regression.

Other studies demonstrated that the number of TNF receptors

on malignant cells increases when they are incubated with gamma interferon (IFN) and that the two agents act synergistically. Cytotoxic activity of TNF can also be enhanced by hyperthermia and conventional chemotherapeutic agents.[99] Consequently, phase II studies were initiated using hyperthermic ILP (40–40.5°C) with melphalan, TNF at a dose of 2–4 mg by bolus arterial injection, and INF given by two preoperative subcutaneous injections and one perfusate injection. Patients were also given prophylactic dopamine and indomethacin.

In their initial report on 19 patients with stage IIIa* or IIIab* melanoma of the extremities, softening of tumours occurred in every cases within 3 days, and a complete response was seen in 18 cases.[101] The median response time was over 9 months. Subsequent reports have confirmed the extremely high response rate.[102] In the latest report on 53 patients with stages IIIa/IIIab/IV* disease, 90% displayed complete remission and 10% partial remission with no failures.[103] The median follow-up time was 26 months and the median response time 14 months. Local recurrence was observed in 21 cases. No patient died as a result of treatment but systemic complications included renal failure, adult respiratory distress syndrome, hepatic dysfunction, leucopenia and thrombocytopenia. All patients experienced fevers lasting several hours.

Other groups have not met with the same success. Vaglini et al reported the results of hyperthermic ILP in 22 patients with stage IIIa–IIIab* melanoma using TNF at a dose of 2–4 mg, melphalan and, in 12 cases, IFN.[104] The dose of TNF was reduced in the 12 cases not given IFN. A complete response rate was achieved in only 58% of cases given TNF and INF and in 70% of those given TNF alone.

Our own experience of ILP with TNF includes 4 cases with advanced (stage IIIa/IV) limb melanomas.[105,106] Because of the risk of systemic leakage during iliac perfusion we used the superficial femoral vessels instead. More importantly, we also used a much lower dose of TNF (250–500 µg bolus) than that used by Lienard and others. All cases nonetheless exhibited complete remission with softening apparent within 48 h of perfusion. None of them had systemic side effects.

The surgery branch of the NCI is currently carrying out a prospective randomized trial comparing ILP with melphalan alone with TNF, IFN and melphalan in patients with two or more satellite or intransit lesions in the perfusion field and no evidence of disease elsewhere. Patients with stage IV* disease or those who have failed to respond to perfusion with melphalan are being given IL-2.[107]

Adjuvant perfusion

The impressive response to ILP in patients with advanced and recurrent melanoma soon led to its use as an adjuvant to surgery.[82,87,108-111] Evaluation of all the early studies is severely limited, however, because tumour thickness was not recognized as an important prognostic parameter. This is a major deficiency as appraisal of adjuvant therapy depends on estimating the risks of relapse, not on measuring an observable clinical response. It is worth noting, even so, that nearly all retrospective studies of ILP in CS-I patients demonstrate a survival advantage and a reduction in locoregional relapse from perfusion.[82, 09] McBride et al. for example reported a 5 year survival rate of 86% (76% disease free) in perfused cases compared with a 70% 5 year survival rate (45% disease free) in non-perfused cases. Similar survival figures for CS-I disease are reported by others.[89] In a review of the literature on ILP in 1988, Lee concluded that the mean 5 year survival rate after ILP in 950 patients with localized disease, derived from 8 reports, was 85% compared with 75% for 9244 non-perfused patients, derived from 11 reports.[112] This overview was not a meta-analysis however.

Evidence of a reduction in loco-regional recurrence was reported by Stehlin and Clark[82] and by McBride et al.[109] In the latter study of 88 cases with CS-I disease perfused with melphalan, 2% developed local recurrence, 3% in-transit metastases and 18% regional node metastases. In a subsequent report on 199 cases local recurrence occurred in 2%, in-transit metastases in 3%, regional metastases in 13% and disseminated disease in 8%.[110] In non-perfused historical controls the rate of local recurrence was 7%, in-transit metastases 10%, and regional lymph node metastases 38%.

Krementz and Ryan reported a 5 year disease-free survival rate of 81% for patients with stage I limb disease and tumours deeper than Clark's level III.[84] All lesions were treated by perfusion with melphalan or thiotepa followed by wide excision and regional node dissection.

Tumour thickness was recorded in a study by Koops et al. in which 31 patients with stage I melanoma of the extremities were perfused with melphalan.[113] Twenty-four of these cases had Clark level IV disease and the 5 year disease free survival for these cases was 75%, higher that reported elsewhere for non-perfused cases. Likewise, Martijn et al. reported a significantly better 10 year survival rate in women with thick (>1.5 mm) stage I melanoma of the extremity treated by excision and ILP when retrospectively compared with a similar group treated by excision alone.[114]

The controversy over the role of adjuvant hyperthermic ILP will hopefuly be resolved shortly. The WHO trial No.15 has completed patient accrual and early results suggest better loco-regional control among perfused patients not having ELND, but no significant survival improvement among those perfused.[115]

Complications of ILP

In a comprehensive review by Lee in 1988 the overall mortality rate from nearly 2000 perfusions was between 0–10% and the complication rate 4–33%.[112] The amputation rate was under 2%. Wound problems were the chief cause of morbidity along with limb oedema.

INTRAARTERIAL INFUSION

Regional intra-arterial infusion therapy was initiated by Bierman in 1950. A higher concentration of cytotoxic agent can be achieved in tumour tissue by this method but passage of the cytotoxic agent into the systemic circulation limits benefit. Early studies showed a 10–30% response rate for melanoma using a variety of agents.[112] Muchmore et al. have recently described a technique of repetitive intra-arterial infusion using combination chemotherapy with excellent results in patients that had failed to respond to ILP.[116]

CARBON DIOXIDE LASER ABLATION

Laser vapourization is a new method of treating multiple cutaneous and superficial subcutaneous metastases less than 1.5 cm in diameter. Our experience in 60 patients with over 4500 lesions convinces us that it is a much better option than ILP for patients with small superficial lesions.[117] Postoperative recovery from ILP can be protracted while long term survival prospects are extremely poor and the duration of response limited. On the other hand, laser ablation can be performed under local or general anaesthesia, depending on the number of metastases. We have treated as many as 450 lesions under general anaesthetic at a single session. Wounds are generally painless and completely healed within 6 weeks, even after previous ILP. The recurrence rate is around 2% but new crops of lesions usually require further treatment within a few months. Of 32 patients with stage IIIa disease, 56% were controlled by 3 or less treatments in one year.

KEY POINTS FOR CLINICAL PRACTICE

- Tumours under 1 mm thick require only 1 cm excision margins. Tumours 1–4 mm thick require only 2 cm excision margins.
- Primary closure without skin grafting should be attempted whenever possible.
- Skin grafts should be taken from the limb from which the tumour is excised.
- Axillary and inguinal block dissection remain standard treatment for established lymphatic metastases. Ilioinguinal block dissection may have advantages.
- Elective block dissection is still controversial and should only be performed in the context of a clinical trial until its value is proven.
- Selective lymphadenectomy after lymphatic mapping and sampling is being evaluated.
- Isolated limb perfusion plays an important role in palliation and perfusion with a combination of cytotoxic agents and cytokines is an exciting advance.
- Laser vapourization under local or general anaesthesia is an alternative way of treating multiple small cutaneous and subcutaneous lesions and is much better tolerated.

REFERENCES

1 Ross MI, Balch CM. The current management of cutaneous melanoma. In Cameron JL ed. Advances in Surgery. Mosby-Year Book, Inc. St Louis 1991: 139–200.
2 Ironside P, Pitt TTE, Rank BK. Malignant melanoma: some aspects of pathology and prognosis. Aust NZ J Surg 1977; 47: 70–75.
3 Epstein E, Bragg K, Linden G. Biopsy and prognosis of malignant melanoma. JAMA 1969; 208: 1369–1371.
4 Bagley FH, Cady B, Lee A, Legg MA. Changes in clinical presentation and management of malignant melanoma Cancer 1981; 47: 2126–2134.
5 Rampen FHJ, Van Houten WA, Hop WCJ. Incisional procedures and prognosis in malignant melanoma. Clin Exp Dermatol 1980; 5: 313–420.
6 Griffiths RW, Briggs JC. Biopsy procedures, primary wide excisional surgery and long term prognosis in primary clinical stage I invasive cutaneous malignant melanoma. Ann R Coll Surg Eng 1985; 67: 75–78.
7 Handley WS. The pathology of melanotic growths in relation to their operative treatment. Lecture I. Lancet 1907; i: 927–933.
8 Handley WS. The pathology of melanotic growths in relation to their operative treatment. Lecture II. Lancet 1907; i: 996–1003.
9 Raven RW. The properties and surgical problems of malignant melanoma. Ann R Coll Surg Engl 1950: 6: 28–55.
10 Pack GT, Scharnagel I, Morfit M. The principle of excision and dissection in continuity for primary and metastatic melanoma of the skin. Surgery 1945; 17: 849–866.
11 Petersen NC, Bodenham DC, Lloyd OC. Malignant melanomas of the skin: a

study of the origin, development, aetiology, spread treatment and prognosis. Br J Plast Surg 1969; 15: 49–94,97–116.

12 Pack GT. End results in the treatment of malignant melanoma: a later report. Surgery 1959; 46: 447–460.

13 Cochran AJ, Histology and prognosis in malignant melanoma. J Pathol 1969; 97: 459–468.

14 Wong CK. A study of melanocytes in the normal skin surrounding malignant melanomata. Dermatologica 1970; 141: 215–225.

15 Fallowfield ME, Cook MG. Epidermal melanocytes adjacent to melanoma and the field change effect. Histopathol 1990; 17: 397–400.

16 Breslow A. Thickness, cross sectional areas and depth of invasion in the prognosis of cutaneous melanoma. Ann Surg 172; 902–908.

17 Day CL, Mihm MC, Sober AJ, Fitzpatrick TB, Malt RA. Narrower margins for clinical stage I melanoma. N Engl J Med 1982; 306: 479–481.

18 Ackerman AB, Scheiner AM. How wide and deep is wide and deep enough? Hum Pathol 1983; 14: 743–4.

19 Breslow A, Macht SF. Optimal size of resection margin for thin cutaneous melanoma. Surg Gynecol Obstet 145: 691–692.

20 Aitken DR, Clausen K, Klein JP, James AG. The extent of primary melanoma excision. Ann Surg 1983; 198: 634–641.

21 Schmoeckel C, Bockelbrink A, Bockelbrink H, Kistler H, Braun-Falco O. Low- and high-risk malignant melanoma–III. Prognostic significance of the resection margin. Eur J Cancer Clin Oncol 1983; 19: 245–249.

22 Lee YM. Loco-regional primary and recurrent melanoma: III. Update of natural history and non-systemic treatments (1980–1987). Cancer Treat Rev 1988: 15: 135–162.

23 Urist MM, Balch CM, Soong SJ, Shaw HM, Milton GW, Maddox WA. The influence of surgical margins and prognostic factors predicting the risk of local recurrence in 3445 patients with primary cutaneous melanoma. Cancer 1985: 1398–1402.

24 Cascinelli N, van der Esch EP, Breslow A, Morabio A, Bufalino R. Stage I melanoma of the skin: the problem of resection margins. Eur J Cancer 1980; 16: 1079–1085.

25 Rampen F. Melanoma of the skin: the problem of resection margins (letter). Eur J Cancer 1981; 17: 589–590.

26 Kelly JW, Sagebiel RW, Calderon W, Murillo L, Dakin RL, Blois MS. The frequency of local recurrence as a guide to reexcision margins for cutaneous malignant melanoma. Ann Surg 1984: 200: 759–764.

27 Welvaart K, Hermans J, Zwaveling A, Ruiter DJ. Prognosis and surgical treat- ment of patients with stage I melanomas of the skin: a retrospective analysis of 211 patients. J Surg Oncol 1986; 31: 79–86.

28 Milton GW, Shaw HM, McCarthy WH. Resection margins for melanoma. Aust NZ J Surg 1985; 55: 225–228.

29 Taylor BA, Hughes LE, A policy of selective excision for primary cutaneous malignant melanoma. Eur J Surg Oncol 1985; 11: 7–13.

30 Veronesi U, Cascinelli N, Adamus J et al. Thin stage I primary cutaneous melanoma. Comparison of excision with margins of 1 or 3 cms. N Engl J Med 1988; 318: 1159–1162.

31 Veronesi U, Cascinelli N. Narrow excision (1cm margin): a safe procedure for thin cutaneous melanoma. Arch Surg 1991; 126: 438–441.

32 Marsden JR. Malignant melanoma excision margins (letter) Lancet 1993; 341: 184.

33 Timmons MJ, Malignant melanoma excision margins: making a choice. Lancet 1992; 340: 1393–1395.

34 Balch CM, Urist MM, Karakousis CP et al. Efficacy of 2 cm surgical margins for intermediate-thickness melanomas (1 to 4 mm). Ann Surg 1993; 218: 262–269.

35 Timmons MJ, Thomas JM. The width of excision of cutaneous melanoma. Eur J Surg Oncol 1993; 19: 313–315.

36 Olsen G. The malignant melanoma of skin. New theories based on a study of 500 cases. Acta Chir Scand (Suppl) 1966; 365: 128–36.

37 Kenady DE, Brown BW, McBride CM. Excision of underlying fascia with a primary malignant melanoma: effect on recurrence and survival rates. Surgery 1982; 615–618.

38 Pritchard GA, Zhang LJ, Hughes LE. Suture or graft? Changing trends in melanoma wound closure. Eur J Surg Oncol 1988: 371–377.

39 Flook D, Horgan K, Taylor BA, Hughes LE. Surgery for malignant melanoma: from which limb should the graft be taken? Br J Surg 1988; 73: 793–795.

40 Park KG. Blessing K, Kernohan NM. Surgical aspects of subungual melanomas. The Scottish Melanoma Group. Ann Surg 1992: 216: 692–695.

41 Krementz ET, Reed RJ, Coleman WP et al. Acral lentiginous melanoma. A clinicopathologic entity. Ann Surg 1982; 195: 632–645.

42 Day CL, Mihm MC, Sober AJ et al. Prognostic factors for melanoma patients with lesions 0.76–1.69 mm in thickness. Ann Surg 1982; 195: 30–43.

43 Cascinelli N, Bufalino R, Morabito A. BANS: a cutaneous region with no prognostic significance in melanoma. Cancer 1986; 57: 441–444.

44 Orr DJA, Hughes LE, Horgan K. Management of malignant melanoma of the head and neck. Br J Surg 1993; 80: 998–1000.

45 Scott RN, McKay AJ. Elective lymph node dissection in the management of malignant melanoma. Br J Surg 1993; 80: 284–288.

46 Balch CM, The role of elective lymph node dissection in melanoma: rationale, results and controversies. J Clin Oncol 1988; 6: 163–72.

47 Milton GW, Shaw HM, McCarthy WH, Pearson L, Balch CM, Soong S. Prophylactic lymph node dissection in clinical stage I cutaneous malignant melanoma: results of surgical treatment in 1319 patients. Br J Surg 1982; 69: 108–11.

48 McCarthy WH, Shae H, Wilton GW. Efficacy of elective lymph node dissection in 2347 patients with clinical stage I malignant melanoma. Surg Obstet Gynecol 1985: 575–580.

49 Veronesi U, Adamus J, Bandiera DC, et al. Delayed regional lymph node dissection in stage I melanoma of the skin of the lower extremities. Cancer 1982; 49: 2420–2430.

50 Crowley NJ, Siegler HF. The role of elective lymph node dissection in the management of patients with thick cutaneous melanoma. Cancer 1990; 66: 2522–2527.

51 Cady B. Lymph node metastases: indicators, but not governors of survival. Arch Surg 1984; 1190: 1067– 72.

52 Cascinelli N, Preda F, Vaglini M et al. Metastatic spread of stage I melanoma of the skin. Tumori 1983; 69: 449–454.

53 Balch CM, Murad T Soong S, Ingals AL, Richards PC, Maddox WA. Tumour thickness as a guide to surgical management of clinical stage I melanoma patients. Cancer 1979; 43: 883–888.

54 Balch CM, Soong S, Milton GW et al. A comparison of prognostic factors and surgical results in 1786 patients with localized (stage I) melanoma treated in Alabama, USA, and New South Wales, Australia. Ann Surg 1982; 196: 766–784.

55 Drepper H, Kohler CO, Bastian B et al. Benefit of elective lymph node dissection in subgroups of melanoma patients. Results of a multicenter study of 3616 patients. Cancer 1993; 72: 741–749.

56 Hein DW, Moy RL. Elective lymph node dissection in stage I malignant melanoma: a meta-analysis. Melanoma Res 1992; 2: 273–277.

57 Veronesi U Adamus J, Baniera DC et al. Inefficacy of immediate node dissection in stage I melanoma of the limbs. N Engl J Med 1977; 297: 627–630.

58 Sim FH, Taylor WF, Ivins JC, Pritchard DJ, Soule EH. A prospective randomized study of the eficacy of routine elective lymphadenopathy in management of malignant melanoma; preliminary results. Cancer 1985; 41: 948–951.

59 Sim FH, Taylor WF, Pritchard DJ, Soule EH. Lymphadenectomy in the management of stage I malignant melanoma: a prospective randomized study. Mayo Clin Proc 1986; 61: 697–705.

60 Balch CM, Wilkerson JA, Murad TM, Soong SJ, Ingals AL, Maddox WA. The prognostic significance of ulceration of cutaneous melanoma. Cancer 1980; 45: 3012–3017.

61 McCarthy WH, Shaw HM, Cascinelli N, Santinami M, Belli F. Elective lymph node dissection for melanoma: two perspectives. World J Surg 1992; 16: 203–213.

62 Morton DL, Wen D, Wong J et al. Technical details of intraoperative lymphatic mapping for early stage melanoma. Arch Surg 1992; 127: 392–399.

63 Uren RF, Howman-Giles RB, Shaw HM, Thompson JF, McCarthy WH. Lymphoscintigraphy in high risk melanoma of the trunk: predicting draining node groups, defining lymphatic channels and locating the sentinel node. J Nuclear Med 1993; 34: 1435– 1440.

64 Berman CG, Norman J, Cruse CW, Reintgen DS, Clark RA. Lymphoscintigraphy in malignant melanoma. Ann Plastic Surg 1992; 28: 29–32.

65 Norman J, Wells K, Kearney R, Cruse CW, Berman C, Reintgen D. Identification of lymphatic drainage basins in patients with cutaneous melanoma. Semin Surg Oncol 1993; 9: 224–227.

66 Alex JC, Krag DN. Gamma-probe guided localization of lymph nodes. Surg Oncol 1993; 2: 137–143.

67 Alex JC, Weaver DL, Fairbank JT Rankin BS, Krag DN. Gamma-probe-guided lymph node localization in malignant melanoma. Surg Oncol 1993; 2: 303–308.

68 McLeod GRC. Elective and therapeutic lymph node dissection. In: Emmett AJJ, O'Rourke MG, eds. Malignant Skin Tumours. Edinburgh: Churchill Livingstone, 1982.

69 Karakousis CP, Stahl L, Moore R, Holyoke ED. Lymph node dissection in malignant melanoma. J Surg Oncol 1980; 13: 245–252.

70 Beitsch P, Balch C. Operative morbidity and risk factor assessment in melanoma patients undergoing inguinal lymph node dissection. Am J Surg 1992; 164: 462–465.

71 Karakousis CP, Hena MA, Emrich LJ, Driscoll DL. Axillary node dissection in malignant melanoma.: results and complications. Surgery 1990; 108: 10–17.

72 Karakousis CP, Goumas W, Rao U, Driscoll DL. Axillary node dissection in malignant melanoma. Am J Surg 1991; 162: 202–207.

73 Kissen MW, Simpson DA, Easton D, White H, Westbury G. Prognostic factors related to survival and groin recurrence following therapeutic lymph node dissection for lower limb malignant melanoma. Br J Surg 1987; 74: 1023–1026.

74 Coit DG, Rogato A, Brennan MF. Prognostic factors in patients with melanoma metastatic to axillary or inguinal lymph nodes. A multivariate analysis. Ann Surg 1991; 214: 627–636.

75 O'Brien CJ, Gianoutsos MP, Morgan MJ. Neck dissection for cutaneous malignant melanoma. World J Surg 1992; 16: 222–226.

76 O'Brien CJ, Coates AS, Petersen-Schaefer K et al. Experience with 998 cutaneous melanomas of the head and neck over 30 years. Am J Surg 1991; 162: 310–314.

77 Ball ABS, Thomas JMT. Management of parotid metastases from cutaneous melanoma of the head and neck. J Laryngol Otol 1990; 104: 350–351.

78 Barr LC Skene AI, Fish S, Thomas JM. Superficial parotidectomy in the treatment of cutaneous melanoma of the head and neck. Br J Surg 1994; 81: 64–65.

79 Rosin D. Isolated limb perfusion: past experience and present studies using a minimal-access approach. Melanoma Res 1994; 4 (Suppl 1): 51–55.

80 Creech O Jr, Krementz ET, Ryan RF, Wimbled JN. Chemotherapy of cancer: regional perfusion utilizing an extracorporeal circuit. Ann Surg 1958; 148: 616–632.

81 Coit DG. Isolation limb perfusion for melanoma: current trends and future directions. Melanoma Res 1994; 4: 57–60.

82 Stehlin JS, Clark RL. Melanoma of the extremities. Experience with conventional treatment and perfusion in 339 cases. Am J Surg 1965; 110: 366–383.

83 McBride CM, Clark RL. Experience with l-phenylalanine mustard dihydrochloride in isolation-perfusion of extremities for malignant melanoma. Cancer 1971; 28: 1293–1296.

84 Krementz ET, Ryan RK. Chemotherapy of melanoma of the extremities by perfusion: Fourteen years clinical experience. Ann Surg 1972; 175: 900–917.

85 Koops HS, Oldhoff J, Van der Ploeg E, Eibergen R, Beekhuis H. Some aspects of the treatment of primary malignant melanoma of the extremities by isolated regional perfusion. Cancer 1977; 39: 27–33.

86 Golomb FM, Solowey AC, Postel AC, Gumport SL, Wright JC. Induced remission of malignant melanoma with actinomycin D: immunologic implications. Cancer 1967; 20: 656–662.

87 Golomb FM. Perfusion of melanoma: 105 isolated perfusions in 92 patients. Oncology 1972; 26: 197–205.

88 McBride CM. Advanced melanoma of the extremities: treatment by isolated-perfusion with a triple drug combination. Arch Surg 1970; 101: 122–126.

89 Stehlin JS, Giovanella BC, de Ipolyi PD, Muenz LR, Anderson RF. Results of hyperthermic perfusion for melanoma of the extremities. Surg Gynecol Obstet 1975; 140: 338–348.

90 Martijn H, Oldhoff J, Koops HS. Regional perfusion in the treatment of patients with a locally metastasized malignant melanoma of the limbs. Eur J Cancer 1981; 17: 471–476.

91 Cavaliere R, Cavaliere F, Deraco M, Di Filippo F, Santinami M, Monica S, Michele A, Vagliri M. Hyperthermic antiblastic perfusion in the treatment of stage IIIA-IIIAB melanoma patients. Comparison of two experiences. Melanoma Res 1994; 4 (Suppl 1): 5–11.

92 Ghussen F, Kruger I, Stutzer H. Hyperthermic perfusion with chemotherapy in melanoma of the extremities. World J Surg 1989; 13: 598–604.

93 Hofstrom L, Rudenstam CM, Blonquist E et al. Regional hyperthermic perfusion with melphalan after surgery for recurrent melanoma of the extremities, J Clin Oncol 1991;

94 Kroon BB, Klaase JM, van Geel BN, Eggermont AM, Franklin HR, vanDongen JA. Results of double perfusion schedule with melphalan in patients with melanoma of tye lower limb. Eur J Cancer 1993; 29A: 325–328.

95 Klaase JM, Kroon BB, van Geel AN, Eggermont AM, Franklin HR, Hart AA. Prognostic factors for tumor response and limb recurrence-free interval in patients with advanced melanoma of the limbs treated with regional isolated perfusion with melphalan. Surgery 1994; 115: 39–45.

96 Vrouenraets BC, Kroon BBR, Klaase JM et al. Regional isolated perfusion with melphalan for patients with subungual melanoma. Eur J Surg Oncol 1993; 19: 37–42.

97 Skene AI, Bulman AS, Williams TR, Thomas TM, Westbury G. Hyperthermic isolated perfusion with melphalan in the treatment of advanced malignant melanoma of the lower limb. Br J Surg 1990; 77: 765–767.

98 Klaase JM, Kroon BB, van Geel AN, Eggermont AM, Franklin HR, van Dongen JA. The role of regional isolated perfusion in the eradication of melanoma micrometastases in the inguinal nodes: a comparison between an iliac and femoral perfusion procedure. Melanoma Research 1992; 2: 402–410.

99 Lejeune FJ, Lienard D, Leyvraz S, Mirimanoff. Regional therapy of melanoma. Eur J Cancer 1993; 29A: 606–612.

100 Lejeune FJ, Mathiew M, Kenis Y, Hyperthermic isolation-perfusion with melphalan: A preliminary appraisal of local and general effects in malignant melanoma. Tumori 1977; 63: 289–298.

101 Lienard D, Ewalenko P, Delmotte JJ et al. High dose recombinant tumor necrosis factor alpha in combination with interferon gamma and melphalan in isolation perfusion of the limbs for melanoma and sarcoma. J Clin Oncol 1992; 10: 52–60.

102 Lienard D, Lejeune F, Ewalenko P. In transit metastases of malignant melanoma treated by high dose rTNFa in combination with interferon-γ and melphalan in isolation perfusion. World Surg 1992; 16: 234–240.
103 Lienard D, Eggermont AMM, Shraffordt Koops H, Kroon BBR, Rosenkaimer F, Autier P, Lejeune FJ. Isolated perfusion of the limb with high-dose tumour necrosis factor-alpha (TNF-α), interferon-gamma (IFN-γ) and melphalan for melanoma stage III. Results of a multi-centre pilot study. Melanoma Res 1994; 4 (Suppl 1): 21–26.
104 Vaglini M, Santinami M, Manzi R et al. Treatment of in-transit metastases from cutaneous melanoma by isolated perfusion with tumour necrosis factor-alpha (TNF-α), melphalan and interferon-gamma (IFN-γ). Dose- finding experience at the National Cancer Institute of Milan. Melanoma Res 1994; 4 (Suppl 1): 35–38.
105 Hill S, Thomas JM. Low-dose tumour necrosis factor- alpha (TNF-α) and melphalan in hyperthermic isolated limb perfusion. Results from a pilot study in the United Kingdom. Melanoma Res 1994; 4 (Suppl 1): 31–34.
106 Hill S, Fawcett WJ, Sheldon J, Soni N, Williams T, Thomas JM. Low-dose tumour necrosis factor α and melphalan in hyperthermic isolated limb perfusion. Br J Surg 1993; 80: 995–997.
107 Fraker DL, Alexander HR. The use of tumour necrosis factor (TNF) in isolated perfusion: results and side effects. The NCI results. Melanoma Res 1994; 4 (Suppl 1): 27–29.
108 Krementz ET, Creech, O Jr, Ryan RF. Evaluation of chemotherapy of cancer by regional perfusion. Cancer 1967; 20: 834–838.
109 McBride CM, Sugarbaker EV, Hickey RC. Prophylactic isolation-perfusion as the primary therapy for invasive malignant melanoma of the limbs. Ann Surg 1975; 182: 316–324.
110 Sugarbaker EV, McBride CM. Survival and regional disease control after isolation-perfusion for invasive stage I melanoma of the extremities. Cancer 1976; 37: 188–198.
111 Krementz ET, Carter RD, Sutherland CM, Campbell M. The use of regional chemotherapy in the management of malignant melanoma. World J Surg 1979; 3: 289–304.
112 Lee YM. Loco-regional recurrent melanoma: II. Non- systemic treatments (1964–1979). Cancer Treat Rev 1988; 15: 105–133.
113 Koops HS, Oldhoff J, Van der Ploeg E, Vermey A, Eibergeu R. Regional perfusion for recurrent malignant melanoma of the extremities. Am J Surg 1977; 133: 221–224.
114 Martijn H, Koops HS, Milton GW et al. Comparison of two methods of treating primary malignant melanomas Clark IV and V, thickness 1.5mm and greater, localized on the extremities. Cancer 1986; 57: 1923–1930.
115 Lejeune F et al. A randomized trial on prophylactic isolation perfusion for safe I high risk (i.e. 1.5 mm thickness) malignant melanoma of the limbs: an interim report. Melanoma Res 1993 ; 3 (Suppl 1): 95.
116 Muchmore JH, Krementz ET, Carter RD, Beg MH. Salvage treatment for patients with limb melanomas failing isolated regional perfusion. Melanoma Res 1993; 3(Suppl 1): 31.
117 Hill S, Thomas JM. Treatment of cutaneous metatases from malignant melanoma using the carbon-dioxide laser. Eur J Surg Oncol 1993; 19: 173–177.

British Medical Bulletin 1995, Vol 51, No. 3 pp. 609–630
©The British Council 1995

Melanoma: chemotherapy

S M Lee, D C Betticher & N Thatcher

CRC Department of Medical Oncology, Christie Hospital NHS Trust, Manchester M20 4BX

The overall median survival of patients with systemic metastasis from melanoma is about 6 months. Survival is dependent on the sites of first metastasis, the resectability of the metastases, and the number of metastases. Patients with non-visceral metastases at first relapse i.e. in skin, subcutaneous tissues, distant lymph nodes, and lung, have a better survival rate than patients with visceral (liver, bone, brain) metastases. Treatment of patients with systemic melanoma should include careful evaluation for the potential role of surgery, radiotherapy, and systemic therapy. The main use of chemotherapy in metastatic melanoma patients remains palliative. The chapter reviews the chemotherapeutic options available for the treatment of malignant melanoma including recent published works on new agents, multi-agent therapy, high dose chemotherapy with autologous bone marrow rescue, adjuvant chemotherapy and regional perfusion chemotherapy.

SINGLE AGENT CHEMOTHERAPY INCLUDING NEW INVESTIGATIONAL AGENTS

Dacarbazine, DTIC

Dacarbazine (DTIC) remains the most active agent used for the treatment of systemic melanoma. The agent was synthesized at the Southern Research Institute in 1959[1] in an attempt to design antagonists of 5 aminoimidazole-4-carboxamide, an intermediate in purine ring synthesis. It was subsequently found to have marked inhibitory activity against L-1210 leukaemia and other rodent solid neoplasms.[2] The response rate in melanoma is about 20% (Table 1). Patients with skin, subcutaneous tissue, lymph node and lung metastases respond more frequently but responses in liver, bone and brain

Table 1   Single agent chemotherapy

Agents	Number of evaluable patients	Number of responders	Overall response rate	Reference number
Alkylators				
Dacarbazine (DTIC)	1920	377	20%	58,86,87
Temozolomide	23	4	17%	88
Dibromodulcitol (Mitolactol)	205	28	14%	35,36,37
Ifosfamide	60	7	12%	89
Nitrosoureas				
Carmustine (BCNU)	122	22	18%	90,91,92
Lomustine (CCNU)	270	35	13%	93,94,95,96
Semustine	347	54	16%	86
Fotemustine	153	37	24%	19,97
Spindle agents				
Vincristine	52	6	12%	98–104
Vinblastine	62	8	13%	105–112
Vindesine	273	39	14%	23–27
Paclitaxel (Taxol)	71	17	24%	41–43
Platinum analogue				
Cisplatin	114	17	15%	27–33
Carboplatin	43	17	16%	34
Purine analogues				
2–chlorodeoxyadenosine	12	0	0%	113,114
Fludarabinephosphate	27	0	0%	115
Miscellaneous				
Piritrexim	31	8	26%	39
Detorubicin	22	8	36%	38

CR - complete response, PR - partial response

metastases are infrequent and survival short (Table 2). The median duration of response is about 5–6 months. Complete responses were observed in about 5% of patients and most of these occurred in subcutaneous and lymph node metastases. Overall about 2% of patients treated with DTIC achieved long term complete remission and remained disease free more than 6 years.[3].

The doses and schedules of DTIC have varied widely and include 2 to 4.5 mg/kg/day intravenously for 10 days, 250 mg/m^2/day for 5 days, and 850–1000 mg/m^2 given in one day. Treatment is usually repeated 3–4 weeks for up to six cycles. Infusion of DTIC over 24 hours has also been evaluated.[4] Although to date there has been no randomised study comparing the different treatment schedules, retrospective data suggest that the prolonged daily administration of DTIC may be slightly more effective in terms of response but

Table 2   Relationship between number and type of metastases and survival in melanoma patients

	Median duration of survival (months)
Number of metastases	
1	7
2	4
3	2
Type of metastases	
Nonvisceral and lung	7–11
Visceral	2–6

Data from 68,116

not survival than with shorter schedules.[5] Because of the ease of administration in an out-patient setting coupled with in-patient bed availability, DTIC nowadays is usually given as a single intravenous treatment over just one day. This one-day scheduling has become much more acceptable given the availability of effective 5HT3 antagonist as antiemetic treatment. The development of 5HT3 antagonists was very important for DTIC and platinum chemotherapy regimens as in the past nausea and vomiting were the most frequent and disabling side effects occurring in the majority of patients. Haematologic toxicity is generally mild and is dose-related. However, significant bone marrow toxicity occurs when more than $1.4g/m^2$ DTIC is given as a single intravenous bolus or the total DTIC dosage exceeds $1g/m^2$ when using the 5-day schedule. Occasionally doses above $1.5 g/m^2$ when given by rapid infusion have been associated with hypotension. Other side effects include local pain at injection sites, a flu like syndrome and malaise lasting several days. Photosensitivity has been reported in several patients, especially after high dose therapy and it is probably related to photodecomposition to toxic intermediates.[6] It has been suggested that patients should avoid strong sunlight for several days after treatment. Headache, facial flushing, alopecia, disturbed hepatic and renal function occur infrequently. Life threatening hepatic veno-occlusive disease as a distinct clinical pathologic entity has been reported in a few cases.[7]

DTIC undergoes metabolic N-demethylation to give the monomethyl triazene, 5-(3-methyl-1-triazeno)imidazole-4-carboxamide (MTIC) which methylates cellular macromolecules including DNA. It is generally believed that the cytotoxic effect of DTIC is related to DNA alkylation, and among the twelve DNA lesions generated, O^6-methylguanine (O^6-MeG) is thought to be the principal cytotoxic product.[8,9] Experimental studies have shown that melanoma cell lines resistant to MTIC accumulated less of the O^6-MeG lesion by being able to remove the toxic product more readily when compared to more sensitive melanoma cell lines.[10,11] One recent clinical study demonstrated wide inter-individual variations in the amount of O^6-MedG formed after DTIC chemotherapy and tumour responses appeared to occur in those patients with the highest O^6-MedG levels. Although the true significance of the observation needs to be confirmed in a larger study.[12]

DTIC analogues

In an attempt to improve the response rate, a number of DTIC analogues have been synthesized recently. CB10-277 {1-(4-carboxylphenyl)-3,3-dimethyltriazene} was synthesized by substituting the imidazole moiety of DTIC with a phenyl ring and carboxylic acid.[13] Despite promising activity demonstrated in experimental models and against metastatic melanoma in a clinical dose finding phase I study, the activity was not confirmed in a subsequent phase II study.[14] Nevertheless like DTIC, it is of interest to note that clinical response appeared to occur in the patients who achieved the highest O^6-MedG levels.[15]

The emergence of temozolomide as an oral monomethyl prodrug with activity against melanoma has lead to the demise of CB10-277.[16] Temozolomide has a number of potentially substantial advantages over DTIC. It is a prodrug form of MTIC which unlike DTIC does not depend on host metabolic activation. Therefore temozolomide bypasses the species and patient differences in metabolic activation that lead to variations in the formation of the active monomethyl metabolite MTIC from DTIC. Indeed, it has been suggested that one possible reason for the low clinical activity of DTIC in patients may be the inefficient metabolic activation relative to experimental animal models.[17] The early studies have confirmed that temozolomide has excellent oral bioavailability. Clinical activity was reported against malignant melanoma when patients were treated with a 5-day schedule.[16] If the activity is confirmed in a larger clinical study, it is anticipated that temozolomide would replace DTIC as the first line treatment for disseminated melanoma given the ease of oral administration, potential for improved clinical activity and its ability to achieve adequate CNS penetration.[18]

Nitrosoureas

The nitrosoureas (BCNU, CCNU, methyl-CCNU and fotemustine) are the second group of anti-tumour agents with activity against melanoma. Response rates range between 10% and 25% (3) Table 1. Alkylation at the O^6-position of guanine also appears to be involved in the cytotoxicity of the nitrosoureas: the O^6-chloroethylguanine generated in the DNA exerts its cytotoxic effect through the formation of DNA interstand cross-links.[8,9] The main limitation of the nitrosoureas is delayed and cumulative bone marrow toxicity, particularly thrombocytopenia. It was thought initially that the lipid soluble nitrosoureas might lead to more frequent response in brain metastases given their ability to cross into central nervous tissue. This unfortunately has not been substantiated, with the possible exception of the new nitrosourea fotemustine.[19] Fotemustine contains a phosphonoalanine carrier grafted to the nitrosourea radical and exhibited activity against melanoma cerebral metastases. In a phase II study of fotemustine in 153 evaluable patients with metastatic melanoma, an overall response of 24% was achieved including patients with cerebral metastases.[19] In another study of 42 patients with cerebral metastases, two complete and nine partial responses were seen on repeat CT scanning giving an overall response rate of 28%.[20]

Tumour resistance

There is increasing experimental evidence to suggest that resistance both to MTIC the active moiety of DTIC and to nitrosoureas in tumour tissues involves the expression of the DNA repair protein O^6-alkylguanine-DNA alkyltransferase (ATase) which transfers the alkyl group from O^6-alkylguanine to an internal residue in an autoinactivating, stoichiometric reaction.[8,9] One approach that can be taken in an effort to improve the therapeutic effect of DTIC and nitrosoureas is centred on identifying agents capable of depleting the ATase repair protein in tumour tissues. The inhibitor, O^6-benzylguanine was recently identified as capable of effectively depleting human ATase.[21] In an attempt to exploit the interaction combinations of O^6-benzylguanine with DTIC and related agents such as temozolomide or with nitrosoureas are now being considered for clinical trials by the National Cancer Institute, USA and Cancer Research Campaign, UK. It is interesting to note that temozolomide exhibits marked schedule dependency and has little activity when given as a single dose in experimental models or indeed clinically. In contrast when temozolomide is given over several consecutive days activity has been observed.[16] The difference in schedule activity has been postulated to be related to the cumulative ATase depletion seen with consecutive daily dose treatment.[22]

Other agents

Anti-melanoma activity has also been reported with a number of other groups of anti-cancer agents (Table 1). Of the vinca alkaloids, vindesine has been most extensively studied producing an overall response rate of 14%. Antitumour activity appears to be schedule-dependent: intermittent bolus was associated with 17% response rate whereas no activity was seen in 45 patients treated with continuous infusion.[23–26] Cisplatin and the related compound carboplatin have also measurable activity against melanoma. Although several complete responses have been noted, the median duration of response is only 3 months.[27–34]

Dibromodulcitol (mitolactol), a halogenated sugar alcohol with alkylating properties, has been shown to have activity in melanoma.[35–37] Of more interest was that responses occurred in patients refractory to DTIC and nitrosoureas. It appears that a daily dose schedule is more effective than an intermittent dose schedule and toxicity is mainly haematological. Two other agents, the semisynthetic anthracycline, detrorubicin,[38] and the dihydrofolate reductase inhibitor piritrexim,[39] have been reported to have activity against melanoma in single phase II trials but these studies need to be confirmed. Preclinical results with the camptothecins, potent plant alkaloid inhibitors of DNA and RNA synthesis, are of interest in that differential activity on malignant melanocytes compared to normal melanocytes have been reported and appropriate clinical trials are awaited.[40]

Taxol, a plant product derived from the Pacific yew tree (*Taxus brevifolia*) represents a new class of anti-cancer agent which promotes microtubule assembly. Five patients responded in a study of 34 patients treated at a dose of 250 mg/m^2 infused over 24-hour. Although most remissions were short, one complete response exceeded 14 months. Toxicities include neutropenia, neuropathy and acute hypersensitivity reactions.[41–43] Unfortunately, these preliminary results have not been followed up by large studies in melanoma to parallel the broad investigations with this new agent reported for ovarian, breast, and lung cancer. Bryostatin is a novel class of anti-cancer agent which probably acts through protein kinase C activator and in the process affects signal transduction pathways within cells. Potent anti-tumour activity has been demonstrated in vitro and in vivo melanoma xenografts.[44,45] Clinical activity against metastatic malignant melanoma was seen in patients in a recently reported phase I study.[46]

COMBINATION CHEMOTHERAPY

The relative ineffectiveness of single agent chemotherapy for metastatic melanoma led many oncologists to combine the more active agents in an attempt to improve the rate and duration of response rate. Table 3 lists some of the recent two-, three- and four-drug

Table 3   Combination chemotherapy

Agents	Number of evaluable patients	Response rate	Median duration of response (months)	Reference Number
Two drug combination				
DTIC + nitrosourea	238	17%	0.5–7	117–118
DTIC + cisplatin	30	37%	7	119
DTIC + VBL	50	40%	10	120
DTIC + Tam	117	29%	12	58
DTIC + fotemustine	60	30%	6	60
Three drug combination				
DTIC + BCNU + hydroxyurea	329	23%	6–7	121–123
DTIC + VDS + cisplatin	119	28%	4–6	124,125
DTIC + CDDP + VBL	50	40%	9	126
DTIC + CDDP + VDS	40	38%	4	127
DTIC + CDDP + BCNU	20	10%	8–9	55
DTIC + CDDP + Tam	74	15%	2–64	128,129
DTIC + CDDP + procarbazine	13	15%	3	130
DTIC + BCNU + VCR	40	43%	4	131
DTIC + dactinomycin + chlorozotocin	30	17%	7	132
CDDP + BLM + CCNU	25	48%	1–20	133
CDDP + BLM + VBL	204	26%		3,86
Four drug combination				
DTIC + BLM + CCNU + VCR	292	32%	4–7	134–138
DTIC + CDDP + BCNU + Tam	141	46%	3–10	52,53,139
DTIC + CCNU + VDS + BLEO	25	45%	6	140
DTIC + CDDP + VCR + procarbazine	13	15%	4	141
DTIC + BCNU + VCR + chlorpromazine	121	22%	10	89

DTIC - dacarbazine, VBL - vinblastine, Tam - tamoxifen, BCNU - carmustine, VDS - vindesine, CDDP - cisplatin, CCNU - lomustine, VCR - vincristine, BLM - bleomycin combinations. Although there is a impression that combination chemotherapy may yield a clinically important increase in the objective response rate, there is little statistical evidence to suggest that the true response rates exceed the response rate observed with DTIC alone.[47,48] Furthermore most of the combination studies are of relatively few patient numbers and were generally associated with increased toxicity with little evidence of improved survival when compared to DTIC alone. Other older combination regimens incorporating DTIC, nitrosourea, vincristine and chlorpromazine gave response rates of 17–22% with median durations of 3–22 months but failed to demonstrate superiority when compared to DTIC alone.[3] Newer combinations of cisplatin, bleomycin and vinblastine were initially reported to induce responses in 35–47% of patients but again in randomised trials of DTIC alone versus combination therapy comparable response rates in both arms of the study, i.e. 14% and 10% respectively, were observed.[49–51] Moreover, patients who responded to DTIC exhibited a trend toward longer survival, longer progression free intervals as well as less toxicity.[51]

Combinations with tamoxifen

Nevertheless, some of the combination regimens are worth noting. The combination of DTIC, BCNU (carmustine), cisplatin and tamoxifen (DBCT) has an overall response rate of 46% and a complete response rate of 11% in 141 patients examined in sequential phase II studies. The regimen was developed by Del Prete et al,[52] who reported a response rate of 55% in twenty patients: four patients obtained complete responses in sites which included visceral disease and seven patients achieved partial response. McClay and co-workers,[53] confirmed and extended the finding reporting ten responders in twenty treated patients. Omission of tamoxifen from the regimen resulted in a decrease in the overall response rate to 10%,[54] but subsequent reincorporation of tamoxifen increased the response rate back up to 50% suggesting that tamoxifen is an important component of the four-drug combination.[55] The improved therapeutic effect is thought to be related to a synergistic effect between tamoxifen and cisplatin. It is difficult to provide an explanation as to why tamoxifen is active in a tumour that rarely expresses oestrogen receptor and why there is potentiation of activity of tamoxifen with some chemotherapeutic agents. Although synergism between tamoxifen and cisplatin has been observed in some human melanoma cell lines in vitro and occasionally of tamoxifen with DTIC, other explanations should be considered. Recently tamoxifen has been shown to enhance levels of transforming growth factor beta (TGF beta) which in turn can inhibit the growth of several cancer cell lines. Tamoxifen also is capable of exerting an anti-cancer effect through inhibition of endothelial cell proliferation. TGF beta also inhibits tumour angiogenesis and therefore tamoxifen may be an active anti-cancer agent even in oestrogen receptor poor tumours such as melanoma by acting as an anti-angiogenic agent. By combining chemotherapy with tamoxifen, not only are tumour proliferating cells damaged but intratumoural endothelial proliferating cells are also affected leading to potentiation of the effect of each agent.[56] However, against this hypothesis is the speed at which responses occur, usually within three weeks of chemotherapy with tamoxifen which suggests that an anti-angiogenic effect is unlikely to be responsible for any synergy in the clinical setting.

As a word of caution however not all the subsequent series have shown a 50% response rate,[57] with DBCT and this four drug combination now warrants a comparative randomised phase III study against DTIC to assess its therapeutic efficacy. It is interesting that an Italian study comparing DTIC alone with DTIC and tamoxifen also noted a significant improved response for the combination arm, 20% response compared with 12% with DTIC alone again suggesting a synergistic effect between DTIC and tamoxifen.[58] However the response reported with single agent DTIC in this study was considerably lower than that generally reported in the literature and the advantage would be lost if the DTIC response approached the usual 20% value.

Tumour resistance

Since there is considerable experimental evidence to suggest that resistance to the two main anti-melanoma drug classes, i.e. DTIC and nitrosoureas may be related to the expression of the DNA repair protein, ATase;[8,9] we and others,[59,60] designed a regimen using sequential DTIC and fotemustine. Fotemustine was given 4 h after DTIC administration, the time which was shown to be associated with maximum ATase depletion induced by DTIC.[61] A nitrosourea administered at the DTIC induced nadir of ATase would be anticipated to have greater cytotoxic effect. Such an enhanced cytotoxic effect was seen in vitro on a number of tumour cell lines and xenografts when nitrosourea was administered after reduction of ATase activity.[62-64] In 60 treated patients, the response rates appeared to be stepwise related to the dosage of DTIC, being 24%, 30% and 40% in patient groups receiving 400, 500 and 800 mg/m^2 DTIC respectively.[60] Whether the response rate can be increased by more effective scheduling in order to completely suppress ATase activity in tumour tissue will require further exploration. Nevertheless, it is anticipated that the introduction of new powerful ATase inhibitors such as O^6-benzylguanine will lead to their incorporation into combinations containing DTIC, its analogues and possibly nitrosoureas in an attempt to improve efficacy.

Chemotherapy with interferon

The combination containing DTIC plus interferon-alpha is also worth noting particularly in view of the occasional durable remissions reported for interferon-alpha alone. However, published randomised trials comparing DTIC with DTIC plus interferon-alpha have produced conflicting results. One study reported an improvement in response rates and survival for the combined arm;[65] a second study did not observe any response rate or survival advantage,[66] whereas a third study reported a significant prolongation of response duration but no response rate nor survival advantage was seen with the combined arm.[67] Addition of interferon to the DBCT regimen described above has also been attempted: studies to date however suggested that the addition of alpha-interferon does not enhance the efficacy of this combination and may be associated with greatly increased toxicity.[68–70] A more complex regimen containing DTIC, vincristine, bleomycin, and lomustine combined with interferon alpha was reported to induce response in 62% of patients (with 13% complete responses) and included patients with metastatic ocular melanoma,[71] but this result again needs confirmatory studies. Other aspects of cytokine therapy in melanoma is the subject of a separate review in this issue.

HIGH DOSE CHEMOTHERAPY

The demonstration of a steep, log-linear dose response curve for alkylating agents generated interest in dose intensification with autologous bone marrow rescue as another approach to improve the response and survival rates in patients with malignant melanoma. The avenue has been explored with several agents, singly and in combination and the results are summarized in Table 4. Most of these studies involved small numbers of patients. Although the overall response rate of 53% appears high, sustained complete remissions and long term survival were rarely seen. High-dose melphalan, BCNU and thiotepa have induced responses in 40% to 60% of

Table 4   High dose chemotherapy with autologous bone marrow rescue

Agents	Number of evaluable patients	CR	PR	Response rate	Median response duration (months)	Reference Number
Melphalan	43	9	19	58%	3–6	142–144
BCNU	29	4	7	38%	6	145
Thiotepa	51	4	25	57%	3	146
DTIC, melphalan	27	5	11	59%	4	147
DTIC, ifosfamide	0	0	2	20	4	147
BCNU, melphalan	8	1	5	75%	4	148
BCNU, cisplatin	7	1	2	43%	3	149
BCNU, CTX	6	0	2	33%	2.5	150
BCNU, cisplatin, CTX	17	1	10	65%	4.7	151
TOTAL	203	25	83	53%		

CR, complete response; PR, partial response; BCNU, carmustine; DTIC, dacarbazine; CTX, cyclophosphamide.

patients (Table 4). The median duration of responses was brief and very similar for all 3 agents ranging from 3 to 6 months. The survival results obtained from high-dose DTIC or BCNU combinations are not better than those obtained for single agents.[47] Toxicity of the regimens is substantial, and are associated with treatment related deaths in up to a third of cases at very high doses. Although advances in haematopoietic growth factor support and peripheral blood stem cell rescue may reduce haematological toxicity, extra-medullary life-threatening toxic reactions will still occur. These include gastrointestinal toxicity with melphalan, cardiac, pulmonary and hepatic toxicity with BCNU and other nitrosoureas and hepatic veno-occlusive disease with dacarbazine.

In the absence of a randomised comparative assessment, this technique therefore must be considered investigational and has no established merit in the routine management of disseminated melanoma. Comparative studies will be required to determine if new high-dose regimens are better than the DBCT regimen described previously. The most likely potential application of high dose chemotherapy with bone marrow rescue is as consolidation therapy in patients who achieve a complete remission with standard dose chemotherapy.

ADJUVANT CHEMOTHERAPY

A number of attempts have been made in the past to develop an effective adjuvant chemotherapy in patients with malignant melanoma at high risk of recurrence following definitive surgery. The definition of high risk varies but for stage I disease includes Clark's level III or greater and Breslow thickness ≥ 1.5 mm. Patients with regional nodal metastases and disseminated disease who are free of disease following surgery have been included in adjuvant trials. To date most randomised prospective studies with an untreated control arm and at least one arm containing chemotherapy have *not* demonstrated a survival benefit.[72-76] Even a recent randomised trial using high-dose combination chemotherapy with autologous bone marrow support in patients with resected nodal metastases failed to demonstrate any survival benefit.[77] Based on these findings, adjuvant chemotherapy cannot be routinely recommended in patients at high risk except in a clinical research setting.

REGIONAL CHEMOPERFUSION

One of the major problems in the treatment of malignant melanoma is locoregional relapse particularly with multiple skin nodules. In this circumstance, effort has been focused upon control of tumour growth, since surgical resection in this situation is of limited value. In addition, tumour reduction is of the utmost importance for enhancing and maintaining quality of life. If the multiple recurrences are localized to the limb and there are no signs of generalized disease, regional chemotherapy may be envisaged. Results have been reported using this technique either alone or in association with hyperthermia.[78,79] The rationale for regional chemotherapy is to achieve a high drug concentration limited to the limb for a period of time without exposing the rest of the body to the drug, thus avoiding, or at least reducing, systemic toxicity. In practice, the following outline protocol has been developed since its early use in 1950.[79] After mobilization of the vessels, suitable vascular catheters are inserted and secured. A tourniquet is tightened proximally to the ends of catheters and venous blood is collected by gravity flow, pumped through an oxygenator, defoamed, in some centres warmed to 38–41°C and finally pumped back into the limb via the artery. When the perfusion system is functioning well, the chemotherapeutic agent is injected. In most trials melphalan has been used in a dose of 0.45–2.0 mg/kg of body weight The perfusion time ranges between 45–120 min. Leakage of the perfusate into the general circulation has been reported to be 400–800 ml, which is about 50% of the entire volume of perfusate and must be borne in mind when discussing side effects. The tumour remission rate of normothermic perfusion ranges from 40 to 80%. The British experience has been reported by Bulman

and Jamieson.[80] Twenty-nine patients with extensive and unresectable local recurrence were treated with melphalan perfusion.
The total response rate ($>50\%$ regression) was 48% and the mean
survival time was 36 months for those patients who responded and
9 months for non-responders. Rosin, also in Britain,[81] reported on
80 patients with locally recurrent melanoma. The response rate was
52% (26% complete remissions) and the 3-year survival rate was
34%. In order to improve the efficacy, hyperthermia was added
based on laboratory observations of enhanced tumour sensitivity to
active drug, increased tumour cell kill and decreased DNA repair.[79]
Although the studies combining melphalan with hyperthermia (39–
41°C) seem to improve the response rate to 85%,[82-85] it has so far
not been resolved in a randomized study whether the use of heat and
drug perfusion together are better than perfusion alone. The median
survival appears to be slightly improved over that of surgical treatment alone when this is feasible,[78,79] but all comparisons have been
retrospective and uncontrolled. Since melanoma is known for its
unpredictable natural evolution in the individual and for the mul-
tiplicity of factors affecting prognosis, comparisons with historical
controls must be made with caution.

The toxicity of regional perfusion chemotherapy with melphalan
has been mostly mild; however, a mortality of 1.2% has been
reported. Complications of significance are temporary paralysis of
neuromuscular function in 3%, oedema of the limb occurs in about
10% and a subsequent amputation has to be performed in 0.7% of
patients. Leukopenia, probably due to the perfusion leakage to the
body circulation occurs in 5% of patients. In conclusion, regional
chemotherapy with melphalan for recurrent cutaneous malignant
melanoma has a high response rate of 40–80% with occasional side
effects. However, to date no study has shown convincing survival
benefit. Controlled randomized clinical studies to establish with cer-
tainty the indications and the definitive value of perfusion chemotherapy are needed.[79]

SUMMARY

The treatment of metastatic malignant melanoma remains a for-
midable problem. DTIC is the standard chemotherapy agent but the
introduction of a new oral analogue, temozolomide may replace its
role because of the ease of administration and potential improved
therapeutic effect. Dibromodulcitol, taxol and bryostatin are promising investigational agents which require further study. High dose
chemotherapy with bone marrow rescue may achieve an improved

short-term response rate but does not appear to lead to durable remission or improved survival and can be associated with life-threatening toxicity. Regional perfusion produces regression of inoperable dermal and subcutaneous metastases confined to an extremity but as yet perfusion or postsurgical adjuvant chemotherapy has not been proven to definitely increase survival.

Improved understanding of the DNA repair mechanisms mediated by ATase following DTIC and nitrosoureas may lead to improved cytotoxic effect by incorporating ATase depleting agents such as O^6-benzylguanine. Older combination chemotherapy regimens did not appear to be superior to DTIC alone. However recent regimens containing DTIC, BCNU, cisplatin particularly when tamoxifen has been incorporated for a synergistic effect produce remissions in over 50% of patients treated. Given the overall poor survival results further clinical investigations in well defined protocols of systemic therapy are clearly needed.

ACKNOWLEDGEMENTS

Dr D C Betticher (Funded by the Swiss National Science Foundation and the Bernese League against Cancer) and E Morgan for secretarial assistance.

REFERENCES

1 Shealy YF, Krauth CA, Montgomery JA. Imidazoles. I. Coupling reactions of 5-diazoimidazole-4-carboxamide. J Org Chem 1962; 27: 2150–2154.
2 Montgomery JA. Experimental studies at Southern Research Institute with DTIC (NSC-45388). Cancer Treat Rep 1976; 60: 125–134.
3 Balch CM, Houghton AN, Peters LJ. Cutaneous melanoma. In: DeVita VT, Hellman S, Rosenberg SA, eds. Cancer: Principles and practice of oncology. Philadelphia: Lippincott, 1993, pp. 1612–1661.
4 Thatcher N, Henderson H, James R, Davenport P, Craig P. Treatment of metastatic melanoma by 24–hour DTIC infusions and hemibody irradiation. Cancer 1985; 57: 2103–2107.
5 McClay EF, McClay MET. Tamoxifen: is it useful in the treatment of patients with metastatic melanoma? J Clin Oncol 1994; 12: 617–626.
6 Buesa JM, Urrechaga E. Clinical pharmacokinetics of high-dose DTIC. Cancer Chemother Pharmacol 1991; 28: 475–479.
7 Marsh JC. Hepatic vascular toxicity of dacarbazine (DTIC): not a rare complication. Hepatol 1989; 9: 790.
8 D'Incalci M, Citti L, Taverna P, Catapano CV. Importance of DNA repair enzyme O^6-alkyltransferase (AT) in cancer chemotherapy. Cancer Treat Rev 1988; 15: 279–292.
9 Pegg AE, Byers TL. Repair of DNA containing O^6-alkylguanine. FASEB 1992; 6: 2302–2310.
10 Parsons PG, Smellie SG, Morrison LE, Hayward IP. Properties of human melanoma cells resistant to 5-(3'-3'-dimethyl-I-triazeno)imidazole-4-carboxamide and other methylating agents. Cancer Res 1982; 42: 1454–1461.
11 Hayward IP, Parsons PG. Comparison of virus reactivation, DNA base damage,

and cell cycle effects in autologous melanoma cells resistant to methylating agents. Cancer Res 1984; 44: 55–58.

12 Lee SM, Margison GP, Thatcher N, O'Connor P, Cooper D. Formation and loss of O^6-methyldeoxyguanosine in human leukocyte DNA following sequential DTIC and fotemustine chemotherapy. Br J Cancer 1994; 69: 853–857.

13 Newell DR, Foster B, Carmicheal J, et al. Clinical studies with the p-carboxyl dimethyl phenyl triazene CB10–277. In: Giraldi T, Connors TA, Cartei G, eds. Triazenes. Chemical, biological, and clinical aspects. New York: Plenum Press, 1990, pp 119–131.

14 Bleehen NM, Calvert AH, Lee SM, et al. A Cancer Research Campaign (CRC) phase II trial of CB10–277 given by 24 hour infusion for malignant melanoma. Br J Cancer 1994; 70: 775–777.

15 Lee SM, O'Connor PJ, Thatcher N, Crowther D, Margison GP, Cooper DP. Relationships between the formation of O^6-methyldeoxyguanosine by 1-p-carboxyl-3,3–dimethylphenyltriazene in DNA and O^6-alkylguanine-DNA alkyltransferase in human peripheral leukocytes. Cancer Research 1994b; 54: 4072–4076.

16 Newlands ES, Blackledge GRP, Slack JA, et al. Phase 1 trial of temozolamide (CCRG 81045: M&B 39831: NSC 362856). Br J Cancer 1992; 65: 287–291.

17 Rutty CJ, Newell DR, Vincent RB, et al. The species dependent pharmacokinetics of DTIC. Brit J Cancer 1983; 48: 140.

18 Stevens MFG, Newlands ES. From triazines and triazenes to temozolomide. Eur J Cancer 1993; 29A: 1045–1047.

19 Jacquillat C, Khayat D, Banzet P, et al. Final report of the French multicenter phase II study of the nitrosourea fotemustine in 153 evaluable patients with disseminated malignant melanoma including patients with cerebral metastases. Cancer 1990a; 66: 1873–1878.

20 Jacquillat C, Khayat D, Banzet P, et al. Chemotherapy by fotemustine in cerebral metastases of disseminated malignant melanoma. Cancer Chemother Pharmacol 1990b; 25: 263–266.

21 Dolan ME, Robert CM, Pegg AE. Depletion of mammalian O^6-alkylguanine-DNA alkyltransferase activity by O^6-benzylguanine provides a means to evaluate the role of this protein in protection against carcinogenic and therapeutic agents. Proc Natl Acad Sci USA 1990; 87: 5368–5372.

22 Lee SM, Thatcher N, Crowther D, Margison GP. Inactivation of O^6-alkylguanine-DNA alkyltransferase in human peripheral mononuclear cells by temozolomide. Br J Cancer 1994; 69: 452–456.

23 Currie WE, Wong PP, Krakoff IH and Young CW. Phase I trial of vindesine in patients with advanced cancer. Cancer Treat Rep 1978; 62: 1333–1336.

24 Quagliana JM, Stephens RL, Baker LH and Costanzi JJ. Vindesine in patients with metastatic malignant melanoma. J Clin Oncol 1984; 2: 316–319.

25 Rumke P, Everall JD, Mulder JH, Rozencweig M, Czarnetzki B and Thomas D. EORTC phase II trial of vindesine in advanced melanoma. Eur J Cancer Clin Oncol 1983; 19: 1173–1174.

26 Wagstaff J, Anderson HA, Shiu W and Thatcher N. Phase II trial of vindesine infusion in visceral metastatic malignant melanoma. Cancer Treat Rep 1983; 67: 839–840.

27 Al-Sarraf M, Fletcher W, Oishi N et al. Cis-platin hydratation with and without mannitol diuresis in refractory disseminated malignant melanoma: A Southwest Oncology Group study. Cancer Treat Rep 1982; 66: 31–35.

28 Goodnight JEJr, Moseley HS, Eilber FR, Sarna G and Morton DL. Cis-dichlorodiammineplatinum (II) alone and combined with DTIC for treatments of disseminated malignant melanoma. Cancer Treat Rep 1979; 63: 2005–2007.

29 Schilcher RB, Wessels M, Niederle N, Seeber S and Schmidt, C.G. Phase II evaluation of fractionated low and single high dose cisplatin in various tumors. J Cancer Res Clin Oncol 1984; 107: 57–60.

30 Glover D, Glick J, Weiler C, Fox K, Turrisi A and Kligerman MM. Phase I/II

trials of WR-2721 and cis-platinum. Int J Radiat Oncol Biol Phys 1986; 12: 1509–1512.
31 Chary KK, Higby DJ, Henderson ES and Swinerton KD. Phase I study of high dose cidichlorodiamminplatinum (2) with forced diuresis. Cancer Treat Rep 1977; 61: 367–370.
32 Mortimer JE, Chestnut T and Higano CS. High dose cisplatin in metastatic melanoma: comparison of two schedules. Proc Am Soc Clin Oncol USA 1988; 7: 254.
33 Kim S, Howell SB, McClay E, Kirmani S, Goel R, Plaxe S, Braly P and Bonetti A. Dose intensification of cisplatin chemotherapy through biweekly administration. Ann. Oncol. 1993; 4: 221–227.
34 Evens LM, Casper ES and Rosenbluth R. Phase II trial of carboplatin in advanced malignant melanoma. Cancer Treat Rep 1987; 71: 171–172.
35 Amato DA, Bruckner H, Guerry D, Ash A, Falkson G, Borden EC, Creech RH, Savlov ED and Cunningham TJ. Phase II evaluation of dibromodulcitol and actinomycin D, hydroxyurea and cyclophosphamide in previously untreated patients with malignant melanoma. Invest New Drugs 1987; 5: 293–297.
36 Medina W and Kirkwood JM. Phase II trial of mitolactol in patients with metastatic melanoma. Cancer Treat Rep 1982; 66: 195–196.
37 Murray N, Silver H, Shah A and Wilson K. Phase II trial of mitolactol in advanced malignant melanoma. Cancer Treat Rep 1985; 69: 723–724.
38 Chawla SP, Legha SS and Benjamin RS. Detorubicin - an active anthracycline in untreated metastatic melanoma. J Clin Oncol 1985; 3: 1529–1534.
39 Feun LG, Gonzalez R, Savaraj N, Hanlon J, Collier M, Robinson WA and Clendeninn NJ. Phase II trial of piritrexim in metastatic melanoma using intermittant low-dose administration. J Clin Oncol 1991; 9: 464–467.
40 Pantazis P, Hinz HR, Mendoza JT, et al. Complete inhibition of growth followed by death of human malignant melanoma cells in vitro and regression of human melanoma xenografts in immunodeficient mice induced by camptothecins. Cancer Res 1992; 52: 3980–3987.
41 Wiernik PH, Schwartz EL, Einzig A, Strauman J, Lipton RB, Dutcher JP. Phase I trial of taxol given as a 24 hour infusion every 21 days: response observed in metastatic melanoma. J, Clin Oncol 1987; 8: 1232–1239.
42 Einzig A, Trump DL, Sasloff J. Phase II pilot study of taxol in patients with malignant melanoma (abst). Proc Am Soc Clin Oncol 1988; 7: 249.
43 Legha SS, Ring S, Papadopoulos N, Raber M, Benjamin RS. A phase II trial of taxol in metastatic melanoma. Cancer 1990; 65: 2478–2481.
44 Schuchter LM, Esa AH, May S, Laulis MK, Pettit GR, Hess AD. Successful treatment of murine melanoma with bryostatin 1. Cancer Res 1991; 51: 682–687.
45 Hornung RL, Pearson JW, Beckwith M, Longo DL. Preclinical evaluation of bryostatin as an anticancer agent against several murine tumour cell lines: *in vitro* vs *in vivo* activity. Cancer Res 1992; 52: 101–107.
46 Philip PA, Rea D, Thavasu P, et al. Phase I study of bryostatin 1: assessment of interleukin 6 and tumor necrosis factor alpha induction *in vivo*. The Cancer Research Campaign Phase I Committee. J Natl Cancer Inst 1993; 85 (22): 1790–1792.
47 Lakhani S, Selby P, Bliss JM, Perren TJ, Gore ME, McElwain TJ. Chemotherapy for malignant melanoma: combinations and high doses produce more responses without survival benefit. Br J Cancer 1990; 61: 330–334.
48 Mulder NH, van der Graaf WTA, Willemse PHB, Schraffordt Koops H, de Vries EGE, Sleijfer DT. Dacarbazine (DTIC)-based chemotherapy or chemo-immunotherapy of patients with disseminated malignant melanoma. Br J Cancer 1994; 70: 681–683.
49 Nathanson L, Kaufman SD, Carey RW. Vinblastine infusion, bleomycin, and cisdichlorodiammine-platinum chemotherapy in metastatic melanoma. Cancer 1981; 48: 1290–1294.
50 National Cancer Institute of Canada Melanoma Group. Vinblastine, bleomycin,

and cis-platinum for the treatment of metastatic malignant melanoma. J Clin Oncol 1984; 2: 131–134.

51 Luikart SD, Kennealey GT, Kirkwood JM. Randomised phase III trial of vinblastine, bleomycin, and cis-dichlorodiammine-platinum versus dacarbazine in malignant melanoma. J Clin Oncol 1984; 2: 164–168.

52 Del Prete SA, Maurer LH, O'Donnell J, Forcier RJ, Lemarbre P. Combination chemotherapy with cisplatin, carmustine, dacarbazine and tamoxifen in malignant melanoma. Cancer Treat Rep 1984; 68: 1403–1405.

53 McClay EF, Mastrangelo MJ, Bellet RE, Berd D. Combination chemotherapy and hormonal therapy in the treatment of malignant melanoma. Cancer Treat Rep 1987; 71: 465–469.

54 McClay EF, Mastrangelo MJ, Sprandio JD, Bellet RE, Berd D. The importance of tamoxifen to a cisplatin-containing regimen in the treatment of metastatic melanoma. Cancer 1989; 63: 1292–1295.

55 McClay EF, Mastrangelo MJ, Berd D, Bellet RE. Effective combination chemo/hormonal therapy for malignant melanoma: experience with three consecutive trials. Int J Cancer 1992; 50: 553–556.

56 Gasparini G. Tamoxifen and chemotherapy in the treatment of metastatic melanoma: are there other possible mechanisms explaining their potentiation? J Clin Oncol 1994; 12, 1994–1996.

57 Saba HI, Cruse CW, Wells KE, Klein CJ, Reintgen DS. Treatment of stage IV malignant melanoma with dacarbazine, carmustine, cisplatin, and tamoxifen regimens: a University of South Florida and H. Lee Moffitt melanoma center study. Ann Plast Surg 1992; 28: 65–69.

58 Cocconi G, Bella M, Calabresi F, et al. Treatment of metastatic malignant melanoma with dacarbazine plus tamoxifen. N Engl J Med 1992; 327: 516–523.

59 Gerard B, Aamdal S, Lee SM, et al. Activity and unexpected lung toxicity of the sequential administration of two alkylating agents-dacarbazine and fotemustine-in patients with melanoma. Eur J Cancer 1993; 29A: 711–719.

60 Lee SM, Margison GP, Woodcock AA, Thatcher N. Sequential administration of varying doses of dacarbazine and fotemustine in advanced malignant melanoma. Br J Cancer 1993; 67: 1356–1360.

61 Lee SM, Thatcher N, Margison GP. O^6-alkylguanine-DNA alkyltransferase depletion and regeneration in human peripheral lymphocytes following dacarbazine and fotemustine. Cancer Res 1991; 51: 619–623.

62 Dempke W, Nehls P, Wandl U, Soll D, Schmidt CG, Osieka R. Increased cytotoxicity of 1-(2-chloroethyl)-1-nitroso-3-(4-methyl)-cyclohexylurea by pretreatment with O^6-methylguanine in resistant but not in sensitive human melanoma cells. J Cancer Res Clin Oncol 1987; 113: 387–391.

63 Dolan ME, Mitchell RB, Mummert C, Moschel RC, Pegg AE. Effect of O^6-benzylguanine analogues on sensitivity of human tumor cells to the cytotoxic effects of alkylating agents. Cancer Res 1991; 51: 3367–3372.

64 Friedman HS, Dolan ME, Moschel RC, et al. Enhancement of nitrosourea activity in medulloblastoma and glioblastoma multiforme. J Natl Cancer Inst 1992; 84: 1925–1931.

65 Falkson CI, Falkson G, Falkson HC. Improved results with the addition of interferon alpha-2b to dacarbazine in the treatment of patients with metastatic malignant melanoma. J Clin Oncol 1991; 9: 1403–1408.

66 Thomson DB, Adena M, McLeod GR. Interferon alpha-2a does not improve response or survival when combined with dacarbazine in metastatic malignant melanoma: results of a multiinstitutional Australian randomized trial. Melanoma Res 1993; 3: 133–138.

67 Bajetta E, Leo AD, Zampino MG, et al. Multicenter randomized trial of dacarbazine alone or in combination with two different doses and schedules of interferon alfa-2a in the treatment of advanced melanoma. J Clin Oncol 1994; 12: 806–811.

68 Feun LG, Gutterman J, Burgess MA, et al. The natural history of resectable metastatic melanoma (stage IVa melanoma). Cancer 1982; 50: 1656–1663.
69 Schultz M, Poo W-J, Buzaid AC. A phase II study of cisplatin (CDDP), dacarbazine (DTIC), carmustine (BCNU), tamoxifen (TM) and interferon α 2B (α-IFN) in metastatic melanoma. Proc Am Soc Clin Oncol 1993; 12: 390.
70 Stark JJ, Schulof R, Wiemann M, Barth N, Honeycutt P, Soori G. Alpha interferon and chemo-hormonal therapy in advanced melanoma: a phase I-II NBSG/MAOP study. Proc Am Soc Clin Oncol 1993; 12: 392.
71 Pyrhonen S, Hahka-Kempinnen M, Muhonen T. A promising interferon plus four-drug chemotherapy regimen for metastatic melanoma. J Clin Oncol 1993; 10: 1919–1926.
72 Banzet P, Jacquillat C, Civatte J, et al. Adjuvant chemotherapy in the management of primary malignant melanoma. Cancer 1978; 41: 1240–1248.
73 Hill GJI, Moss SE, Golomb FM, et al. DTIC and combination therapy for melanoma: III. DTIC (NSC 45388) Surgical Adjuvant Study COG Protocol 7040. Cancer 1981; 47: 2556–2562.
74 Fisher RI, Terry WD, Hodes RJ, et al. Adjuvant immunotherapy or chemotherapy for malignant melanoma. Surg Clin North Am 1981; 61: 1267–1277.
75 Veronesi U, Adamus J, Aubert C, et al.. A randomised trial of adjuvant chemotherapy and immunotherapy in cutaneous melanoma. N Engl J med 1982; 307: 913–916.
76 Balch CM, Murray D, Presant C, Bartolucci AA. Ineffectiveness of adjuvant chemotherapy using DTIC and cyclophosphamide in patients with resectable metastatic melanoma. Surgery 1984; 95: 454–459.
77 Meisenberg BR, Ross M, Vredenburgh JJ, et al. Randomised trial of high-dose chemotherapy with autologous bone marrow support as adjuvant therapy for high-risk, multi-node-positive malignant melanoma. J Natl Cancer Inst 1993; 85: 1080–1085.
78 Cumberlin R, De Moss E, Lassus M, Friedman M. Isolation perfusion for malignant melanoma of the extremity: a review. J Clin Oncol 1985; 3: 1022–1031.
79 Hafström L, Mattsson J. Regional chemotherapy for malignant melanoma. Cancer Treat Rev 1993; 19: 17–28.
80 Bulman AS, Jamieson CW. Isolated limb perfusion with melphalan in the treatment of malignant melanoma. Br J Surg 1980; 224: 1031–1036.
81 Rosin RD, Westburg G. Isolated limb perfusion for malignant melanoma. Practitioner 1980; 224: 1031–1036.
82 Lejeune FJ, Deloof T, Ewalenko P, et al. Objective regression of unexcised melanoma in-transit metastases after hyperthermic isolation perfusion of the limbs with melphalan. Recent Results Cancer Res 1983; 46: 1849–1854.
83 Skene AI, Bulman AS, Williams TR, Meirion TJ, Westbury G. Hyperthermic isolated perfusion with melphalan in the treatment of advanced malilgnant melanoma of the lower limb. Br J Surg 1990; 77: 765–767.
84 Westbury G. Regional cancer chemotherapy. Br J Surg 1967; 54: 824–827.
85 Storm FK, Morton LD. Value of therapeutic hyperthermic limb perfusion in advanced recurrent melanoma of the lower extremity. Am J Surg 1985; 150: 32–35.
86 Mastrangelo MJ, Bellet RE, Kane MJ, Berd D. Chemotherapy of melanoma. In: Perry, MC ed. The chemotherapy source book. Baltimore: Williams and Wilkins 1992; pp. 886–907.
87 Pritchard KI, Quirt IC, Cowan DH, Osoba D, Kutas GJ. DTIC therapy in metastatic malignant melanoma: a simplified dose schedule. Cancer Treat Rep 1980; 64: 1123–1126.
88 O'Reilly SM, Newlands ES, Stevens MF. Temozolomide (CCRG 81045; M and B 39831; NSC 362856): a new oral cytotoxic agent with activity against melanoma, mycosis fungoides and high-grade glioma. Proc Ann Meet Am Assoc Cancer Res 1992; 33: A1267.

89 Varini M. Ifosfamide in tumour therapy – an overview. Contrib Oncol 1987; 26: 12–21.
90 Ramirez G, Wilson W, Grage T, Hill G. Phase II evaluation of 1,3–bis(2chloroethyl)-1-nitrosourea (BCNU; NSC-409962) in patients with solid tumors. Cancer Chemother Rep 1972; 56: 787–790.
91 DeVita VT, Carbone PP, Owens AH, Gold GL, Krant MJ, Edmonson J. Clinical trials with 1,3,-bis(2–chloroethyl)-1–nitrosourea, NSC-409962. Cancer Res 1965; 25: 1876–1881.
92 Ahmann DL. Nitrosoureas in the management of disseminated malignant melanoma. Cancer Treat Rep 1976; 60: 747–751.
93 Beretta G, Pancera G, Locatelli C. Lomustine (CCNU) and epirubicin as alternative treatments to dacarbazine (DTIC) for advanced malignant melanoma. Proceedings of the first International Conference on Skin Melanoma 1985; 1: 148.
94 Hoogstraten B, Gottlieb JA, Caoili E, Tucker WG, Talley RW, Haut A. CCNU (1-(2-chloroethyl)-3-cyclohexyl-1-nitrosourea, NSC-79037) in the treatment of cancer. Phase II study. Cancer 1973; 32: 38–43.
95 Wasserman TH, Slavik M, Carter SK. Methyl-CCNU in clinical cancer therapy. Cancer Treat Rev 1974; 1: 251–269.
96 Amann DL, Hahn RG, Bisel HF. Comparative study of 1-(2-chloroethyl)-3-syclo-exyl-1-nitrosurea (NSC-79037) and imidazole carboxamide (NSC-45388) with vincristine (NSC-67574) in the palliation of disseminated malignant melanoma. Cancer Res 1972; 32: 2432.
97 Khayat D, Lokiec F, Bizzari JP, et al. Phase I clinical study of the new amino acid-linked nitrosourea S 10036 administered on a weekly schedule. Cancer Res 1987; 47: 6782–6785.
98 Rumke P. The use of chemotherapy in the management of patients with malignant melanoma. Clinics Oncol 1994; 3: 555–570
99 Costa G, Hreshchyshyn MM, Holland JF. Initial clinical studies with vincristine. Cancer Chemother Rep 1962; 24: 39–44.
100 Holland JF, Scharlau C, Gailani S, et al. Vincristine treatment of advanced cancer: a cooperative study of 392 cases. Cancer Res 1964; 33: 1258–1264.
101 Gubisch NJ, Norena D, Perlia CP, Taylor SG. Experience with vincristine in solid tumors. Cancer Chemother Rep 1963; 32: 19–22.
102 Shaw RK, Brunner JA. Clinical evaluation of vincristine (NSC-67574). Cancer Chemother Rep 1964; 42: 45–48.
103 Reitemeier RJ, Moertel CG, Blackburn CM. Vincristine (NCS-67574) therapy of adult patients with solid tumors. Cancer Chemother Rep 1964; 34: 21–23.
104 Smart CR, Ottoman RE, Rochlin DB, Hornes J, Silva AR, Goepert H. Clinical experience with vincristine (NSC-67574) in tumors of the central nervous system and other malignant disease. Cancer Chemother Rep 1968; 52: 733–741.
105 Frei E, Franzino A, Shnider BI, et al. Clinical studies of vinblastine. Cancer Chemother Rep 1961; 12: 125–129.
106 Armstrong JG, Dyke RW, Fouts PJ, Gahiner JE. Hodgkin's disease, carcinoma of the breast and other tumors treated with vinblastine sulfate. Cancer Chemother Rep 1962; 18: 49–71.
107 Bond WH, Rohn RJ, Bates LH, Hodes ME. Treatment of neoplastic diseases with an improved oral preparation of vinblastine sulfate. Cancer 1966; 19: 213–219.
108 Hodes ME, Rohn RJ, Bond WH, Yardley JM, Corpening WS. Vincaleukoblastine IV. A summary of two and one half years experience in the use of vinblastine. Cancer Chemother Rep 1962; 16: 401–406.
109 Hill JM, Loeb E. Treatment of leukemia, lymphoma, and other malignant neoplasms with vinblastine. Cancer Chemother Rep 1961; 15: 41–61.
110 Wright TL, Hurley J, Korst DR, et al. Vinblastine in neoplastic disease. Cancer Res 1963; 23: 169–179.
111 Smart CR, Rochlin DB, Nahum AM, Silva A, Wagner D. Clinical experience

with vinblastine sulfate (NSC-49842) in squamous cell carcinoma and other malignancies. Cancer Chemother Rep 1964; 34: 31–45.

112 Bleehan NM, Jelliffe AM. Vinblastine sulphate in the treatment of malignant disease. Br J Cancer 1965; 19: 268–273.

113 Saven A, Kawasaki H, Carrera CJ, et al. 2–chlorodeoxyadenosine dose escalation in nonhematologic malignancies. J Clin Oncol 1993; 11: 671–678.

114 Saven A, Waltz T, Carrera CJ, et al. Phase I study of 2–chlorodeoxyadenosine (2–CDA) in nonhematologic malignancies. Proc Am Soc Clin Oncol USA 1992; 11: 119.

115 Kish JA, Kopecky K, Samson MK, et al. Evaluation of fludarabine phosphate in malignant melanoma. A Southwest Oncology Group study. Invest New Drugs 1991; 9: 105–108.

116. Balch CM, Soong S, Murad TM, Smith JW, Maddox WA, Durant JR. A multifactorial analysis of melanoma. IV. Prognostic factors in 200 melanoma patients with distant metastases (stage III). J Clin Oncol 1983; 1: 126–134.

117 Joensuu H. Association between chemotherapy response and rate of disease progression in disseminated melanoma. Br J Cancer 1991; 63: 154–156.

118 Costanza ME, Nathanson L, Lenhard R, et al. Therapy of malignant melanoma with an imidazole carboxamide and bis-chloroethyl nitrosurea. Cancer 1972; 30: 1457–1461.

119 Fletcher WS, Green S, Fletcher JR, Dana B, Jewell W, Townsend RA. Evaluation of cis-platinum and DTIC combination chemotherapy in disseminated melanoma. Am J Clin Oncol 1988; 11: 589–593.

120 Legha SS, Ring S, Papadopoulos N, Plager C, Chawla S, Benjamin R. A prospective evaluation of a triple-drug regimen containing cisplatin, vinblastine, and dacarbazine (CVD) for metastatic melanoma. Cancer 1989; 64: 2024–2029.

121 Costanzi JJ, Vaitkevicius VK, Quagliana JM, Hoogstraten B, Coltman CA, Delaney FC. Combination chemotherapy for disseminated malignant melanoma. Cancer 1975; 35: 342–346.

122 Carter RD, Krementz ET, Hill GJ, et al. DTIC (NCS-45388) and combination therapy for melanoma. I. studies with DTIC, BCNU (NCS-409962), CCNU (NCS-79037), vincristine (NCS-67574), and hydroxyurea (NCS-32065). Cancer Treat Rep 1976; 60: 601–609.

123 Costanzi JJ, Fletcher WS, Balcerzak SP, et al. Combination chemotherapy plus levamisole in the treatment of disseminated malignant melanoma. A Southwest Oncology Group study. Cancer 1984; 53: 833–836.

124 Grundersen S. Dacarbazine, vindesine, and cisplatin combination chemotherapy in advanced malignant melanoma: a phase II study. Cancer Treat Rep 1987; 71: 997–999.

125 Verschraegen CF, Kleeberg UR, Mulder J, et al. Combination of cisplatin, vindesine, and dacarbazine in advanced malignant melanoma. A phase II study of the EORTC Malignant Melanoma Cooperative Group. Cancer 1988; 62: 1061–1065.

126 Legha S, Ring S, Balch C, et al. Induction chemotherapy using cisplatin, vinblastine, and DTIC (CVD) for stage-II melanoma. Sixth International Conference on Adjuvant Therapy of Cancer. 1990; 40.

127 Ringborg U, Jungnelius U, Hansson J, Strander H. Dacarbazine-vindesine-cisplatin in disseminated malignant melanoma. A phase I-II trial. Am J Clin Oncol 1990; 13: 214–217.

128 Buzaid AC, Murren JR, Durivage HJ. High-dose cisplatin with dacarbazine and tamoxifen in the treatment of metastatic melanoma. Cancer 1991; 68: 1238–1241.

129 Ferri W, Agarwala SS, Kirkwood JM, et al. Carboplatin (C) and dacarbazine (D) ± tamoxifen (T) for metastatic melanoma. Proc Am Soc Clin Oncol USA 1994; 13: 394(A1341).

130 Karakousis CP, Getaz EP, Bjornsson S, Henderson ES, Irequi M, Martinez L. Cis-dichlorodiammineplatinum (II) and DTIC in malignant melanoma. Cancer Treat Rep 1979; 63: 2009–2010.

131 Cohen SM, Greenspan EM, Ratner LH, Weiner MJ. Combination chemotherapy of malignant melanoma with imidazole carboxamide, BCNU and vincristine. Cancer 1977; 39: 41–44.

132 Samson MK, Baker LH, Cummings G, Talley RW, McDonald B, Bhathena DB. Clinical trial of chlorozotocin, DTIC, and dactinomycin in metastatic malignant melanoma. Cancer Treat Rep 1982; 66: 371–373.

133 Cohen SM, Ohnuma T, Ambinder EP, Holland JF. Lomustine, bleomycin and cisplatin in patients with metastatic malignant melanoma. Cancer Treat Rep 1986; 70: 688–689.

134 Seigler HF, Lucas VSJr, Pickett NJ, Huang AT. DTIC, CCNU, bleomycin and vincristine (BOLD) in metastatic melanoma. Cancer 1980; 46: 2346–2348.

135 Ahn SS, Giuliano A, Kaiser L. The limited role of BOLD chemotherpay for disseminated malignant melanoma. Proc Am Soc Clin Oncol USA 1983; 2: 228.

136 Jose DG, Minty CCJ, Hillcoat BL. Treatment of patients with disseminated malignant melanoma with bleomycin, oncovin, lomustine and DTIC (BOLD). First International Conference on Skin Melanoma 1985; A151.

137 York RM, Foltz AT. Bleomycin, vincristine, lomustine, and DTIC chemotherapy for metastatic melanoma. Cancer 1988; 61: 2183–2186.

138 The Prudenete Foundation Melanoma Study Group. Chemotherapy of disseminated melanoma with bleomycin, vincristine, CCNU, and DTIC (BOLD regimen). Cancer 1989; 63: 1676–1680.

139 Richards JM, Gilewski TA, Ramming K, Mitchel B, Doane LL, Vogelzang NJ. Effective chemotherapy for melanoma after treatment with interleukin-2. Cancer 1992; 69: 427–429.

140 Young DW, Lever RS, English JS, MacKie RM. The use of BELD combination chemotherapy (bleomycin, vindesine, CCNU and DTIC) in advanced malignant melanoma. Cancer 1985; 55: 1879–1881.

141 McKelvey EM, Luce JK, Vaitkevicius K, et al. Bis chloroethyl nitrosourea, vincristine, dimethyl triazeno imidazole carboxamide and chlorpromazine combination chemotherapy in disseminated malignant melanoma. Cancer 1977; 39: 5–10.

142 Lazarus HM, Herzig RH, Wolff SN, et al. Treatment of metastatic malignant melanoma with intensive melphalan and autologous bone marrow transplantation. Cancer Treat Rep 1985; 69: 473–477.

143 McElwain TJ, Hedley DW, Burton G, et al.. Marrow autotransplantation accelerates haematological recovery in patients with malignant melanoma treated with high-dose melphalan. Br J Cancer 1979a; 40: 72–80.

144 McElwain TJ, Hedley DW, Gordon MY, Jarman M, Millar JL, Pritchard J. High dose melphalan and non-cryopreserved autologous bone marrow treatment of malignant melanoma and neuroblastoma. Exp Hematol 1979b; 7(Suppl 5): 360–371.

145 Philips GL, Fay JW, Herzig GP, et al.. Intensive 1,3-bis (2-chloroethyl)-1-nitrosourea (BCNU), NSC 4366650 nd cryopreserved autologous marrow transplantation for refractory cancer. A phase I-II study. Cancer 1983; 52: 1792–1802.

146 Wolff SN, Herzig RH, Fay JW. High-dose thiotepa with autologous bone marrow transplantation for metastatic malignant melanoma: results of phase I-II studies of the North American Bone Marrow Transplantation Group. J Clin Oncol 1989; 7: 245–249.

147 Thatcher N, Lind M, Morgenstern G, et al.. High-dose double alkylating agent chemotherapy with DTIC melphalan or ifosphamide and marrow rescue for metastatic malignant melanoma. Cancer 1989; 63: 1296–1302.

148 Thomas MR, Robinson WA, Hartmann D, Glode LM, Koppler H, Morton NJ. Treatment of advanced malignant melanoma with high dose chemotherapy and autologous bone marrow transplantation. Preliminary results. Am J Clin Oncol 1982; 5: 611–622.

149 Ciobanu N, Dutcher J, Gucalp R, et al. High dose chemotherapy with autologous bone marrow transplantation (ABMT) for malignant melanoma after failure of interleukin-2 (IL2) and lymphokine activated killer (LAK) cells. Proc Am Soc Clin Oncol 1989; 8: 281.

150 Slease RB, Benear JB, Selby GB, et al. High dose combination alkylating agent therapy with autologous bone marrow rescue for refractory solid tumors. J Clin Oncol 1988; 6: 1314–1320.

151 Antman K, Eder JP, Elias A, et al. High-dose combination alkylating agent preparative regimen with autologous bone marrow support: the Dana Farber Cancer Institute/Beth Israel Hospital experience. Cancer Treat Rep 1987; 71: 119–125.

British Medical Bulletin 1995, Vol 51, No. 3 pp. 631–646
©The British Council 1995

Active specific immunotherapy of melanoma

M S Mitchell

Centre for Biological Therapy and Melanoma Research, University of California at San Diego Cancer Centre La Jolla CA, USA

Active specific immunotherapy, or the use of tumor 'vaccines', attempts to stimulate the patient to reject his or her tumor. Nowhere has this approach been utilized more than in melanoma, often with encouraging results. The best results have occurred in the setting of minimal residual disease after resection of the primary tumor and involved lymph nodes, but responses have also been obtained in disseminated disease. Prolonged survivals of several years have been achieved in both settings, particularly the former, with little toxicity attributable to the treatment. Genetic and biochemical approaches promise considerably improved preparations of 'vaccines', with defined components and improved activity within the immediate future.

An area of great promise for the treatment of cancer, alone or in combination with other forms of immunotherapy, is active specific immunization. The materials used in this form of treatment are usually called 'vaccines', but since they are now used solely as therapy for established cancers they should be distinguished from the prophylactic vaccines, such as those used to prevent viral infections. Thus, in this review we will often use the term '*therapeutic vaccines*', to emphasize their therapeutic intent. Since the ultimate goal of many immunologists is to prevent cancer through immunization, it may soon be unnecessary to draw this distinction.

AUTOLOGOUS VACCINES

Autologous melanoma cells with or without hapten

From the human serological studies of Old and co-workers in the 1980's,[1] it appeared that many, if not most, melanomas had specific antigens that were unique to the individual and not shared by other tumors of the same melanomas. Thus, it seemed necessary to use the patient's own melanoma cells. The best '*match*' between HLA phenotypes would also be obtained by this strategy. More recent data, including those with therapeutic allogeneic vaccines, call these points into question. Nevertheless, the impetus towards autologous vaccination from those studies was considerable.

Mastrangelo, Berd and their co-workers have emphasized autologous immunization for melanoma for many years. In several studies they obtained evidence for clinical activity. Laucius et al.[2] noted 2 complete remissions (CR) and 2 partial responses (PR) among 18 patients given autologous tumor cells and BCG. Responses lasted 2–4 months, and were achieved mainly in soft tissue sites, such as lymph nodes and skin. In a more recent study, Berd et al.[3] elicited 4 CR and 1 PR in 40 evaluable patients (12.5%) treated with autologous tumor cells combined with BCG. The responses were again mainly in the skin, lymph nodes and lung, and possibly the liver, with a median duration of response of 10 months. They have also attempted to improve immunogenicity of autologous preparations by making them more '*foreign*' to the host through the addition of a hapten, dinitrophenyl. A considerable increase in local inflammatory responses to subcutaneous tumors was elicited in 20 of 46 patients. A prominent CD8 T cell infiltrate was noted, with evidence of activation (CD69+, HLA DR+), although the CD25 (Tac receptor) was absent, and IFN-γ was also found in the tissues by polymerase chain reaction analysis. In this advanced disease setting, 5/46 patients (5/20 who had inflammatory responses) had a PR.[4]

The most encouraging data come from Phase II studies of Stage III patients with minimal residual disease, after removal of the primary tumor and involved lymph nodes. There was a 2-year disease-free survival of 78% for patients receiving haptenized melanoma cells and BCG, whereas 50% would have been expected to relapse by 18 months from historical data.[4] If these results are confirmed, it would be a significant improvement in the use of autologous immunization for melanoma. It would also correlate with the results obtained with allogeneic preparations in the same early setting of disease, which also deserve randomized trials as confirmation.

The most obvious limitations of this form of treatment are the necessity for an accessible tumor nodule of sufficient size to provide tumor cells in sufficient number to serve as autologous immunogens. The inherently weak immunogenicity of an autologous tumor is also a problem, perhaps now addressed by haptenization. Since it is now clear that there are antigens shared by many if not all melanomas, it is not necessary to use autologous immunization. Finally, although some degree of matching similarity between the HLA alleles of cytotoxic T lymphocytes (CTL) and the target melanoma is necessary in vitro to permit rejection, whether an analogous HLA matching between the vaccinating tumor cells and the host is essential has not been resolved.

ALLOGENEIC VACCINES

Irradiated whole cells

Morton and colleagues have recently reported encouraging results in their institutional Phase II trial. Survival was improved in a cohort of 68 patients with metastatic melanoma given irradiated whole melanoma cells and BCG.[5] The response rate in the first 27 patients was only 19% (5/27), but in the expanded group there was a median duration of survival of 23.1 months, with a 5-year survival of 26%. This is in contrast to the usual 7 to 12 month survival expected in disseminated melanoma, and an expected 5-year survival of less than 10%. It is obviously impossible to study patients not given any therapy as a concomitant control, but a randomized trial of this regimen versus chemotherapy would be an interesting comparison.

Lysates

Viral oncolysates

The observation that selected viruses could enhance the immunogenicity of tumor cells ultimately led to clinical trials of therapeutic vaccines composed of such virally transformed tumor cells. Some of the earliest trials were performed by Cassel and his colleagues at Emory University. In patients with measurable, advanced melanoma they saw evidence of tumor shrinkage in skin nodules and lymph nodes in 7 of 13 patients treated with Newcastle disease virus-induced melanoma cell lysates.[6]

Most studies using this approach have been conducted in the surgical adjuvant setting i.e. after surgical removal of all visible or otherwise detectable tumor. Hersey et al reported that a lysate derived from a vaccinia-treated melanoma cell line, given alone with no immune stimulant over a 2 year period to 96 patients led to a median survival of approximately 5 years, exceeding the 2 year median survival of historical and concomitant nonrandomized controls (personal calculations made from the author's data).[7] Cyclophosphamide appeared to lessen the effectiveness of the oncolysates in Hersey's subsequent Phase II study. Wallack has reported a similar improvement in disease-free survival and overall survival with vaccinia viral oncolysates in a Phase II trial.[8] In a recent multi-institutional Phase III trial of 250 patients, Wallack found a 10% improvement in overall survival (non statistically significant) in the viral lysate-treated group versus vaccinia placebo. However, a subset of 20 male patients, aged 44–57, with <5 lymph nodes had a 50% improvement in survival versus placebo-matched controls (Sivanandham M and Wallack MK, personal communication, 1994). A randomized trial in this subset is anticipated to examine this difference.

Mechanical lysates

We have treated patients with disseminated melanoma with a therapeutic vaccine composed of mechanically disrupted melanoma cells from 2 cell lines, together with the adjuvant DETOX™.[9,10] We have also used (on an empirical basis) a low dose of cyclophosphamide (300 mg/m^2) before the course of treatment in approximately one-half of the patients. An increase in precursors of CTL against one of the melanoma cell lines in the lysate was noted in the blood of 50% of the patients between 2 and 6 weeks after beginning immunization. CTL clones were also derived from immunized patients with strong reactivity against autologous and allogeneic melanoma cells. CR and PR were noted in these patients as well, always in those who developed an increase in CTL in their blood. Serum antibodies were also developed in nearly 50% of the patients, but did not correlate with clinical response.

Our personal experience, now extending over a period of 9 years, shows 5 CR and 15 PR (19%) in 106 patients, with the responding sites including lung, lymph nodes, subcutaneous tissue, breast, liver and small intestines.[11] The median duration of these responses on the therapeutic vaccine treatment was 21 months. Although many of these patients went on to other treatments, such as IFN-α, IL-2, or chemotherapy after the vaccine, their survival dating from the start of treatment was striking. Thus, the cohort of responders had a median survival of 46 months.

We have recently calculated the survival of all 154 patients who received various batches of our melanoma therapeutic vaccine, including 2 batches prepared at Ribi ImmunoChem Research (Hamilton, MT, USA) (Groshen S and Mitchell MS, unpublished data, 1994). The median survival was 12.2 months, at the upper end of the expected range of survival for Stage IV melanoma patients. However a cohort of 15 responding patients (10% of the entire group) has formed a 'tail' to the curve, with survivals beginning at 23 months and extending beyond 8 years (Fig. 1). Four patients treated exclusively with the vaccine, all given periodic maintenance injections following induction, have lived for more than 4 years, with the longest responders now living more than 8 years and more than 9 years, respectively. All but one has no evidence of disease, with the fourth having a persistent, stable small liver lesion on CT scans. The patient with the longest response had a brain metastasis in 1988 that was resected, and has had no further central nervous system (CNS) recurrences since. It is entirely possible that her monthly vaccinations have helped to prevent recurrences, even though they failed to prevent her single, large metastasis 1 year after she began the treatment.

A multicenter trial involving 139 patients given Ribi's preparation of our vaccine (Melacine™), showed a much lower objective response rate (3% CR, 5% PR), but minor responses were found in 4% and stable disease for over 6 months, in 23%. More encouragingly, the median survival for all 120 patients actually treated with

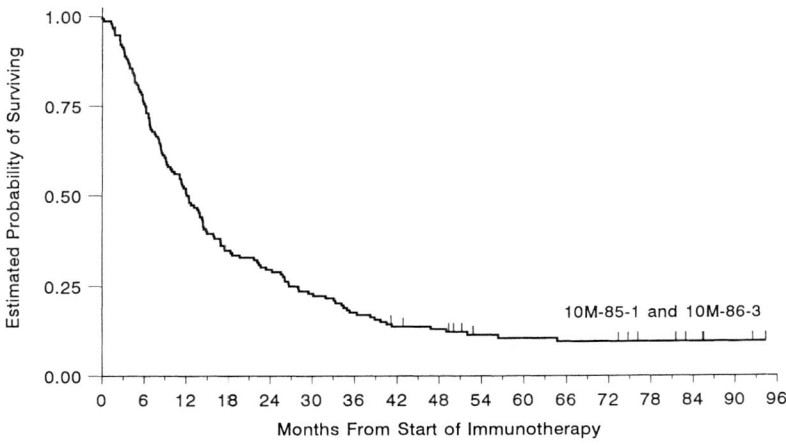

Fig. 1 Survival of 154 patients treated with various lots of therapeutic melanoma vaccine that we have treated over the course of 9 years. Note the 'tail' indicating a subgroup with a profound response lasting at least 23 months to over 8 years in one instance.

Melacine™ was 23 months, with an improvement in survival found for those patients who had stable disease or better.[12]

An analysis of our patients given the therapeutic vaccine with minimal residual disease likewise shows encouraging results. Fifty patients with deeply invasive skin disease (Stage Ib-II) or lymph nodes (Stage III) have had a 90% 1 year survival and 80% 2 year survival. More strikingly, 29 patients with minimal residual Stage IV disease, after resection of a single skin or lung nodule on recurrent lymph nodes, have had the same survival, with a maximum follow-up of 33 months (Figs 2 and 3).

A recently concluded randomized Phase III trial comparing Mel-acine™ with 4-drug chemotherapy in 2 groups of 70 patients each found survival to be equivalent in the two groups, but with far fewer reportable adverse events attributable to the vaccine (133) than chemotherapy (593) (Von Eschen K, personal communication, 1994). The response rate was lower (2 CR, 1 PR, 5 stable) in the vaccine group than in our institutional studies, and lower than that achieved by chemotherapy (2 CR, 11 PR, 23 stable). Whether there is a subgroup of patients who will have a prolonged survival is uncertain from the early analysis.

It is of interest that a primary melanoma has been treated with active immunotherapy. We treated a primary choroidal melanoma, which responded on 2 separate occasions over the course of more than 4 years in an elderly gentleman who eventually died of old age. The diminution in size was documented by serial ultrasound

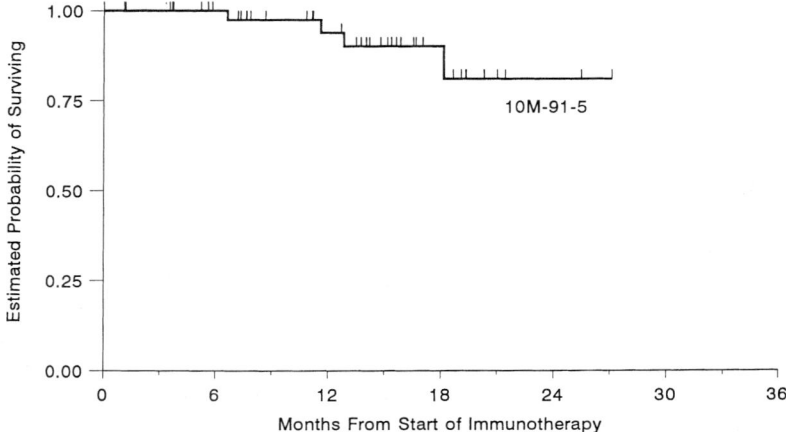

Fig. 2 Survival of 50 patients with Stage II b or III disease, resected, who were then given melanoma vaccine over the course of 48 weeks (10 injections). Follow-up period, 33 months.

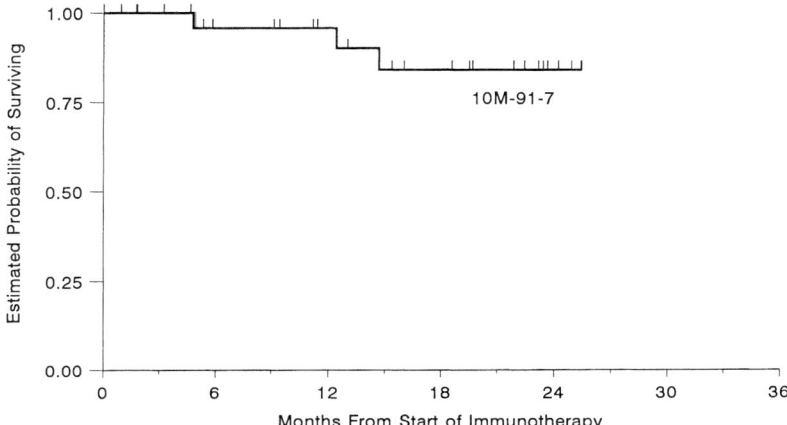

Fig. 3 Survival of 29 patients with a single metastasis to lung or skin or recurrent lymph nodes (Stage IV, resected) treated with a melanoma vaccine over the course of 48 weeks (10 injections). A survival similar to that of the Stage II b and III patients is noted thus far, after a 33 months follow-up.

measurements, and no metastases were ever detected by periodic CT scans.[13] The value of this case may be less in demonstrating our ability to treat a primary tumor, for which the opportunities will be very limited, but in the possibility of preventing metastases. It also demonstrated in vivo what we had found in vitro: that there are antigens in common between skin and ocular melanomas, such that a vaccine preparation from skin metastases could successfully cause shrinkage of choroidal melanoma cells.

Extracts

Bystryn and colleagues have treated nearly 400 patients with a melanoma vaccine composed of antigens shed by cultured melanoma cell lines. They elicited one PR and one long-term stability in 13 patients in an early trial,[14] but results have been far more encouraging in earlier stages of the disease. They have obtained an improved survival in Stage III melanoma after resection, in patients who developed a DTH reaction to the vaccine (>38 months) versus those who did not (13.5 months).[15] Moreover, there appeared to be a relationship between the intensity of DTH and length of survival, with more than 4 years difference of a strong DTH response compared with non-responders.

Defined vaccines

Gangliosides

Livingston et al. have used the melanoma-associate gangliosides GM2 and GD2 with the adjuvant BCG to try to immunize melanoma patients with minimal residual disease.[16] They have successfully generated IgM antibodies in those patients, indicative of a primary response, and more recently IgG antibodies, signifying a secondary response. However, cell-mediated immunity (CTL or T helper cells) has not yet been demonstrated. This group has noted in a recent randomized trial that GM2 immunization together with the adjuvant BCG improved disease-free interval by 23% and survival by 14% in melanoma patients with resected Stage III disease.[17] When comparisons were made of the 'as randomized' groups rather than 'as treated', the differences were not significant, but were still 18% and 11% respectively. While conclusive proof of the potency of previous ganglioside preparations is still lacking, newer constructs of GM2 attached to an immunogenic carrier molecule, and combined with a more potent adjuvant, offer the potential of a better clinical effect.

Anti-idiotype vaccines

Mimicry of melanoma antigens is a clever scientific expedient at a time when we do not know most of the critical tumor-associated antigens, and have isolated only one or two of them. Anti-idiotype vaccines rely on the property of a small subset of anti-antibodies to mimic the eliciting antigen, either by their structure or through their effect on the immune system. Antibody 1 is generated against the antigen; antibody 2 (anti-idiotype) is generated by immunizing an animal with antibody 1. A subset of antibody 2 reacts with the hypervariable region of antibody 1, and a subset of that group mimics the antigen.

In animals, Kohler and colleagues have shown that anti-idiotype vaccines have potent antitumor prophylactic effects. They have emphasized, however, that one must be careful to choose the proper anti-idiotype or risk either having no effect or, worse, suppressing immunity.[18] Ferrone and colleagues have demonstrated in humans that anti-idiotype vaccine mimicking a high molecular weight melanoma antigen induced IgG as well as IgM antibodies, showing the involvement of T helper cells. No cytolytic T cells specific for that antigen have yet been demonstrated. Some regression of disease has been noted in patients, as well as prolongation of survival. Whether the mechanism involved DTH or antibody-mediated immunity was not resolved,[19] but DTH to a very similar anti-idiotype was not found by other investigators.[20]

We treated 25 patients with advanced melanoma with an anti-idiotypic vaccine (at that time called IMelPg2), together with the adjuvant SAF-M (containing muramyl dipeptide), both from IDEC Pharmaceuticals. Responses were noted in 3 patients, of whom one has just had a CR during 3–4-monthly maintenance injections after 2.5 years of a PR, in lung and liver. That patient had a brain metastasis resected just before starting treatment, again suggesting as with our allogeneic lysates, that active specific immunotherapy may help to prevent CNS recurrences at least in some cases (Quan WDY and Mitchell MS, data to be published, 1994).

GENETICALLY ENGINEERED VACCINES

Cytokines

Cytokines have been genetically inserted into tumor cells in animals, to see whether they can enhance immunity in vivo. Originally it was thought that only GM-CSF, somewhat unexpectedly, had that property – judging from a melanoma B16 syngeneic system in C57 BL/6 mice.[21] Subsequent reports have clearly shown that other cytokines, including IL-2, are effective in improving immunogenicity of tumor vaccines in animals, by attracting macrophages and T lymphocytes to the site of injection and activating them there.[22,23]

Insertion of cytokines into human melanoma cells is just beginning, but may prove to be an important stride in the perfection of vaccines. GM-CSF, IL-2, IL-4, IL-7, and IFN-γ are among the cytokines with promise, judging from the animal models. These experiments should indicate which cytokines are most important in immune responses to tumor antigens. However, as a practical issue, it remains to be shown, in preclinical or clinical trials, whether the insertion of cytokines offers a real improvement over the admixture of adjuvants, which improve immunity by eliciting cytokines in their milieu.

Accessory molecules

The interaction of CTL with tumor cells is primarily through their T cell receptor, which recognizes the tumor epitope as presented by the HLA Class I molecule. There are other interactions between the two cells that are of importance, some of which improve the apposition of the two, and others that also transduce second signals into the T cells leading to their activation. ICAM-1, which interacts with the LFA-1 molecule on CTL, is an example of an accessory molecule that improves apposition. B7, which interacts with CD28 on lymphocytes, is a prime example of a molecule that causes transduction of a second signal, through its interaction with CD28/CTLA4 on lymphocytes. B7 is ordinarily found on macrophages, where it assists in their interaction with T helper cells. When put into B16 tumor cells, B7 permits the vaccinated melanoma cells interact directly with CD8 cells, even in the absence of CD4 cells, and makes the weakly immunogenic cells into a potent protective vaccine.[24,25]

Human trials with melanoma cells transduced with B7 will soon begin at several institutions. In our laboratory, Wang has shown that B7 transduced human melanoma cells are 3 times more potent at stimulating CTL lines to proliferate in vitro than parental melanoma cells, and also cause a selective increase in anti-melanoma cytotoxicity by these lines (H Wang, D Kohn and MS Mitchell, data to be published). The killing of parental melanoma cells by the CTL under these circumstances is equivalent to that of genetically altered cells, which suggests that the autochthonous tumor will be attacked more effectively after vaccination with B7-containing melanoma cells.

SYNTHETIC PEPTIDE VACCINES

Methods of obtaining immunogenic peptides

For the production of synthetic peptide vaccines, it will be necessary to isolate those peptides either from the melanoma cells or from genes obtained from those cells. The group at the University of Virginia[26] have used the former approach to isolate melanoma peptides that act as targets for CTL, and can render autologous B cells susceptible to CTL. Their ability to sequence the picogram quantities of peptide isolated by these methods, by mass spectrometry, has been a crucial factor in their success. Other groups have also used elution, with considerable success in identifying immunogenic peptides, but have not yet published sequence information.[27]

The alternative genetic approach has been taken by Boon and his collaborators.[28] They have isolated a gene and antigen called MAGE-1 (melanoma antigen-1) that sensitizes cells to killing by CTL, as measured by TNF-α release from the CTL. This was the first tumor-associated antigen to be isolated by any method, and is the forerunner of a series of antigens from this group. Nevertheless, it should be noted that MAGE-1 is not unique to melanomas, being found in

40% of breast cancers, on other cancers, and in normal tissues. It is HLA-A1 restricted, and is present in only 40% of those melanomas. Yet in those patients its increased expression in the melanoma may make it a good target for CTL in vivo after vaccination with the peptide. A series of MAGE genes have now been isolated, and several of the antigens have been expressed. Others in the series may prove to have greater specificity and applicability to human immunization than MAGE-1 itself. MAGE-3, found on 70% to 80% of melanoma lines and on lung cancer cells lines (both small cell and non-small cell), will shortly undergo clinical trial admixed with incomplete Freund's adjuvant (Weber J, personal communication, 1994).

Other genes encoding antigens have recently been described, to which patients with melanoma react and generate CTL. There is a family of differentiation antigens including tyrosinase, gp100 and Melan-A/Mart-1, cloned by Boon's and Rosenberg's groups.[29,30] Parmiani and his collaborators in Milano have initiated clinical trials with HLA A2 compatible, Melan-A/Mart-1+, IL-2-transduced, irradiated melanoma cells. IL-2 released from those cells generate LAK and CTL-mediated killing, the latter directed against Melan-A/Mart-1 antigen (Parmiani G, personal communication, 1994). Clinical results from the trial are still preliminary.

By subtractive hybridization, our group has isolated 9 genes that originally had novel sequences,[31] two of which have been more fully sequenced. One of them encodes a peptide that stimulates proliferation of T cell from melanoma patients, while the other is identical with PMP-22, lately isolated from Schwann cells, whose immunogenicity is still uncertain (Uchiyama C et al, data to be published).[32,33]

What will be necessary to create potent vaccines from peptides?

Even when we have a large number of synthetic peptides from melanoma antigens, it will still be necessary to make them maximally immunogenic to patients. That is not a small task, because peptides have been far less immunogenic than whole proteins in other systems, such as malarial immunization. The geometric configuration of the peptides, such as in a cluster, or on the surface of inert particles of cell size (pseudocells), may be an important determinant. This will allow direct interaction with CD8 or CD4 T cells, as desired. Potent adjuvants are now available for investigational use, and may also be a critical part of vaccines containing synthetic peptides. Perhaps the construction of antigen-presenting cells displaying the peptide on its surface, together with appropriate accessory molecules and cytokines, will be an optimal approach to this issue, replacing the tumor cell. It is likely in any event that more than one peptide will prove necessary, because it is improbable that all melanoma patients will respond to the same immunodominant epitope.

COMBINATION THERAPIES

While one must first study each new treatment by itself, to see exactly what its strengths and weaknesses are, it is combinations of agents that offer the most promise in cancer treatment. Combinations of different types of immunotherapy are not only possible, because of the absence of additive toxicity, but desirable because of theoretical complementarity. The addition of CTL and/or cytokines to vaccines, are methods that have already been tested in patients.

Combinations of autologous vaccine and adoptive immunotherapy

In an interesting series of studies Shu, Chang, and colleagues[34] have obtained lymphocytes from lymph nodes draining the sites of injection of vaccines in animals, re-educating them in vitro and then using them as more specific effector cells in reinfusion experiments. This strategy has begun to be tested in patients by this and other groups, with evidence of transfer of DTH against the tumor and several early tumor responses. Whether the transferred cells are more potent than tumor-infiltrating lymphocytes, or simply peripheral blood lymphocytes from the same patients, remains to be proved.

Combinations of allogeneic vaccine and cytokines

We have reported[35] that patients who were treated with IFN-α after having received a therapeutic melanoma vaccine had a 45% response rate (8 of 18 patients), including site-specific CR in 5 of the 8. The median survival was extended, to 36 months, and 3 patients remain alive after more than 4 years. The probability of surviving more than a year was 70% in responding patients evaluated at 4 months, when responses were clear in all patients. In contrast, by this landmark analysis, that likelihood was only 13% for the clinical non-responders. Patients with a variety of HLA phenotypes responded to the IFN-α, in contrast to our experience with the vaccine alone, where 3 alleles (HLA-A2/28, B12/44/45 and C3) were critical determinants of response.[36] IFN-α can upregulate tumor antigens and HLA Class I molecules, and may have exerted its clinical effect on our patients by this means – making the patients' tumor more recognizable to the immune system and permitting the augmented immune response to act effectively on metastatic sites of the tumor. Expanded clinical trials at our institution and nationally in the United States are planned for 1995.

We previously combined IL-2 (Roche) and the vaccine in 18 patients, but perhaps at a schedule that was suboptimal. The IL-2 was given from the outset of vaccine treatment, which may have skewed the response away from CTL towards activated NK (LAK) cells. Nonetheless, we noted several responding patients: 1 PR and 1 mixed response in each of the groups (6 and 3 patients, respectively) receiving the highest doses of IL-2 (approximately 11.25 and 15 million international units/m^2). Toxicity was prohibitive however, with abrupt losses of consciousness in 4 of 9 patients at these dose levels, which forced the study to be discontinued.[37] A more logical use of the two types of immunotherapy may be sequential, with immunization first and then IL-2 to increase specific CTL.

THE PROBLEM OF BRAIN METASTASES

Brain metastases have been the principal complication of attempts to cure melanoma patients with immunotherapy. Improved responses with vaccines and IL-2, and other types of immunotherapy, have translated into improved survival in some cases, but responders have often succumbed to CNS metastases[38] reinforcing the concept of a blood-brain barrier. Eradication of visceral metastases by vaccines or any other means will be of little benefit unless this problem is solved. 75% of melanoma patients have brain metastases, as determined by autopsy studies. If we extend survival without eradicating the brain metastases, the patients will simply live long enough to develop clinical disease in the CNS. While in mice prior vaccination has prevented CNS metastases,[39] treatment of established metastases has been far less successful. Intensive regional treatment with cytokines is under exploration in several centers as an approach to this important issue.

CONCLUSIONS ABOUT VACCINES

Several tentative conclusions may be drawn from the cumulative experience with therapeutic vaccines. Foremost, although our perspective is undoubtedly somewhat biased, the weight of evidence points to some degree of effectiveness of active immunization against melanomas, most strikingly when used in the setting of minimal residual disease.[40] Even vaccines that have shown little effect with

644   MELANOMA: CUTANEOUS AND OCULAR

measurable lesions appear to have prolonged survival after lymph node resection. Since bulky tumors may exert immunosuppressive influences over the host, e.g. by their secretion of downregulatory cytokines, that makes them far more difficult to treat than microscopic deposits of tumor cells. The sheer numbers of tumor cells to be eradicated is another obvious reason for the poorer results obtained in that setting.

The therapeutic effects from cancer vaccines have been elicited without significant systemic toxicity. Most of the toxicity noted was at the sites of injection, due to the adjuvant, or was due to cyclophosphamide pretreatment. Anaphylactic reactions were absent, as were serious autoimmune phenomena, with only a patchy vitiligo occasionally noted in responding patients. Regressions of melanoma metastases have been noted in only 10–20% of all patients, but a significant proportion of the responding patients lived for years rather than simply months. Thus, we believe that the results justify further attempts to develop this easily tolerated form of treatment for both residual and metastatic melanoma.

PERSPECTIVES

Several approaches are in fact already in process, in the continued development of a vaccine approach to human melanoma. Combinations of active immunotherapy with cytokines, such as IFN-α, or adoptive immunotherapy will be explored in the immediate future. Genetically-engineered vaccines, at first whole cell-based, will be a major focus of investigation, and should soon lead to a better formulation for synthetic vaccines. Since synthetic peptides lack the immunogenicity of whole proteins, it will be essential to pay attention to their formulation as therapeutic materials, including the choice of potent adjuvants. The most important element of exploration will be of the immune response itself, to determine how one can manipulate antigen-presentation networks to best advantage, perhaps transducing genes for antigens, accessory molecules and cytokines into antigen-presenting cells as the ultimate vaccine for prevention of melanoma.

REFERENCES

1 Old LJ. Cancer immunology: the search for specificity. GHA Clowes Memorial Lecture. Cancer Res 1981; 41: 361–375.
2 Laucius JF, Bodurtha AJ, Mastrangelo MJ, Bellett RE. A phase II study of autologous irradiated tumor cells plus BCG in patients with metastatic malignant melanoma. Cancer 1977; 40: 2091–2093.

3 Berd D, Maguire HC Jr, McCue P, Mastrangelo JM. Treatment of metastatic melanoma with an autologous tumor cell vaccine: clinical and immunological results in 64 patients. J Clin Oncol 1990; 8: 1858–1867.

4 Berd D, Sato T, Lattime ED, Maguire HC Jr, Mastrangelo MJ. Immunization with hapten-modified tumor cells: a strategy for the treatment of human melanoma. Am Assoc Cancer Res 1994; 35: 667–668.

5 Morton DL, Foshag LJ, Hoon DSB, et al. Prolongation of survival in metastatic melanoma after active specific immunotherapy with a new polyvalent melanoma vaccine. Ann Surg 1992; 216: 463–482.

6 Cassel WA, Murray DR, Phillips HS. A phase II study on the postsurgical management of stage II malignant melanoma with a Newcastle disease virus oncolysate. Cancer 1983; 52: 856–886.

7 Hersey P. Vaccinia viral lysates in treatment of melanoma. In: Mitchell MS, ed. Biological approaches to cancer treatment: Biomodulation. New York: McGraw-Hill, 1992: 302–325.

8 Wallack MK, Bash J, Bartolucci A. Improvement in disease-free survival of melanoma patients in conjunction with serologic response in a phase Ia/Ib Southeastern Cancer Study Group trial of vaccinia melanoma oncolysate. Am Surg 1989; 55: 243–247.

9 Mitchell MS, Kan-Mitchell J, Kempf RA, Harel W, Shau H, Lind S. Active specific immunotherapy for melanoma: Phase I trial of allogeneic lysates and a novel adjuvant. Cancer Res 1988; 48: 5883–5893.

10 Mitchell MS. Active specific immunotherapy of cancer: therapeutic vaccines ('theraccines') for the treatment of disseminated malignancies. Biological approaches to cancer treatment: Biomodulation. New York: McGraw Hill, 1992: 326–351.

11 Mitchell MS, Harel W, Kan-Mitchell J et al. Active specific immunotherapy of melanoma with allogeneic cell lysates. Rationale, results, and possible mechanisms of action. Ann NY Acad Sci 1993; 690: 153–166.

12 Elliott GT, McLeod RA, Perez J, Von Eschen KB: Interim results of a phase II multicenter clinical trial evaluating the activity of a therapeutic allogeneic melanoma vaccine (theraccine) in the treatment of disseminated malignant melanoma. Semin Surg Oncol 1993; 9: 264–272.

13 Mitchell MS, Liggett PE, Green RL et al. Sustained regression of a primary choroidal melanoma under the influence of a therapeutic melanoma vaccine (melanoma theraccine). J Clin Oncol 1993; 12: 396–401

14 Bystryn JC, Jacobsen S, Harris M, et al. Preparation and characterization of polyvalent human melanoma antigen vaccine. J Biol Response Mod 1986; 5: 211–224.

15 Bystryn JC. Immunogenicity and clinical activity of a polyvalent melanoma antigen vaccine prepared from shed antigens. Ann NY Acad Sci 1993; 690: 190–203.

16 Livingston PO. Approaches to augmenting the IgG antibody response to melanoma ganglioside vaccines. In: Bystryn JC, Ferrone S, Livingston P, eds. Specific immunotherapy of cancer with vaccines. Ann. NY Acad. Sci 1993; 690: 276–291.

17 Livingston PO, Wong GY, Adluri S et al. Improved survival in stage III melanoma patients with GM2 antibodies: a randomized trial of adjuvant vaccination with GM2 ganglioside. J Clin Oncol 1994; 12: 1036–44.

18 Anderson DR, Kohler H, Muller S. Biomodulation with network epitopes. In: Mitchell MS, ed. Biological approaches to cancer treatment: Biomodulation. New York: McGraw-Hill, 1992: 155–171.

19 Ferrone S. Human tumor-associated antigen mimicry by anti-idiotypeic antibodies. Ann NY Acad Sci 1993; 690: 214–224.

20 Livingston PO, Sucharita A, Raychaudhuri S, Hughes MH, Calves MJ, Merritt JA. Phase I trial of immunological adjuvant SAFm in melanoma patients vaccinated with antiidiotype antibody MELIMMUNE-1. Vaccine Res 1994; 3: 71.

21 Pardoll DM, Golumbeck P, Levitsky H, Jaffee L. Molecular engineering of the anti-tumor immune response. Bone Marrow Transplant 1992; 9 (Suppl 1): 182–186.

22 Gansbacher B, Zier B, Daniels K, Cronin R, Bannerji R, Gilboa E. Interleukin-2 gene transfer into tumor cells abrogates tumor: genicity and induces protective immunity. J Exp Med 1990; 172: 1217–1224.

23 Musiani P, Modesti A, Brunetti M, et al. Nature and potential of the reactive response to mouse mammary adenocarcinoma cells engineered with interleukin-2, interleukin-4, or interferon-gamma genes. Natural Immun 1994; 13(2–3): 93.

24 Townsend SE, Allison JP. Tumor rejection after direct costimulation of CD8 + T cells by B7-transfected melanoma cells. Science 1993; 259: 368–370.

25 Chen L, Ashe S, Brady WA, et al. Dostimulation of antitumor immunity by the B7 counter receptor for the T lymphocyte molecules CD28 and CTLA-4. Cell 1991; 71: 1093–1102.

26 Cox AL, Skipper J, Chen Y et al. Identification of a peptide recognized by five melanoma-specific human cytotoxic T cell lines. Science 1994; 264: 716–719.

27 Storkus WJ, Zeh HJ 3d, Maeurer MJ, Salder RD, Lotze MT. Identification of human melanoma peptides recognized by class I restricted tumor infiltrating T-lymphocytes. J Immun 1993; 151(7): 3719–27.

28 Van der Bruggen C, Traversari C, Chomez P, Boon T. A gene encoding an antigen recognized by cytolytic T lymphocytes on a human melanoma. Science 1991; 254: 1643–1647.

29 Kawakami Y, Eliyahu S, Delgado CH, et al. Cloning of the gene coding for a shared human melanoma antigen recognized by autologous T cells infiltrating into tumor. Proc Natl Acad Sci USA 1994; 91: 3515–3519.

30 Coulie PG, Brichard V, Vanpel A, Wolfel T, et al. A new gene coding for a differentiation antigen recognized by autologous cytolytic T lymphocytes on HLA-A2 melanomas. J Exp Med 1994; 180: 35–42.

31 Hutchins JT, Deans RJ, Mitchell MS, Uchiyama C, Kan-Mitchell J. Novel gene sequences expressed by human melanoma cells identified by molecular substraction. Cancer Res 1991; 51: 1418–1425.

32 Snipes GJ, Suter U, Welcher AA, Shooter EM. Characterization of a novel peripheral nervous system myelin protein (PMP-22/SR13). Cell Biol 1992; 117: 225–238.

33 Hayasaka K, Himoro M, Nanao K, et al. Isolation and sequence determination of cDNA encoding PMP-22 (PAS-II/SR13/GAS-3) of human peripheral myelin. Biochem Biophys Res Commun 1992; 186: 827–831.

34 Chang AE, Yoshizawa H, Sakai K, Cameron MJ, Sondak VK, Shu S. Clinical observations on adoptive immunotherapy with vaccine-primed T-lymphocytes secondarily sensitized to tumor in vitro. Cancer Res 1993; 53(5): 1043–1050.

35 Mitchell MS, Jakowatz J, Harel W, Dean G, Spears L, Groshen S. Increased effectiveness of interferon-alfa-2b following active specific immunotherapy for melanoma. J Clin Oncol 1994; 2: 402–411.

36 Mitchell MS, Harel W, Groshen S. Association of HLA phenotype with response to active specific immunotherapy of melanoma. J Clin Oncol 1992; 10: 1158–1164.

37 Mitchell, MS. Chemotherapy in combination with biomodulation: a 5-year experience with cyclophosphamide and interleukin-2. Semin Oncol 1992; 19: 80–87.

38 Mitchell MS. Relapse in the central nervous system in melanoma patients successfully treated with biomodulators. J Clin Oncol 1989; 7: 121–129.

39 Staib L, Harel W, and Mitchell MS. Protection against experimental cerebral metastases of murine melanoma B16 by active immunization. Cancer Res 1993; 53: 1113–1121.

40 Bysnyn JC, Ferrone S, Livingston P, eds. Specific immunotherapy of cancer with vaccines. Ann NY Acad Sci, 1993: 690.

British Medical Bulletin 1995, Vol 51, No. 3 pp. 647–655
©The British Council 1995

Targeted gene therapy

I R Hart

Richard Dimbleby Department of Cancer Research, Rayne Institute, St Thomas' Hospital, London, UK

R G Vile

ICRF Laboratory of Cancer Gene Therapy, Rayne Institute, St. Thomas' Hospital, London, UK

Melanin biosynthesis is limited to melanocytes partly as a consequence of transcriptional regulation of the enzymes involved in this pathway. Promoter sequences of these enzyme genes may be utilised to drive expression of complementary DNA coding for therapeutic genes so as to provide transcriptional targeting. We have used the 5'-flanking sequences of the murine tyrosinase or tyrosinase-related protein 1 (TRP-1) genes to show that such transcriptional targeting can be achieved both in vitro and in vivo. Using IL-2 as an example of an immunostimulatory gene and Herpes Simplex Virus thymidine kinase (HSVtk) as an example of a prodrug-activating gene we have shown, in murine model systems, that substantial anti-tumour effects can be achieved by targeted gene therapy approaches. The stage now is set for initial clinical evaluations in human patients.

IN VIVO GENE TRANSFER

Gene therapy approaches for cancer treatment are being developed and tested in the clinic.[1] Many of these protocols are based upon the removal ex vivo of either the neoplastic or immune effector cells, their genetic manipulation in vitro and subsequent return to the patient.[2] Some of the ways of using these techniques to develop vaccination protocols are covered elsewhere in this volume (*see* Mitchell, this issue). There are significant limitations to such manipulations including the fact that these rather cumbersome and technically-demanding procedures probably will be limited to specialised centres. Their application to widespread use is unlikely both on the grounds of cost and available technology. An alternative strategy, which has several conceptual advantages, would be the direct modification *in situ* of cancer cells with novel genetic material (Fig. 1). Such direct gene transfer recently has been shown to be achievable in humans using cutaneous malignant melanoma.[3] Thus Nabel and his colleagues were able to introduce the human HLA-B7 gene into subcutaneously located melanoma deposits of HLA-B7-negative patients using the direct injection of DNA complexed with liposomes.[3] Not only was the procedure shown to be safe in the 5 patients evaluated but also between 1–10% of the tumour cells around the site of injection were shown to express protein derived from the transduced gene. This seminal paper established the fact that direct genetic modification of tumour cells is possible in man using injected DNA. That such in vivo transduction also might occur in human tumours as a consequence of retrovirally-mediated gene transfer has been the basis of alternative strategies.[4] Based upon the demonstration that *in situ* retrovirally mediated gene transfer has proved feasible in the treatment of brain tumours in rats[5] clinical evaluations are underway to assess the response of brain tumour patients to the implantation of virus-producing lines.[4] While formal proof of viral integration in the human neoplastic cells has not yet been published it seems likely, from the rodent model, that such an event indeed is occurring.

The capacity to transduce and to genetically modify human cells *in situ* therefore already exists and the refinement of these procedures over the next few years should enhance the efficiency of this phenomenon considerably. What genes though should be introduced into such recipient cells? At the present time the genes available appear to fall into one of three broad categories:

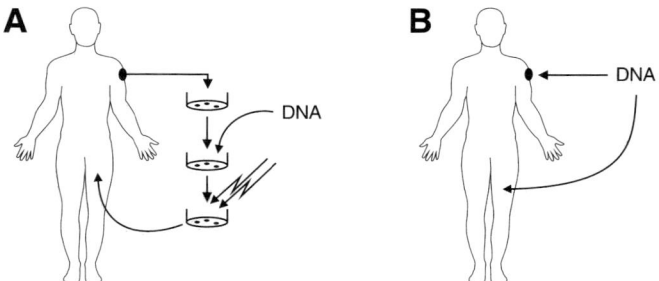

Fig. 1 A. In ex vivo genetic modification protocols, the tumour cells are removed from the host, modified genetically in vitro, irradiated and returned to the host in the form of a vaccine. **B.** In vivo genetic modification protocols rely upon the introduction of DNA either directly into the tumour mass or into muscle tissue to produce their anti-tumour effects.

1. Those which correct genetic changes responsible for the acquisition and progression of the malignant phenotype and thereby arrest tumour development.
2. Those which evoke or amplify an immune response.
3. Those which render cells sensitive to subsequently delivered drugs by coding for enzymes capable of converting harmless prodrugs to active cytotoxics.

The utilisation of the genes represented in category 1 is beset by two major difficulties. Firstly, in a process as extended as tumour development and progression, identification of the major underlying genetic aberrations/lesions is not always clearcut. In hereditary melanoma, for instance, the p16 (CDKN2) gene located at chromosome 9p21 may be a candidate for introduction of a normal wild-type gene.[6,7] The fact though that even in melanoma patients, mutations in this gene are not frequent, relative to unaffected members of families showing linkage to 9p21,[7] calls in to question the generality of the involvement of p16. That the product of the p16 (CDKN2) gene inhibits an enzyme involved in regulating the cell cycle serves to underscore the second difficulty associated with attempts at correctional therapy in cancer. This approach requires the delivery of the corrective gene to every neoplastic cell, or at least every neoplastic stem cell. Failure to correct the deficiency in any one such stem cell might lead to the rapid overgrowth of an 'unreversed' clone. Accordingly, our efforts have focused upon the utilisation of genes from categories 2 and 3. Clearly there are theoretical advantages to be gained during the use of genes from either category 2 or 3 in restriction of their expression to tumour cells alone. The currently available physical transfer techniques and viral vectors do not possess the necessary degree of specificity to ensure that this occurs. The use of tumour cell-specific promoters to direct expression of the therapeutic gene is one approach to overcoming these limitations; non-specific delivery vehicles would be tolerable because specific expression would occur only in the neoplastic cells. This approach was pioneered by Huber and co-workers,[8] using the alphafetoprotein promoter to direct expression to hepatocellular carcinoma, and led us to examine similar possibilities in malignant melanoma.

MELANIN BIOSYNTHESIS PATHWAY AND TYROSINASE REGULATION

The pigment cell exists to synthesise melanin and this capacity frequently is retained and often elevated in tumours arising from this cell type. The key regulatory steps in the melanin biosynthesis pathway centre around control of the activity of the copper-binding enzyme tyrosinase. Thus the rate-limiting step is the oxidation of tyrosine to dopa and that of dopa to dopaquinone.[9] Several other proteins associated with melanogenesis have been identified including proteins related to tyrosinase e.g. TRP-1[10] and TRP-2.[11] Although post-transcriptional control of expression does contribute to cell type regulation the specificity of melanin synthesis is due, in large part, to melanocyte-specific transcription of both TRP-1[10] and tyrosinase[12] genes. The transcribing of a gene in this tissue-specific fashion depends on achieving expression in the appropriate cell type and repression in other tissues.[13] Using β-galactosidase as a reporter gene we showed that as little as 769 base pair of the 5′ flanking region of the murine tyrosinase and 1.4 kb pair of the murine TRP-1 genes were sufficient to direct expression to both human and murine melanocytes and melanoma cells in vitro.[14] Thus high levels of activity were observed in 12 of 14 human and murine melanoma lines tested but basal levels only, similar to that obtained with promoterless constructs, in a panel of 12 other cell types.[14] Direct injection of DNA into melanoma or control non-melanoma tumours resulted in transduction of up to 10% of tumour cells within the melanoma but no expression was seen in the control cancer.[14] The reporter gene was expressed in some normal melanocytes but not in other surrounding normal tissues.[14] These results showed that it was possible, using the transcriptional specificity of a melanocyte-specific promoter, to direct expression of genes to melanocyte-derived cells (Fig. 2).

TARGETING OF IMMUNITY-ENHANCING GENES

Melanoma always has been the human malignancy considered most likely to be immunogenic based upon rather indirect immunological assays and its somewhat capricious clinical behaviour.[15,16] The recent demonstration that this is the human tumour type from which a number of tumour peptide antigens, restricted by class I molecules of the major histocompatibility complex (MHC), can be isolated serves to confirm biochemically these earlier suspicions.[17] Thus the MZ2-E antigen (product of the MAGE-1 gene), for example, is expressed by many melanomas, as well as other tumour types, but not by normal tissues (apart from the testis)[18] and represents a potential vaccination target (more of this below). Why such tumour-specific neoantigens are not recognised by T cells from the tumour-bearing patients is not immediately apparent. Pardoll[17] has suggested that

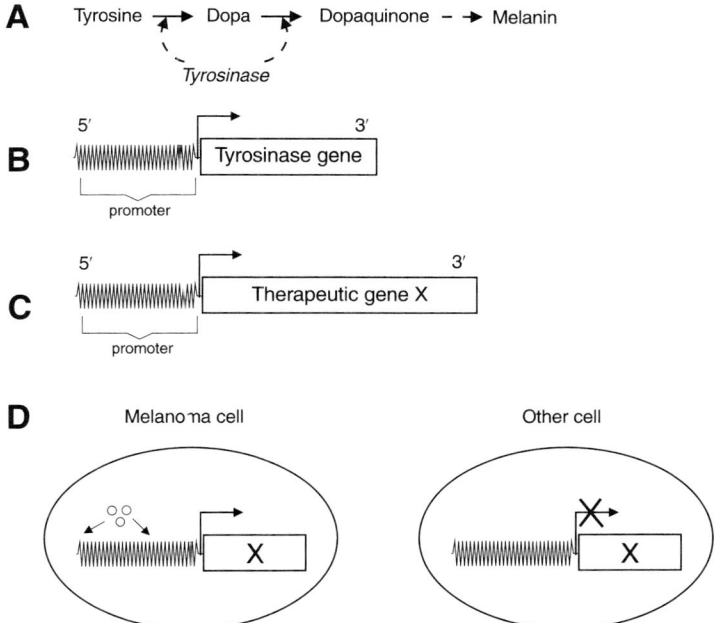

Fig. 2 The gene for the enzyme tyrosinase is transcribed specifically in melanocytic cells. Isolation of the 5′ promoter region of the tyrosinase gene allows it to be fused to an heterologous therapeutic gene (X). If DNA is introduced into melanocyte-derived cells then specific transcription factors will bind to the promoter sequence and initiate transcription, whereas when DNA is introduced into non-melanocytic cells the absence of specific transcription factors means the promoter remains inactive and the gene is not transcribed.

tolerance of the neoantigen may be comparable to that of a tissue-specific antigen and relate to the efficiency of epitope processing and presentation. Additionally the tumours may lack the necessary levels of MHC class 1 or additional co-stimulatory molecules (see below) and thus be safe from cytotoxic T lymphocyte recognition.

Such considerations raise a number of possibilities for therapy. The costimulatory molecule B7 binds to the CD28 and CTLA-4 receptors on T cells and results in optimal activation of these cyto-toxic effectors. Introduction of the B7 gene into murine melanoma cells has led to the rejection of murine melanoma cells.[19,20] Restricted delivery of the B7 molecule to melanoma cells using the transcriptional control of tissue-specific promoters, could result in effective immune stimulation. Recently we have shown (Chong, Hart and Vile, unpublished observations) that expressionof the B7 gene driven by the tyrosinase promoter makes expressing melanoma cells highly immunogenic.

A theoretical advantage to this type of immunostimulatory approach is the release from the necessity to deliver genes to disseminated cancer deposits. Activated cytolytic T cells should themselves be capable of recirculating and homing to distant growths. Since such effectors can kill more than a single tumour cell it also may not be necessary to deliver immune-stimulating genes to more than a relatively small percentage of target tumour cells. The finding that established $B7^{-ve}$ micrometastases were eliminated by the immune response generated by the subcutaneous inoculation of $B7^{+ve}$ transfected tumour cells supports this argument[19]. Various cytokine cDNAs may be introduced into tumour cells to amplify the number of responding T-cells and other immune effector cells. While such approaches frequently have been undertaken in the quest for more immunogenic vaccine material[21] there is every reason to suppose that the local production of such cytokines *in situ* may have a beneficial effect.[22] Again transcriptional targeting may enhance the efficacy of such *in situ* modification by bringing the stimulated proliferating T cells into close juxtaposition with the cytokine-expressing tumour cells. An obvious caveat is that the cytokine cDNA chosen to be inserted into the tumour cells should not represent a gene whose product already is produced by these cells nor, obviously, should such cells possess the cognate receptor and respond in an autocrine growth fashion to cytokine stimulation. Using IL-2 and IL-4 as examples of cytokines we have shown that direct injection of cDNAs, expressed from the tyrosinase promoter, into established B16 melanoma results in gene expression within the melanoma cells[23] and a significant number of tumour regressions (RG Vile and IR Hart, unpublished observations).

TARGETING OF PRODRUG ACTIVATING GENES

The use of genes capable of converting an inert prodrug to an active cytotoxic is an area of intense research interest at this time. There are a number of such genes, frequently referred to as 'suicide' genes, but two have received the greatest amount of attention. The bacterial cytosine deaminase gene encodes an enzyme that converts 5-fluorocytosine into 5-fluorouracil. The HSVtk gene encodes a kinase which phosphorylates ganciclovir, a guanosine analogue, to an intermediate which, after further phosphorylation by cellular kinases, disrupts DNA synthesis. The transfer of prodrug activation-based gene therapy from the laboratory to the clinic is likely to be expedited by the fact that considerable clinical experience has been accumulated with both ganciclovir as an anti-viral and 5-fluorocytosine as an antifungal agent. We have shown that direct injection of HSVtk cDNA, under the control of the tyrosinase promoter, followed by systemic treatment with ganciclovir produced a significant reduction in tumour size but no evidence of adverse cellular effects elsewhere in the body.[24] Part of this reduction in tumour bulk probably is attributable to the so-called 'bystander' phenomenon. This effect, which probably depends on the transfer of toxic metabolites, means that not every cell requires transduction with DNA and has the practical implication that efficiencies of gene transfer considerably lower than 100% may be effective. Thus when a clone of B16 cells stably transduced with HSVtk (E26) was admixed with parental, untransduced B16 cells, refractory to the toxic effects of ganciclovir, in varying proportions and cultured in 1 μg/ml ganciclovir there was substantial killing of the parent cells; at a 50:50 mix of trans-fected:untransfected cells over 90% of the total cell population was killed.[24]

The problem of course with all the direct injection routes of administration of prodrug-activating genes, as distinct from immunity modulating genes, is the relatively limited extent of any field effect. The central conundrum remains how such genes are to be delivered to viscerally located tumours. Our own efforts in murine model systems have centred very much upon the use of recombinant retro-viral vectors as systemic delivery agents where tissue-specific expression is maintained by incorporating the 5' promoter of the murine tyrosinase gene.[25] While the use of such vectors in human patients is unlikely to be sanctioned we recently have obtained some dramatic results in animals which, we believe, have profound implications for future gene therapy approaches. We found that the number of recently established lung metastases of murine melanoma in syngeneic mice was reduced markedly in animals treated with ganciclovir compared to controls after multiple intravenous injections of high titre retroviral supernatant encoding the HSVtk gene.[26] The reduction in lung tumour nodules exceeded the anticipated extent of transduction and was taken to be indicative of a marked bystander effect. The magnitude of this reduction was not obtained in athymic immunodeficient mice, suggesting that an immune component was somehow involved in this bystander effect. In support of this concept we demonstrated that, whereas the parental cells were only poorly immunogenic, a partial but effective anti-tumour immune response was generated following killing of neoplastic cells in vivo as a result of treatment with ganciclovir.[26] This combination of direct killing leading to an augmented immune response, possibly as a consequence of the liberation of some of the tumour neoantigens described earlier, might mean that prodrug activation by gene therapy could play some part in the therapy of metastatic melanoma.

It is the refractoriness of late-stage malignant melanoma to conventional treatment regimes which fuels the search for novel therapeutic approaches. This tumour type possesses distinct immunological and biochemical properties which offer the prospect of targeting selectively any gene therapy modalities and the exploitation of such characteristics could provide therapeutic gains in forthcoming years.

REFERENCES

1 Culver KW, Blaese RM. Gene therapy for cancer. Trends Genet 1994; 10: 174–178.
2 Vile RG, Russell SJ. Gene transfer technologies for the gene therapy of cancer. Gene Ther 1994; 1: 88–98.
3 Nabel GJ, Nabel EG, Yang Z-Y et al. Direct gene transfer with DNA-liposome complexes in melanoma: Expression, biologic activity, and lack of toxicity in humans. Proc Natl Acad Sci USA 1993; 90: 11307–11311.
4 Oldfield EH, Ram Z, Culver KW, Blaese RM, De Vroom HL, Anderson WF. Clinical protocol: Gene therapy for the treatment of brain tumours using intratumoral transduction with the thymidine kinase gene and intravenous ganciclovir. Hum Gene Ther 1993; 4: 39–69.
5 Ram Z, Culver KW, Walbridge S, Blaese RM, Oldfield EH. In situ retroviral mediated gene transfer for the treatment of brain tumors in rats. Cancer Res 1993; 53: 83–88.
6 Kamb A, Gruis NA, Weaverfeldhaus J et al. A cell-cycle regulator potentially involved in genesis of many tumor types. Science 1994; 264: 436–440.
7 Kamb A, Shattuckeidens D, Eeles R et al. Analysis of the p16 gene (cdkn2) as a candidate for the chromosome 9p melanoma susceptibility locus. Nature Genet 1994; 8: 22–26.
8 Huber BE, Richards CA and Krenitsky TA. Retroviral-mediated gene therapy for the treatment of hepatocellular carcinoma: an innovative approach for cancer therapy. Proc Natl Acad Sci USA 1991; 88: 8039–8043.
9 Korner A, Pawelek J. Mammalian tyrosinase catalyses three reactions in the biosynthesis of melanin. Science 1982; 217: 1163–1165.
10 Jackson IJ, Chambers DM, Budd PS, Johnson R. The tyrosinase related protein-1 gene has a structure and promoter sequence very different from tyrosinase. Nucl Acids Res 1991; 19: 3798–3804.
11 Tsukamoto K, Jackson IJ, Urabe K, Montague PM, Hearing VJA. Second tyrosinase related protein, TRP-2, is a melanogenic enzyme termed DOPAchrome tautomerase. EMBO J 1992; 11: 519–526.
12 Kluppel M, Beermann F, Puppert S, Schmid E, Hummler E, Schutz G. The mouse tyrosinase promoter is sufficient for expression in melanocytes and in the pigmented epithelium of the retina. Proc Natl Acad Sci USA 1991; 88: 3777–3781.
13 Yavuzer U, Goding CR. Melanocyte-specific gene expression: Role of repression and identification of a melanocyte-specific factor, MSF. Mol Cell Biol 1994; 14: 3494–3508.
14 Vile RG, Hart IR. In vitro and in vivo targeting of gene expression to melanoma cells. Cancer Res 1993; 53: 962–967.
15 Carrell S, Johnson JP. Immunologic recognition of malignant melanoma by autologous T lymphocytes. Curr Opin Oncol 1993; 5: 383–389.

16 Crowley NJ, Seigler HF. Possibilities of immunotherapy and gene therapy for malignant melanoma. Semin Surg Oncol 1993; 9: 273–278.

17 Pardoll DM. Tumour antigens: a new look for the 1990s. News and Views. Nature 1994; 369: 357–358.

18 Van der Bruggen P, Traversari C, Chomez P et al. A gene encosing an antigen recognized by cytolytic T lymphocytes on a human melanoma. Science 1991; 254: 1643–1647.

19 Chen L, Ashe S, Brady WA et al. Costimulation of antitumour immunity by the B7 counter-receptor for the T lymphocyte molecules CD28 and CTLA-4. Cell 1992; 71: 1093–1102.

20 Townsend SE, Allinson JP. Tumor rejection after direct costimulation of CD8 + cells by B7-transfected melanoma cells. Science 1993; 259: 368–370.

21 Gansbacher B, Houghton A, Livingston, P et al. Clinical protocol: A pilot study of immunization with HLA-A2 matched allogeneic melanoma cells that secrete interleukin-2 in patients with metastatic melanoma. Hum Gene Ther 1992; 3: 677–690.

22 Plautz GE, Yang ZY, Wu BY, Gao X, Huong L, Nabel GJ. Immunotherapy of malignancy by in vivo gene transfer into tumors. Proc Natl Acad Sci USA 1993; 90: 4645–4649.

23 Vile RG, Hart IR. Targeting of cytokine gene expression to malignant melanoma cells using tissue specific promoter sequences. Anna Oncol 1994; 5 (Suppl. 4): S59–S65.

24 Vile RG, Hart IR. Use of tissue-specific expression of the Herpes Simplex Virus thymidine kinase gene to inhibit growth of established murine melanomas following direct intratumoural injection of DNA. Cancer Res 1993; 53: 3860–3864.

25 Vile RG, Miller N, Hart IR. Retroviral vectors for the gene therapy of malignant melanoma. Gene Ther 1994; 1: 307–316.

26 Vile RG, Nelson JA, Castleden S, Chong H, Hart IR. Systemic gene therapy of murine melanoma using tissue specific expression of the HSVtk gene involves an immune component. Cancer Res (In Press).

British Medical Bulletin 1995, Vol 51, No. 3 pp. 656–677
©The British Council 1995

Biological response modifiers in melanoma

J A Bridgewater and M E Gore

Department of Medicine, Royal Marsden Hospital, London, UK

Immunotherapy for cancer comprises the enhancement of the immune and cytokine systems to modulate host immunity to tumour in order to overcome an implicit anergy of self to tumour. This expanding field includes the use of cytokines, antibodies, modified T-lymphocytes and tumour vaccines, and their use in combination with conventional cytotoxic chemotherapy.

Expansion in their use has occurred since the late 1970's for several reasons. The isolation of cytokines, originally the interferons, led to an elucidation of their potent anti-proliferative effects and the demonstration of efficacy in many animal tumour models.[1] The concurrent development of recombinant biotechnology has made available sufficient quantities of cytokine for use in human malignancy and other specialities. Attempts to combine biological agents with conventional chemotherapy have followed initial demonstrations of efficacy in phase I and II trials. The combination of biological and conventional agents is particularly attractive because of the opportunities for synergy and diversity of toxicity, allowing an optimum dosage of both types of agents. The success of immunotherapy in advanced disease has led to investigation of its value as an adjuvant treatment.

Immunotherapy differs in its mode of action from conventional chemotherapy in several ways. A response may take a long time to develop, particularly with interferons, in keeping with the time course of cellular immunity. Kirkwood describes a remarkable case of metastatic melanoma where despite initial progression of disease, continuation of IFN-α led eventually to a durable complete response.[2] A corollary to this observation is that stable disease may exist for a long period as modulated host immunity holds tumour in immunological check. Stable disease may not count towards better results, but for the patient, may provide valuable palliation with minimal toxicity. Similarly, the demonstration of durable complete responses as opposed to the short term complete responses seen in conventional chemotherapy, intuitively reflects the power of enhanced host immunity. The use of immunotherapy as adjuvant treatment reflects an expectation of advantage against small volume disease.

Much of the following discussion will concern metastatic melanoma. This tumour is a good candidate for immunotherapy for many reasons. There is currently no standard treatment for metastatic melanoma,[3] an increasingly common condition.[4] Melanoma is intrinsically immunogenic: spontaneous remissions are well documented and there is much in vitro data documenting the incidence of specific host anti-tumour responses following immune modulation in patients responding to immunotherapy. It is thus a logical treatment strategy to enhance intrinsic immunogenicity.

Differences in the inherent immunogenicity of some tumours has several drawbacks for the investigator. Variability within a patient sample and thus unrandomised data are difficult to interpret but because of the experimental nature of new modalities, randomisation is often inappropriate or not feasible. Immunological heterogeneity will also occur within the tumour itself. A differential response between primary tumour and metastasis is well documented and probably reflects clonal variation within the tumour. This clonal variation is demonstrated by recent data which suggests expansion of differing yet specific cytotoxic T cell clones in different tumour sites.[5] Thus a mixed response to treatment, that is, response in some sites but progressive disease in others, is a common observation amongst our patients treated with chemoimmunotherapy.

The following chapter describes the experimental and clinical development of biological response modifiers for melanoma, followed by a brief appraisal of immunotherapy as an adjuvant for metastatic melanoma.

Interferon in metastatic melanoma

A large body of experimental data demonstrate the biological activity of interferons (IFN) and their efficacy in animal tumour models[1]. The main potential advantages of interferons include their antiproliferative activity, ability to stimulate natural killer (NK) cell and cytotoxic T-lymphocytes (CTL) and their ability to up-regulate cell surface antigens on tumour in vitro, in particular major histocompatability complex (MHC) I and II (Fig 1). These molecules are responsible for the presentation of tumour antigen on the cell surface: in association with MHCI on antigen presenting cells and MHCII on tumour cells. Boon has elegantly demonstrated the loss of expression of MHC on spontaneous human tumours, rendering them less able to present tumour antigen for recognition.[6] A reversal of this

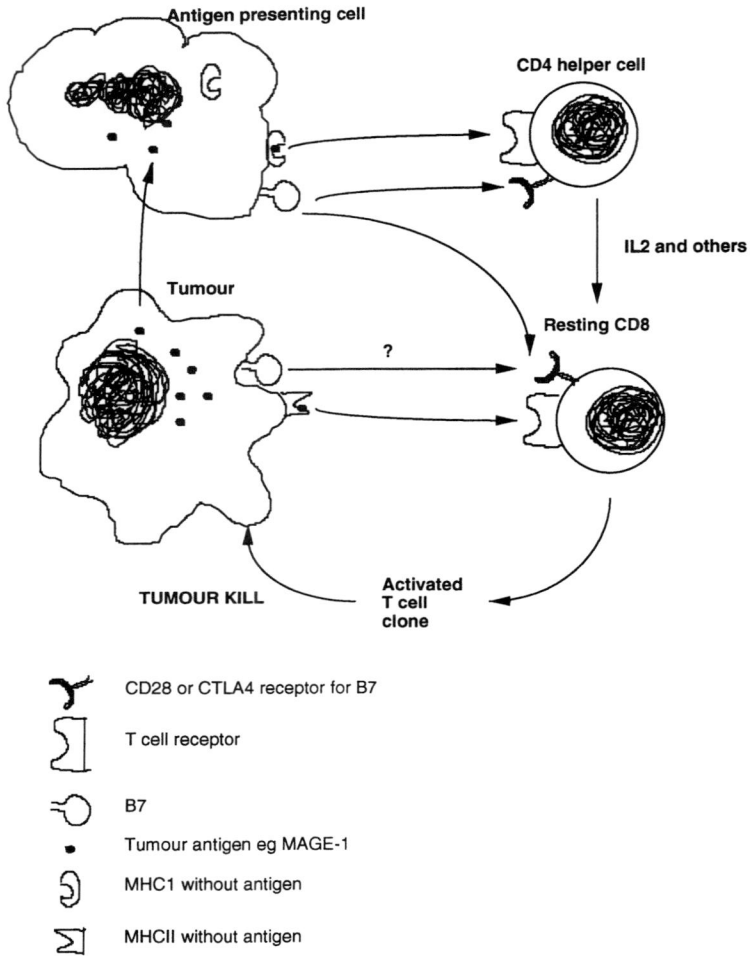

Fig. 1 Cell mediated tumour immunity. Tumour antigen, for instance MAGE-1, is released and is taken up by the antigen presenting cell. Antigen is processed and presented to T-helper and resting cytotoxic T-cells, a stimulus that is relatively specific for antigen and T-cell, and requires the co-stimulatory cell surface molecule B7 to avoid anergy. In the presence of IL-2 and other lymphokines, probably IL-4 and IL-12m cytotoxic T cells are activated and recognise antigen presented by the tumour cell by MHCII. Points of intervention includ enhancement of MHC, B7 or antigen, stimulation with cytokines or the piecemeal replacement of antigen presenting cells or lymphocytes.

anergy may allow antigen presentation and recognition of tumour as foreign. Numerous murine models have demonstrated regression of tumour following exogenous administration of IFN. More recently, the transduction of tumour cells with IFN-γ[7] has been used as a strategy to confer immunogenicity in animal models as a tumour vaccine.

Early human trials of interferon in metastatic melanoma (MM) used purified human interferon. Results were poor[8,9] probably because the extract used contained only 2% interferon and it was only with the development of recombinant interferons that efficacy was demonstrated (Table 1[10–20]). Overall response rates (OR) to interferon-α are approximately 16% in MM with 1 in 20 patients experiencing a durable complete response (CR). Good prognosis groups for response are similar to those for chemotherapy: good performance status, soft tissue, skin and lymph node disease. Toxicity was generally mild, the only grade III or greater toxicity being flu-like symptoms, leading to some dose modification in approximately 50% of all patients. Other common toxicities, grade II or less were leucopenia, derangement of liver function, gastrointestinal symptoms and pruritius. Schedules with intermittent administration[12] tend to be less successful than those with continuous administration[10]: most protocols have given treatment for 3 or more months.

Experience with IFN-γ has been disappointing[21] despite good in vitro data of increased MHCII expression and IL-2 activation.[7] Dosage of IFN-γ given to date has been arguably suboptimal, but overall response rates are 5% or less. In addition IFN-γ appeared to negate the documented IFN-α response when the two agents were given in parallel.[22] Studies with IFN-β have proven similarly disappointing, in particular when in combination with IFN-γ.[22] Phase I trials of other cytokines have not offered new opportunities: tumour

Table 1   Interferon alpha in metastatic melanoma

Investigator	IFN/dose/Schedule	Evaluable	CR/PR	OR (%)
Creagan (1984)[10]	Alpha-2a 12 MU/m^2/TIW	30	1/5	20
Creagan (1984)[11]	Alpha-2a 50 MU/m^2/TIW	31	3/4	23
Coates (1986)[12]	Alpha-2a 20 MU/m^2/OD	15	0/0	0
Hersey (1985)[13]	Alpha-2a 50 MU/m^3/TIW	18	1/1	11
Legha (1987)[14]	Alpha-2a 3–36 MU/m^2/OD-TIW	62	0/5	8
Elasser-Beile (1993)[15]	Alpha-2a 18 MU/m^2/OD-TIW	21	3/1	14
Steiner (1987)[16]	Alpha-2a 18 MU/m^2/OD	12	1/0	8
Kirkwood (1994)[2]	Alpha-2b 10–100 MU/m^2/OD	23	3/2	22
Dorval (1992)[17]	Alpha-2b 10 MU/m^2/TIW	22	2/4	27
Robinson (1986)[18]	Alpha-2b 30 MU/m^2/TIW	40	4/6	25
Sertoli (1989)[19]	Alpha-2b 10 MU/m^2/TIW	21	0/3	14
Mughal (1991)[20]	Alpha-2b 10 MU/m^2/TIW	51	4/6	20

necrosis factor[23,24] and IL-4[25] have performed poorly. Current prospects for IFN include combination with other cytokines and chemotherapy as well as a role in adjuvant disease (see below).

Interferon in combination with chemotherapy

There is little evidence that chemotherapy affects long term survival for MM, which remains at 6–9 months. Thus chemotherapy has been used primarily for palliation and more complex experimental programmes of treatment reserved for research institutions.[3] The most effective single agent chemotherapy for MM at present is dacarbazine (DTIC) with response rates between 15–25%.[3] There is evidence that combinations of chemotherapy with carmustine or platinum agents alter response rate,[26] but undoubtedly add to toxicity (*see* Thatcher this issue).

It was in an attempt to improve this dismal prognosis that IFN was introduced to chemotherapy. The toxicity profiles between IFN and chemotherapy differ thus both agents could be administered at greater dosages than would otherwise have been possible. IFN-α 2a and 2b were introduced into several programmes for MM in the late 1980's (Table 2[27–32]). Response rates were promising but the value of adding IFN required large randomised studies to evaluate fully any potential advantage. The variability between studies evident from the following description gives some indication of the inherent variability of melanoma.

Kirkwood and colleagues[27] combined conventional doses of both DTIC and IFN-α 2a and was randomised against DTIC alone and IFN-α 2a alone. Response rates were 23%, 24% and 4% respectively but the study was terminated prematurely for administrative reasons. The study size was small with only 24, 23 and 21 patients in the chemotherapy, IFN and combination arms respectively. The response rate for IFN alone was unusually poor and although there was no advantage shown for the combination, the small sample size makes these data difficult to interpret. A study from South Africa[29] used similar doses of DTIC and IFN-α 2b but in contrast showed a dramatic survival advantage for the combination group of 30 patients, documenting 12 CR and 4 partial response (PR) with an overall response rate of 53% against 20% for the DTIC arm alone. Again, the study numbers were small: 60 patients in total although patients were well matched for disease sites and performance status. Subsequently, larger randomised studies[31,30] have failed to show survival advantage for the DTIC/IFN combination, although there is an

Table 2   Interferon alpha and dacarbazine (DTIC) in metastatic melanoma

Investigator	Interferon/dose/ schedule	Dacarbazine	Evaluable	CR/ PR	OR (%)
Kirkwood (1990)[+ 27]	IFN alpha-2b 10 MU/m²/TIW	DTIC 250 mg/m²/DI-5 in 21d	21	4	19
McLeod (1990)[28]	IFN alpha-2a 3–9 MU/m²/OD	DTIC 200 mg/m²/21d	43	6/7	30
McLeod (1990)[28]	IFN alpha-2a 9 MU/m²/OD	DTIC 800 mg/m²/TIW in 21 d	76	6/14	26
	18 MU/m²/OD	As above	30	2/5	23
Falkson (1991)[+ 29]	IFN alpha-2b 10 MU/m²/TIW	DTIC 200 mg/m²/DI-5 in 28d	28	12/4	53
Thomson (1993)[+ 30]	IFN alpha-2a 9 MU/m²/OD-TIW	DTIC 800 mg/m²/21d	87	5/10	21
Bajetta (1994)[31]	IFN alpha-2a 3 MU/m²/TIW	DTIC 800 mg/m²/21d	84	6/13	23
	9 MU/m²/TIW	As above	76	6/15	28
ICG* (1992)[32]	IFN alph-2a 9–3 MU/m²/TIW	800 mg/m²/21D	79	6/19	25

[+] Randomised trials against DTIC alone: see text.
[*] Italian Cooperative group.

overall trend towards increased disease free survival. Toxicities tend to be greater for those treated with IFN but not more severe than grade II: most patients complete 70% or more of intended IFN dose.

Combinations of IFN with other chemotherapeutic and immunomodulatory agents have been disappointing. Cimetidine,[33] cyclophosphamide,[34] carmustine,[35] difluoromethylornithine,[36] and others have shown response rates of less than 10%. An exceptions has been the early study of Creagan using IFN and cimetidine (overall response rate 24%) although this was unrandomised data and does not seem significantly different from concurrent response rates to IFN alone. New treatment options were to involve combinations of IFN with interleukin-2 (IL-2) and chemotherapy.

Interleukin-2

As the role of IL2 in the generation of the cellular immune response was elucidated, ways of harnessing the important role of IL2 were devised. IL2 has many functions, the most central of which include the ability to stimulate natural killer cell and specific cytotoxic T cell expansion (Fig 1). NK or lymphokine activated killer (LAK) cell stimulation was linked to tumour eradication and cure in animal models, thus the first human trials of intravenous IL2 ran concurrently with those using LAK cells.[37] This involved extracorporeal expansion (with cytokines and other growth factors) of leukophoresed lymphocytes which were returned to the patient following IL2 administration in an attempt to enhance adoptive immunity.

These trials were performed by Steven Rosenberg and his unit at the National Institute of Health in the early 1980's. The results were reported initially in 1985 and had a dramatic impact for several reasons. High dose bolus IL2 was extremely toxic: there were 3 deaths secondary to treatment in Rosenberg's original group of 157 patients (all tumours), with hypotension requiring support in 123 of 180 courses and respiratory distress requiring intubation in 18 of 180 courses. Renal and hepatic toxicity was common but reversible, returning to normal 3–4 days after completing treatment. Cardiac toxicity was initially a problem: 2 of the 3 deaths were from myocardial infarction in the first year of the regimen. Subsequent patients were screened for cardiac disease and no further myocardial infarction or cardiac toxicity was encountered. Sepsis was common and responsible for 1 death. Septic episodes were found to be secondary to common organisms, related in part to indwelling central venous catheters[38] and early difficulties were resolved with the liberal use of antibiotics. There were no further septic deaths.

There were some dramatic individual responses to treatment including some complete responses in a group of patients with a mixed range of tumours, many of whom had been heavily pre-treated. The response rate for metastatic melanoma was 21% with LAK cells and 24% without, giving a combined response rate of 22% including 4 CR all of whom had received LAK cells. Durable CR was not a feature of IL-2 given alone, although responses to treatment were similar. In a recent review of the mature data from those patients treated with IL2 alone,[39] Rosenberg describes a 7% CR and 14% PR rate (OR 21%) in 134 patients with metastatic melanoma. Of the 9 patients (7%) with CR, 8 are alive without disease (9–91+ months) and one patient is alive with disease. Of note is that all of these patients had pulmonary, lymph node or cutaneous disease, known to be good prognostic indicators for response to treatment. Solitary central nervous system relapse was noted, suggesting that the CNS may be protected from immune modulation by this protocol.

Many centres subsequently undertook similar trials (Table 3[40-44] and 4[40-48]) to confirm this work and to determine the efficacy of a less toxic regimen of IL2 with or without LAK cells given as a continuous infusion (CI). Although the original study of West[48] suggested that CI was effective (50% OR), subsequent data suggested a lower response rate than that of bolus treatment of between 10-15%, despite experimental data that continuous infusion achieved similar immune modulation to high dose administration.[49]

Table 3   IL2: infusional and bolus

Investigator	Dose and schedule	Eval	CR/PR	OR (%)
Rosenberg (1989)[40]	600,000 IU/kg TID D1–5, 14–18	42	0/10	24
Parkinson (1990)[41]	600,000 IU/kg TID D1–5, 15–19	46	2/8	21
Whitehead (1991)[42]	36 MU/m^2/day CI D1, 3, 5, weekly	46	0/4	9
Mitchell (1988)[43]	21.6 MU/m^2/day CI D4–9, 12–16	27	1/5	23
Dorval (1992)[17]	20 MU/D1–5, 5–8, 29–31 CI Then monthly until relapse	24	0/8	33
Vlasveld (1994)*[44]	1.8 MU/m^2/day D1–5, 12–6 Short infusion	15	0/0	0

* As outpatient.

Table 4   IL2 and LAK cells for metastatic melanoma

Investigator	IL2 Dose/schedule	LAK dose schedule	Eval	CR/PR	OR (%)
Rosenberg (1989)[40]	600,000 IU/kg TID D1–5, 11–15	7.5×10^{10} D12, 13, 15	48	4/6	21
Dutcher (1989)[45]	600,000 IU/kg TID D1–5, 12–16	8.9×10^{10} D12, 13, 15	32	1/5	17
Bar (1990)[46]	600,000 IU/kg TID D1–5 1800,000 IU/kg TID D9–15	8.3×10^{10} D9, 10, 12	50	1/6	14
Gaynor (1990)[47]	18–27 × 10^6 IU/m^2/day CI D1–5, 11–16	15×10^{10} D11, 12, 14	30	0/1	3
Dutcher (1989)[45]	18 × 10^6 IU/m^2/day CI	15×10^{10} D11, 12, 14	33	0/1	3
West (1987)[48]	6–42 × 10^6 IU/m^2/day CI D1–5, 10–15, 20–25		10	0/5	50

Data from trials using infused IL-2 without LAK cells show a similar activity (Table 3). Again, infused IL-2 seems less effective than bolus doses and there are a disappointingly small number of CR's with infused treatment. The absolute value of LAK cells is in doubt after the NIH published randomised data showing no advantage for a LAK group over an IL-2/LAK group[50] (Table 4). The clinical and experimental data for tumour infiltrating lymphocytes (TIL) are more convincing. In experimental systems, TIL have been shown to be 100 times more specific in their antitumour action than LAK[51] and there is some correlation with clinical activity[52]. Clinical trials give response rates in the range of that of LAK cells but absolute clinical efficacy of TIL has yet to be shown formally in a randomised study. Furthermore, TIL cell generation is laborious, expensive and time consuming, as well as incurring further morbidity through necessary tissue biopsy. Currently, the NIH are pursuing a programme using TIL genetically modified to produce TNF in order to enhance local toxicity of adoptive therapy.[53]

Interferon in combination with interleukin-2

There is good theoretical evidence why synergy might exist between IFN and IL-2: increased antigen presentation through IFN mediated MHC up-regulation may render tumour targets more susceptible to recognition by IL-2 stimulated lymphocytes. This was demonstrated in several tumour models at doses of cytokine lower than those expected for single agent efficacy thus the experimental precedents for synergy between 2 active agents in human malignancy were good.[54] The first human trials were encouraging (Table 5[40, 55-60]). Using a range of IFN and bolus IL-2 doses, an overall response rate of 33% was achieved,[40] and has prompted the introduction of a series of trials with an overall response rate between 5-30%. A phase III study randomised between bolus IL-2 and bolus IL-2 with IFN-α from the NIH was published as an interim analysis after the accrual of 85 patients.[57] There was no difference in response rate (6% OR), no CR's, no difference in response duration (10 months) and no survival advantage for the combination treatment. In addition toxicity was considerable, with 12 of the 85 patients not receiving full planned treatment. There were 3 deaths, probably cardiac in nature, and 15% of all patients had a rise in creatinine phosphokinase. The addition of IFN did not seem to add to toxicity apart from elevation in transaminase to 20 times normal, which occurred in one half of those receiving IFN. This trial was terminated prematurely as there was no significant response in the combined therapy arm. No expla-

Table 5   Interferon alpha and interleukin-2 in metastatic melanoma

Investigator	IFN dose/schedule	IL2 dose/schedule	Eval	CR/ PR	OR (%)
Lee (1989)[55]	IFN alpha-2a 5–10 MU/m^2/DI–28	3 MU/m^2/DI 1–4 TID bolus	16	1/3	25
Rosenberg (1989)[40]	3–6 MU/m^2/OD	1–4.5 MU/m^2/DI–5 TID bolus	39	3/10	33
Keilholz (1993)[56]	10 MU/m^2/D1–5	1–4 mg/m^2/D1–5	54	4/12	30
Sparano (1993)*[57]	3 MU/m^2/D1–5, 15–19 TID bolus	6 MU/m^2/D1–5, 15–19 TID bolus	41	0/4	10
		As above	44	0/2	5
Atzpodien (1991)[58]	IFN alpha-2b 5 MU/m^2/TIw	9 MU/m^2/BID SC D1–5 then 1.8 MU/m^2/D1–5 each week for 6 weeks	7	0/0	0
Sznol (1993)*[59]	IFN alpha-2a 12 MU/m^2/TIW	3–6 MU/m^2 D0–5, 11–16	40	0/8	20
Whitehead (1993)[60]	IFN alpha 6 MU/m^2/BIW	21 MU/m^2 D1–4, 8–12, 15–8, 22–5	14	0/0 0	

* LAK cells and immunomodulatory cyclophosphamide and doxorubicin given.

nation was evident for the discrepancy between results for bolus IL-2 from this study and those previously achieved by Rosenberg using a very similar protocol.

The predominantly European experience with subcutaneous IL2 in combination with IFN, has been disappointing for MM.[58,61] Most of these regimes were given as outpatient protocols and were well tolerated, however responses have been very few. This is despite clear changes amongst treated patients of recognised immunological parameters such as CD56+ cell numbers, and synergy between IL2 and IFN.[54] Combination of IL2 with TNF, and other combinations have proven disappointing despite in vitro data for synergy.[59]

Interleukin-2 in combination with chemotherapy and interferon

Interleukin-2 has been used in combination with chemotherapy in an attempt to enhance response through synergistic effects. Several phase II trials (Table 6[62–65]) have demonstrated response rates of between 24–41%, although the data require confirmation in a randomised study.

The most recent series of chemoimmunotherapy trials have con-

Table 6   IL2 and chemotherapy in metastatic melanoma

Investigator	IL2 dose/schedule	Other agents	Eval	CR/ PR	OR (%)
Dillman (1990)*[62]	18 MU/m²/D1–5, 12–17, CI	DTIC 1200 mg/m²	27	2/5	26
Stoter (1991)[63]	18 MU/m²/D1–5, 12–17 CI	DTIC 850 mg/m²	25	2/4	24
Demchak (1991)[64]	600,000 U/kg/D1–5, 15–19 Bolus TID	Cisplatin 135–150 mg	27	3/7	37
Flaherty (1993)[65]	24 MU/m²/D12–16, 19–23 Short Infusion OD	Cisplatin 100 mg/m² DTIC 750 mg/m²	32	5/8	41

centrated on intensive regimes using more than one chemotherapeutic agent in addition to both IL-2, given mostly as an infusion, and subcutaneous IFN (Table 7[66–69]). Khayat et al in Paris[69] have used infusional IL-2 with pulsed cisplatin on the basis of the moderate single agent activity of cisplatin and its favourable toxicity profile. Patients were biased for sites of disease towards favourable response sites: skin, lymph node and lung, with only 13% of patients

Table 7   Interferon, interleukin-2 and chemotherapy for metastatic melanoma

Investigator	IL2/IFN/dose/ schedule	Other agents	Eval	CR/ PR	OR (%)
Legha (1993)[66]	IL2 9 MU/m²/D6–10, 17–20, CI IFN alpha 5 MU/D6–10, 17–21	DTIC 800 mg/m² P 20 mg/m²/D2–5 VB 1.6 mg/m²/D1–5	30	6/12	57
Richards (1992)[67]	IL2 1.5–3.9 MU/m²/D4–8 TID IFN alpha 6 MU/m²/D4–8	BCNU 150 mg/m² P 25 mg/m²/D1–3, 22–25 DTIC 220 mg/m²/D1–3, 22–25 Tamoxifen 10 mg bd	42	10/14	57
Khayat (1993)[69]	IL2 18 MU/m²/ D3–6, 17–21 IFN alpha 9 MU/m²/TIW	P 100 mg/m²	39	5/16	54
Ron (1994)[68]	IL2 4.8 MU/m²/D1–5 SC IFN alpha-2a 6 MU/m²/TIW SC Weeks 5–11	CB 400 mg/m²/D1, 8 DTIC 750 mg/m²/D1, 8 Rapid infusions	16	0/6	37.5

BCNU = Carmustine, DTIC = Dacarbazine, CB = Carboplatin, P = Cisplatin having bone disease. Toxicity was most marked for IFN, and resulted in the most changes to regimen, only 42% of all IFN was given. This comprised thrombocytopenia and malaise: there were no life threatening toxicities. Interestingly, there was a borderline advantage for patients showing vitiligo during treatment, suggesting shared immunogenicity in antitumour immunity. The overall response rate was 54%, with 3 durable complete responders amongst 39 patients.

Richards et al.[67] employed the BCDT regime (BCNU, cisplatin, dacarbazine and tamoxifen) previously reported to have a response rate of 50% in MM[26] in combination with IL-2 and IFN. Chills and rigors were universal and overall toxicity was increased, but there was no sepsis or life threatening hypotension. Again autoimmune phenomena developed in several patients and in particular, vitiligo was associated with response to treatment (see later for discussion). The benefit of adding cytokines to chemotherapy requires confirmation with a randomised trial.

Monoclonal antibodies

Monoclonal antibody therapy for melanoma has been directed against molecules on the cell surface. The most widely used targets are the gangliosides, in particular, GD2 and GD3, and a series of phase I trials using anti-ganglioside monoclonal antibodies in metastatic melanoma are listed in Table 8.[70-74] These antibodies confer toxicity through eliciting a complement mediated cell lysis. Other antibodies have used a ricin chain attached to the Fc portion to confer cytotoxicity (XMMME-001-RTA). The overall response rate of studies involving monoclonal antibodies is less than 10%, but individual study sizes are small.

Toxicity can be considerable. The most commonly used antibodies are murine and a human anti-mouse antibody develops in most cases following the first cycle of treatment unless immunosuppression is

Table 8 Monoclonal antibodies in metastatic melanoma

Investigator	Therapy	Evaluable patients	CR	PR
Schroff (1987)[70]	Anti-mCSP	32	0	6(23%)
Houghton (1985)[71]	Anti-GD3	21	0	4(20%)
Bajorin (1992)[72]	Anti-GD3	8	0	0
Murray (1994)[73]	Anti-GD2	11	0	0
Selvaggi (1993)[74]	XOMAZYME-Mel*	9	0	0

* IgG2a murine monoclonal against antigens conjugated to Ricin-A.

simultaneously administered. The use of FAb fragments, human monoclonal antibodies[75] or the concomitant use of cyclosporine[76] may avert such complications. Anaphylaxis, with weight gain and oedema is common but transient. Dramatic hypertension is thought secondary to a tissue specific effect on adrenal tissue, releasing levels of adrenaline compatible with phaeochromocytoma.[70] Neurological symptoms, in particular pain and paraesthesaie, are likely to be secondary to the crossreactivity of anti-GD2 antibodies to antigens on peripheral nerves and were dose limiting toxicity in Murray's study.[73] Future prospects centre on the development of antibodies composed of mouse anti-antigen sequences in conjunction with human non-binding sequences through genetic recombination,[75] and the development of more tumour specific antibodies.

Adjuvant interferon

Following the poor record of adjuvant chemotherapy,[77] an adjuvant role for IFN in high risk melanoma has been investigated. High risk melanoma comprises deep primary lesions: greater than 1.5 mm in depth, resected locoregional nodal disease and in some studies, resected metastatic disease. Unrandomised trials are of no value: Table 9[78] details the randomised trials to date, most of which have

Table 9   Randomised trials of adjuvant interferon in high risk melanoma

Investigator (Trial group)	Interferon Dose/schedule	Duration	Evaluable	Stage
Meyskens (SWOG)	IFN gamma 0.2 mg/m²/TIW	1 year	133	I(> 1 mm), II
Kirkwood (ECOG 1684)	IFN alpha-2b 20 MU/m²/5 × weekly 4 weeks then 10 MU/m² TIW	1 year	287	T4 or N+
Kirkwood (ECOG 1690)	IFN alpha-2b 20 MU/m² 5 × weekly 4 weeks then 3 MU TIW	2 years	430	T4 or N+
Eggermont (EORTC 18871)	IFN alpha-2b	1 year	400	I(> 3 mm), II
Grob (FCG)	IFN alpha-2b 3 MU/TIW	18 months	440	I(1.5 mm), II
Creagan (NCCTG)	IFN alpha-2b 3 MU/m²/TIW	3 months	262	I(> 4 mm), II
Cascinelli (WHO16)	IFN alpha-2a 3 MU/TIW	3 years	426	II

completed recruitment in the past 3 years and have yet to reach publication stage. The data are not all mature but trends are present. Compliance to treatment has been poor: most patients studied are young and it is difficult to maintain a treatment for up to 3 years which can bring on malaise and fatigue in otherwise normal individuals. All the trials have randomised against an observation only arm following surgery.

The first ECOG (Eastern Cooperative Oncology Group) study (ECOG1684) has demonstrated a trend towards survival advantage for patients with resected loco-regional disease at preliminary analysis although final analysis has yet to be undertaken. However, this was at the expense of considerable toxicity during the induction phase and compliance was poor with the high dose of $10MU/m^2$ for 1 year being given. The current ECOG1690 study employs a lower dose of IFN for 2 years in an attempt to lessen withdrawal secondary to toxicity. Interim analyses of the study by the French Cooperative Group (FCG) have shown no significant difference. Creagan et al have shown a non-significant advantage for patients with resected locoregional lymph node metastasis but not stage I at interim analysis. Analysis of the WHO trial (in which only patients with resected locoregional lymph node metastasis were studied) at 2 years demonstrates a survival advantage for the treatment group, with 2 year survival of 46% versus 27% for the observation arm[78]. Subgroup analysis showed increased benefit for males above 50 years of age and females less than 50. Meyskens (South Western Oncology Group, SWOG) has preliminary data showing an adverse effect for IFN-γ but no other trials have investigated the adjuvant value of IFN-γ.

Overall the data suggest a survival benefit for those receiving interferon in the adjuvant setting. However many of the trials await final analysis. Furthermore interferon is a toxic therapy and use of interferon as an adjuvant cannot be justified outside a clinical trial. An observation arm must be intrinsic to such trials, indeed many feel it unethical not to compare any treatment against an observation only arm. Important questions include the value of a more intensive induction period and the duration of treatment.

Toxicity in immunotherapy

The toxicity of high dose IL-2 has already been described. Overall, toxicity from infection and cardiovascular complications has decreased with increasing experience of using IL-2 and with prophylactic measures such as antibiotics and vasopressors. Screening of patients for cardiovascular risk factors may avoid cardiac toxicity.

The use of less toxic regimes such as infusional IL-2 may decrease toxicity and some regimes are being administered in part as outpatient regimes. IL-2 toxicity is reversible on stopping treatment thus all regimes should concentrate on supporting the patient through the treatment with the least intervention and the maximum dose of treatment.

The main toxicities with interferon are malaise and thrombocytopenia. Malaise is the most dose limiting toxicity: in some studies less than 50% of total intended dose has been given because of withdrawal. Thrombocytopenia may be a problem when combined with cytotoxic agents, in particular, cisplatin and BCNU.[67] Autoimmune thrombocytopenia is discussed below. Overall, with increasing experience of using immunotherapy, toxicities have become manageable and treatment related death is rare.

Autoimmune phenomena in immunotherapy

Thrombocytopenia, thyroid disturbance and hypopigmentation are well described in immunotherapy. Thrombocytopenia[67] with the development of positive antibodies in the absence of administration of blood products has been described and may contribute to transient treatment related thrombocytopenia, particularly with IFN. Autoimmune thrombocytopenia, like hypothyroidism and hypopigmentation, may be permanent. Autoimmune thyroiditis develops in some 15% of patients receiving IL-2, typically presenting as hypothyroidism 8–10 weeks after initiating treatment.[79] Transient hyperthyroidism is common and abnormalities resolve spontaneously some 8–11 months following cessation of treatment. It is more common in those receiving IFN in addition to IL-2 and in those with a history of autoimmune disease. Although antithyroid antibodies develop, there is no clear relationship to response.

Hypopigmentation in immunotherapy suggests the development of immunity, cellular or humoral against melanocytes, which may coincide with the simultaneous development of a response of the tumour to treatment.[80,67] Candidates for common antigens include part of the tyrosinase complex and other recently detected cell surface targets.[81,82] Unlike thrombocytopenia and hypothyroidism, hypopigmentation, or melanoma associated hypopigmentation (MAH) is associated with an improved response to therapy.[80] It does not fully resemble vitiligo clinically and may be a pathologically distinct entity, determined by cellular rather than humoral mechanisms as are thought to exist for vitiligo.[88]

Experimental and clinical correlations in immunotherapy

Changes in lymphocyte subset populations with bolus, infused and subcutaneous IL-2 have been well documented. NK (CD56+) cell numbers increase with associated non-specific killing in all modalities.[49,54] There is however no tumour specific killing, and no correlation of CD56+ cell stimulation with response. Aebersold et al.[52] have shown correlation of TIL tumour specific killing with response, but although promising, it is difficult to be certain that this observation can be extrapolated from the highly artificial situation of an in vitro cytotoxic lymphocyte killing assay to the clinic. The data for a role of tumour specific cytotoxic T-cell clones derived from peripheral blood or tumour in tumour kill are more convincing, but such specific killer cells have yet to be used therapeutically.[5] Moreover, expansion of such cells, as for TIL, will be an extremely labour intensive and costly exercise and unlikely to become common clinical practice.

Response to treatment with chemoimmunotherapy has been correlated to performance status, number of disease sites, tumour load and the site of metastasis: patients with disease in visceral sites, bone and liver in particular, fare worse than those patients with skin, lymph node and pulmonary disease.[66,67,69,83] An intuitive immunological explanation exists for the failure of immunotherapy in patients with a larger tumour load. Immune suppression by tumour is well documented[84]: local production of immunosuppressive cytokines is thought to play a major role.[85] It follows that the greater tumour load indicates increased immunosuppression and thus less likelihood of success with immunotherapy. No correlation has been observed with age, site of primary, depth of primary, previous treatment and response to previous treatment, thus there is no specific contraindication to immunotherapy for the older patient who has failed first line treatment.

Future directions in immunotherapy

A major concern still surrounds the poor therapeutic index of cytokines in systemic treatment. Strategies to overcome this include local production of cytokine, as in tumour vaccine protocols,[7] or the reduction of toxicity, in particular, IL-2 toxicity.[86] Much of this toxicity is thought to be secondary to production of TNF[87] and possibly IL-1. Strategies involving the use of anti-TNF antibodies, competitive inhibition of IL-1 and dexamethasone to counteract TNF induced shock have been demonstrated experimentally. IL-4 has been shown in vitro to define a more specific cytotoxic lymphocyte through its synergistic action with IL-2 and stimulation of macrophage stimulating factor. Prospective use in synergy with IL-2 may yield significant advantages.

The definition and mass production of a more specific anti-tumour lymphocyte as a means of focusing adoptive therapy is being investigated.[5] The NIH protocol to develop TIL that secrete TNF locally will also aim to increase the local rather than systemic toxicity in an attempt to overcome systemic toxicity.[53]

CONCLUSION

There has been a resurgence of interest in immunotherapy with the advent of powerful new techniques in molecular immunology. However, dramatic successes where conventional treatment has failed tend to be individual cases rather than the rule: the overall response to treatment is still poor and often associated with severe toxicity. In addition, there is little effect on overall long term survival, and systemic chemoimmunotherapy for MM must remain a research based treatment. Experience with the use of IL-2 has improved the therapeutic index but there is much progress to be made.

Critical questions concerning the value of immunotherapy have not been answered. In particular, there is no randomised study demonstrating the absolute value of IL-2 in addition to chemotherapy alone in response rate or overall survival. In addition, there are no randomised data demonstrating the absolute value of adoptive therapy. Adjuvant therapy using IFN is being addressed and there are promising early data.

KEY POINTS FOR CLINICAL PRACTICE

- There is no standard immunotherapy for metastatic melanoma. All treatments should be undertaken in a specialist centre as part of a clinical trial.
- Toxicity from immunotherapy can be life threatening although increased experience has led to controllable and acceptable morbidity.
- More recent schedules, for instance, those using subcutaneous and infusional administration of cytokine, are associated with both a reduction in toxicity and response rate.
- Data suggest that response relates only to performance status and disease site, although randomised data are limited. Thus age, prior

therapy and previous lack of response are not contraindications for further treatment.

• Early data suggest that IFN may be useful in an adjuvant context and patients with fully resected but high risk stage I disease or fully resected locoregional nodal disease should be referred for randomisation into one of the many current trails.

ACKNOWLEDGEMENTS

JAB is a Cancer Research Campaign Clinical Research Fellow.

REFERENCES

1 Klein J. Immunolcgy, 1st edn. Oxford: Blackwell, 1990.
2 Kirkwood JM. The role of interferons in the therapy of melanoma. Immunol Ser 1994; 61: 239.
3 MacKie RM, Guerry-D. IV. Melanoma and other skin neoplasms: Editorial overview. Curr Opin Oncol 1993; 5.2: 353.
4 La-Vecchia C, Lucchini F, Negri E, Boyle P, Maisonneuve P, Levi, F. Trends of cancer mortality in Europe, 1955–1989: II, respiratory tract, bone, connective and soft tissue sarcomas, and skin. Eur J Cancer 1992; 28.2–3: 514.
5 Weidmann E, Elder EM, Trucco M, Lotze MT, Whiteside, TL. Usage of T-cell receptor V beta chain genes in fresh and cultured tumor-infiltrating lymphocytes from human melanoma. Int J Cancer 1993; 54.3: 383.
6 Boon T, Snick JV, Pel AV, Uyttenhove C, Marchand M. Immunogenic variants obtained by mutagenesis of mouse mastocytoma P815. II. T lymphocyte mediated cytolysis. J Exp Med 1980; 152: 1184.
7 Gansbacher B, Bannerji R, Daniels B, Zier K, Cronin K, Gilboa E. Retroviral vector mediated g-interferon gene transfer into tumour cells generates potent and long lasting antitumour immunity. Cancer Res 1990; 50: 7820.
8 Krown SE, Burk MW, Kirkwood JM, Kerr D, Morton DL, Oettgen HF. Human leukocyte (alpha) interferon in metastatic malignant melanoma: The American cancer society phase II Trial. Cancer Treat Rep 1984; 8.5: 723.
9 Retsas S. Adjuvant interferon in melanoma [letter]. Lancet 1994; 343.8911: 1498.
10 Creagan ET, Ahmann DL, Green SJ et al. Phase II study of low-dose recombinant leukocyte A interferon in disseminated malignant melanoma. J Clin Oncol 1984; 2.9: 1002.
11 Creagan ET, Ahmann DL, Green SJ et al. Phase II study of recombinant leukocyte A interferon (rIFN-alpha A) in disseminated malignant melanoma. Cancer 1984; 54.12: 2844.
12 Coates A, Rallings M, Hersey P, Swanson C. Phase-II study of recombinant alpha-2-interferon in advanced malignant melanoma. J Interferon Res 1986; 6.1: 1.
13 Hersey P, Hasic E, MacDonald M et al. Effects of recombinant leukocyte interferon (rIFN-alpha A) on tumour growth and immune responses in patients with metastatic melanoma. Br J Cancer 1985; 51.6: 815.
14 Legha SS, Papadopoulos NE, Plager C et al. Clinical evaluation of recombinant interferon alfa-2a (Roferon-A) in metastatic melanoma using two different schedules [published erratum appears in J Clin Oncol 1987 Nov;5(11):1858]. J Clin Oncol 1987; 5.8: 1240.
15 Elsasser-Beile U, von-Kleist S, Stahle W, Schurhammer-Fuhrmann C, Monting JS, Gallati H. Cytokine levels in whole blood cell cultures as parameters of the

cellular immunologic activity in patients with malignant melanoma and basal cell carcinoma. Cancer 1993; 71.1: 231.

16 Steiner A, Wolf C, Pehamberger H. Comparison of the effects of three different treatment regimens of recombinant interferons (r-IFN alpha, r-IFN gamma, and r-IFN alpha + cimetidine) in disseminated malignant melanoma. J Cancer Res Clin Oncol 1987; 113.5: 459.

17 Dorval T, Mathiot C, Chosidow O et al. IL-2 phase II trial in metastatic melanoma: analysis of clinical and immunological parameters. Biotechnol Ther 1992; 3.1-2: 63.

18 Robinson WA, Mughal TI, Thomas MR, Johnson M, Spiegel RJ. Treatment of metastatic malignant melanoma with recombinant interferon alpha 2. Immunobiology 1986; 172.3-5: 275.

19 Sertoli MR, Bernengo MG, Ardizzoni A et al. Phase II trial of recombinant alpha-2b interferon in the treatment of metastatic skin melanoma. Oncology 1989; 46.2: 96.

20 Mughal TI, Thomas MR, Robinson, WA. Role of recombinant alpha-interferon in the treatment of advanced cutaneous malignant melanoma. Oncology 1991; 48.5: 365.

21 Creagan ET, Ahmann DL, Long HJ, Frytak S, Sherwin SA, Chang, MN. Phase II study of recombinant interferon-gamma in patients with disseminated malignant melanoma. Cancer Treat Rep 1987; 71.9: 843.

22 Creagan ET, Loprinzi CL, Ahmann DL, Schaid DJ. A phase I-II trial of the combination of recombinant leukocyte A interferon and recombinant human interferon-gamma in patients with metastatic malignant melanoma. Cancer 1988; 62.12: 2472.

23 Creagan ET, Kovach JS, Moertel CG, Frytak S, Kvols LK. A phase I clinical trial of recombinant human tumor necrosis factor. Cancer 1988; 62.12: 2467.

24 Feldman ER, Creagan ET, Schaid DJ, Ahmann DL. Phase II trial of recombinant tumor necrosis factor in disseminated malignant melanoma. Am J Clin Oncol 1992; 15.3: 256.

25 Margolin K, Aronson FR, Sznol M et al. Phase II studies of recombinant human interleukin-4 in advanced renal cancer and malignant melanoma. J Immunother Emphasis Tumor Immunol 1994; 15.2: 147.

26 De-Pretre SA, Maurer LH, O'Donell J et al. Combina tion chemotherapy with cisplatin, carmustine, dacarbazine and tamoxicfen in metastatic melanoma. Cancer Treat Rep 1984; 68: 1403.

27 Kirkwood JM, Ernstoff MS, Guiliano A et al. Interferon alpha-2a and dacarbazine in melanoma. J Natl Cancer Inst 1990; 82: 1062.

28 McLeod GR, Thomson DB, Hersey P. Clinical evaluation of interferons in malignant melanoma. J Invest Dermatol 1990; 95.6(Suppl).

29 Falkson CI, Falkson G, Falkson HC. Improved results with the addition of interferon alfa-2b to dacarbazine in the treatment of patients with metastatic malignant melanoma. J Clin Oncol 1991; 9.8: 1403.

30 Thomson DB, Adena M, McLeod GR et al. Interferon-alpha 2a does not improve response or survival when combined with dacarbazine in metastatic malignant melanoma: results of a multi-institutional Australian randomized trial. Melanoma Res 1993; 3.2: 133.

31 Bajetta E, Di-Leo A, Zampino MG et al. Multicenter randomized trial of dacarbazine alone or in combination with two different doses and schedules of interferon alfa-2a in the treatment of advanced melanoma. J Clin Oncol 1994; 12.4: 806.

32 Italian C, Group. Phase II study of interferon alfa-2a and dacarbazine in advanced melanoma. Biological Response Modifiers in Melanoma (BREMIM) Italian Cooperative Group. Eur J Cancer 1992; 28A.held: 1719.

33 Creagan ET, Ahmann DL, Green SJ, Long HJ, Frytak S, Itri, LM. Phase II study of recombinant leukocyte A interferon (IFN-rA) plus cimetidine in disseminated malignant melanoma. J Clin Oncol 1985; 3.7: 977.

34 Wadler S, Einzig AI, Dutcher JP, Ciobanu N, Landau L, Wiernik PH. Phase

II trial of recombinant alpha-2b-interferon and low-dose cyclophosphamide in advanced melanoma and renal cell carcinoma. Am J Clin Oncol 1988; 11.1: 55.

35 Creagan ET, Kovach JS, Long HJ, Richardson, RL. Phase I study of recombinant leukocyte A human interferon combined with BCNU in selected patients with advanced cancer. J Clin Oncol 1986; 4.3: 408.

36 Creagan ET, Long HJ, Ahmann DL, Schaid DJ. Phase II assessment of recombinant leukocyte A interferon with difluoromethylornithine in disseminated malignant melanoma. Am J Clin Oncol 1990; 13.3: 218.

37 Rosenberg SA, Lotze MT, Yang JC et al. Combination therapy with interleukin-2 and alpha-interferon for the treatment of patients with advanced cancer. J Clin Oncol 1989; 7.12: 1863.

38 Vlasveld LT, Rodenhuis S, Rutgers EJ et al. Catheter-related complications in 52 patients treated with continuous infusion of low dose recombinant interleukin-2 via an implanted central venous catheter. Eur J Surg Oncol 1994; 20.2: 122.

39 Rosenberg SA, Yang JC, Topalian SL et al. Treatment of 283 consecutive patients with metastatic melanoma or renal cell cancer using high-dose bolus interleukin 2 [see comments]. JAMA 1994; 271.12: 907.

40 Rosenberg SA, Lotze MT, Yang JC et al. Combination therapy with interleukin-2 and alpha-interferon for the treatment of patients with advanced cancer. J Clin Oncol 1989; 7: 1863.

41 Parkinson DR, Abrams JS, Wiernik PH et al. Interleukin-2 therapy in patients with metastatic malignant melanoma: a phase II study. J Clin Oncol 1990; 8.10: 1650.

42 Whitehead RP, Kopecky KJ, Samson MK et al. Phase II study of intravenous bolus recombinant interleukin-2 in advanced malignant melanoma: Southwest Oncology Group study. J Natl Cancer Inst 1991; 83.17: 1250.

43 Mitchell MS, Kempf RA, Harel W et al. Effectiveness and tolerability of low-dose cyclophosphamide and low-dose intravenous interleukin-2 in disseminated melanoma [corrected] [published erratum appears in J Clin Oncol 1988 Jun;6(6):1067]. J Clin Oncol 1988; 6.3: 409.

44 Vlasveld LT, Horenblas S, Hekman A et al. Phase II study of intermittent continuous infusion of low-dose recombinant interleukin-2 in advanced melanoma and renal cell cancer. Ann Oncol 1994; 5.2: 179.

45 Dutcher JP, Creekmore S, Weiss GR et al. A phase II study of interleukin-2 and lymphokine-activated killer cells in patients with metastatic malignant melanoma. J Clin Oncol 1989; 7.4: 477.

46 Bar MH, Sznol M, Atkins MB et al. Metastatic malignant melanoma treated with combined bolus and continuous infusion interleukin-2 and lymphokine-activated killer cells [see comments]. J Clin Oncol 1990; 8.7: 1138.

47 Gaynor ER, Weiss GR, Margolin KA et al. Phase I study of high-dose continuous-infusion recombinant interleukin-2 and autologous lymphokine-activated killer cells in patients with metastatic or unresectable malignant melanoma and renal cell carcinoma. J Natl Cancer Inst 1990; 82.17: 1397.

48 West WH, Tauer KW, Yannelli JR et al. Constant-infusion recombinant interleukin-2 in adoptive immunotherapy of advanced cancer. N Engl J Med 1987; 316.15: 898.

49 Vlasveld LT, Hekman A, Vyth-Dreese FA et al. A phase I study of prolonged continuous infusion of low dose recombinant interleukin-2 in melanoma and renal cell cancer. Part II: Immunological aspects. Br J Cancer 1993; 68.3: 559.

50 Rosenberg SA, Lotze MT, Yang JC et al. Prospective randomized trial of high-dose interleukin-2 alone or in conjunction with lymphokine-activated killer cells for the treatment of patients with advanced cancer [published erratum appears in J Natl Cancer Inst 1993 Jul 7;85(13):1091]. J Natl Cancer Inst 1993; 85.8: 622.

51 Rosenberg SA, Packard BS, Aebersold PM et al. Use of tumor-infiltrating lymphocytes and interleukin-2 in the immunotherapy of patients with metastatic melanoma. A preliminary report [see comments]. N Engl J Med 1988; 319.25: 1676.

52 Aebersold P, Hyatt C, Johnson S et al. Lysis of autologous melanoma cells by tumor-infiltrating lymphocytes: association with clinical response. J Natl Cancer Inst 1991; 83.13: 932.

53 Rosenberg SA, Aebersold P, Cornetta K et al. Gene transfer into humans— immunotherapy of patients with advanced melanoma, using tumor-infiltrating lymphocytes modified by retroviral gene transduction [see comments]. N Engl J Med 1990; 323.9: 570.

54 Atzpodien J, Kirchner H, Korfer A et al. Expansion of peripheral blood natural killer cells correlates with clinical outcome in cancer patients receiving recombinant subcutaneous interleukin-2 and interferon-alpha-2. Tumour Biol 1993; 14.6: 354.

55 Lee KH, Talpaz M, Rothberg JM et al. Concomitant administration of recombinant human interleukin-2 and recombinant interferon alpha-2A in cancer patients: a phase I study. J Clin Oncol 1989; 7.11: 1726.

56 Keilholz U, Scheibenbogen C, Tilgen et al. Interferon-alpha and interleukin-2 in the treatment of metastatic melanoma. Comparison of two phase II trials. Cancer 1993; 72.2: 607.

57 Sparano JA, Fisher RI, Sunderland M et al. Randomized phase III trial of treatment with high-dose interleukin-2 either alone or in combination with interferon alfa-2a in patients with advanced melanoma. J Clin Oncol 1993; 11.10: 1969.

58 Atzpodien J, Kirchner, H. The out-patient use of recombinant human interleukin-2 and interferon alfa-2b in advanced malignancies. Eur J Cancer 1991; 27 Suppl 4.held: S88.

59 Sznol M, Thurn A, Aronson FR. Interleukin-2 in combination with other biological agents. In: Atkins MB, Meir JW, eds. Therapeutic applications of interleukin-2. New York: Dekker, 1993: 233.

60 Whitehead RP, Figlin R, Citron ML et al. A phase II trial of concomitant human interleukin-2 and interferon-alpha-2a in patients with disseminated malignant melanoma. J Immunother 1993; 13.2: 117.

61 Castello G, Comella P, Manzo T et al. Immunological and clinical effects of intramuscular rIFN alpha-2a and low dose subcutaneous rIL-2 in patients with advanced malignant melanoma. Melanoma Res 1993; 3.1: 43.

62 Dillman RO, Oldham RK, Barth NM et al. Recombinant interleukin-2 and adoptive immunotherapy alternated with dacarbazine therapy in melanoma: a National Biotherapy Study Group trial. J Natl Cancer Inst 1990; 82.16: 1345.

63 Stoter G, Aamdal S, Rodenhuis S et al. Sequential administration of recombinant human interleukin-2 and dacarbazine in metastatic melanoma: a multicenter phase II study. J Clin Oncol 1991; 9.9: 1687.

64 Demchak PA, Mier JW, Robert NJ et al. Interleukin-2 and high-dose cisplatin in patients with metastatic melanoma: a pilot study. J Clin Oncol 1991; 9.10: 1821.

65 Flaherty LE, Robinson W, Redman BG et al. A phase II study of dacarbazine and cisplatin in combination with outpatient administered interleukin-2 in metastatic malignant melanoma. Cancer 1993; 71.11: 3520.

66 Legha SS, Buzaid AC. Role of recombinant interleukin-2 in combination with interferon-alfa and chemotherapy in the treatment of advanced melanoma. Semin Oncol 1993; 20.6 Suppl 9: 27.

67 Richards JM, Mehta N, Ramming K, Skosey, P. Sequential chemoimmunotherapy in the treatment of metastatic melanoma. J Clin Oncol 1992; 10.8: 1338.

68 Ron IG, Mordish Y, Eisenthal A, Skornick Y, Inbar MJ, Chaitchik S. A phase II study of combined administration of dacarbazine and carboplatin with home therapy of recombinant interleukin-2 and interferon-alpha 2a in patients with advanced malignant melanoma. Cancer Immunol Immunother 1994; 38.6: 379.

69 Khayat D, Borel C, Tourani JM et al. Sequential chemoimmunotherapy with cisplatin, interleukin-2, and interferon alfa-2a for metastatic melanoma. J Clin Oncol 1993; 11.11: 2173.

70 Schroff RW, Morgan A Jr, Woodhouse CS et al. Monoclonal antibody therapy

in malignant melanoma: factors effecting in vivo localization. J Biol Response Mod 1987; 6.4: 457.

71 Houghton AN, Mintzer D, Cordon-Cardo C et al. Mouse monoclonal IgG3 antibody detecting G(D3) ganglioside: A phase I trial in patients with malignant melanoma. Proc Natl Acad Sci USA 1985; 82.4: 1242.

72 Bajorin DF, Chapman PB, Wong GY et al. Treatment with high dose mouse monoclonal (anti-GD3) antibody R24 in patients with metastatic melanoma. Melanoma Res 1992; 2.5-6: 355.

73 Murray JL, Cunningham JE, Brewer H et al. Phase I trial of murine monoclonal antibody 14G2a administered by prolonged intravenous infusion in patients with neuroectodermal tumors. J Clin Oncol 1994; 12.1: 184.

74 Selvaggi K, Saria EA, Schwartz R et al. Phase I/II study of murine monoclonal antibody-ricin A chain (XOMAZYME-Mel) immunoconjugate plus cyclosporine A in patients with metastatic melanoma. J Immunother 1993; 13.3: 201.

75 Yeilding NM, Gerstner C, Kirkwood JM. Analysis of two monoclonal antibodies against melanoma. Int J Cancer 1992; 52.967-73 .

76 Ledermann J, A, Begent RHJ, Bagshawe KD et al. Repeated antitumour antibody therapy in man with supression of the host response by cyclosporin A. Br J Cancer 1988; 58: 654.

77 Aapro MS. Advances in systemic treatment of malignant melanoma. Eur J Cancer 1993; 28A.held: 613.

78 Cascinelli N, Bufalino R, Morabito A, Mackie R. Results of adjuvant interferon study in WHO melanoma programme [letter]. Lancet 1994; 343.8902: 913.

79 Kruit WHJ, BR, Goey SH, Jansen RLH et al. Interleukin-2-induced thyroid dysfunction is correlated with treatment duration but not with tumour response. J Clin Oncol 1993; 11: 921.

80 Duhra P, IA. Prolonged survival in metastatic malignant melanoma associated with vitiligo. Clin Exp Dermatol 1991; 16: 303.

81 Brichard V, Van-Pel A, Wolfel T et al. The tyrosinase gene codes for an antigen recognized by autologous cytolytic T lymphocytes on HLA-A2 melanomas. J Exp Med 1993; 178.2: 489.

82 Anichini A, MC, Mortarini R, Salvi S et al. Melanoma cells and normal melanocytes share antigens recognised by HLA-A2 restricted cytotoxic T cell clones from melanoma patients. J Exp Med 1993; 177: 989.

83 Jones M, Philip T, von der Masse H et al. The impact of interleukin-2 on survival in renal cancer: a multivariate analysis. Cancer Biother 1993; 8: 275.

84 Vose M, Moore M et al. Suppressor activity of lymphocytes infiltrating human lung and breast tumours. Int J Cancer 1979; 24: 579.

85 de-Waal-Malefyt R, YH, Roncarlo M-G, Spits H, de Vries J. Interleukin 10. Curr Opin Immunol 1992; 4: 314.

86 Meir JW. Abrogation of IL-2 toxicity. In: Atkins MB, Meir JW, eds. Therapeutic applications of Interleukin-2. New York: Dekker, 1993: 455.

87 Economou JS, Hoban M, Lee JD et al. Production of tumor necrosis factor alpha and interferon gamma in interleukin-2-treated melanoma patients: correlation with clinical toxicity. Cancer Immunol Immunother 1991; 34.1: 49.

88 Salter J, Maclennan K, Bridgewater JA et al. The histopathological appearance of hypopigmentation following chemoimmunotherapy. Melanoma Res 1995; In press.

British Medical Bulletin 1995, Vol 51, No. 3 pp. 678–693
©The British Council 1995

Pathology of ocular melanomas

A C E McCartney

Ophthalmic Pathology, UMDS, St Thomas' Hospital, London, UK

Primary ocular melanomas usually arise in the uvea, in the choroid and ciliary body. They metastasize primarily and initially exclusively, to the liver. Metastasis and survival is determined by the maximum tumour dimension, the number of epithelioid cells present within the tumour, vascular patterns within the tumour and nucleolar size and activity. Ganglioside and integrin profiles differ from cutaneous melanomas.

Iris melanocytic lesions tend not to metastasize, most being naevi of varying degrees of aggressiveness which may cause glaucoma and corneal decompensation.

Conjunctival melanoma is a rare unilateral tumour arising either in primary acquired melanosis or *de novo* rather than within a naevus. Survival of the patient depends on the location of the tumour and the histological subtype. Tumours not arising in the bulbar or limbal conjunctiva have a much poorer prognosis as do eyelid (cutaneous) melanomas if they involve the lid margin.

Uveal melanomas are the commonest primary malignant tumour within the eye and they differ substantially in their incidence and biological behaviour from cutaneous melanoma. In the following sections some of the current controversies that surround these capricious tumours will be reviewed.

Malignant melanoma may affect the eye as a primary or secondary disease. Primary disease can arise in the skin of the lids, within the conjunctiva, which is also derived from surface ectoderm and from the pigmented uveal components, the iris, ciliary body and choroid. Metastatic cutaneous melanoma can also occur within the richly vascularised choroid and has occasionally been reported within the vitreous cavity.[1] Both primary and metastatic melanomas have been reported within the orbit, with blood borne spread from ocular or cutaneous lesions and direct spread from the conjunctiva, nose or sinuses.

Melanomas arise within the neural crest derived dendritic melanocytes. Retinal, iris and ciliary body pigment epithelial cells, the other melanin producing cells of the eye, which are derived from the neuroectodermal outpouching that forms the eye, form hyperplastic masses or tumours which are very rarely, if ever, malignant.[2] These tumours do not metastasise, in contrast to uveal malignant melanoma, which has a marked predilection for metastasis to the liver. Patients dying from disseminated disease always have liver metastases and the liver is almost invariably the first organ to be involved in metastatic spread.[3]

Uveal melanoma occurs in pale skinned populations and although reported, is very rare in blacks or Asians. Conjunctival melanoma also tends to occur in the same geographic and ethnic groupings but is a much less common disease. Melanoma of the eyelids which can have a poor prognosis,[4] particularly if it involves the lid margins,[5] is luckily rarer still.

NAEVI

Most of the melanocytic lesions in and around the eyes can be classified as naevi. These include skin naevi of usual and atypical types, iris naevi (found in 50% of adults),[6] and choroidal naevi and melanocytomas. In the conjunctiva, in addition to frank naevi, primary acquired melanosis may be benign or show varying degrees of atypia in the premalignant phase corresponding to skin conditions such as lentigo maligna. Malignant transformation of a previously benign naevoid lesion gives rise to some conjunctival melanomas but the majority arise either *de novo* or in the context of primary acquired melanosis with atypia.[7]

True iris melanomas do occur, but the majority of iris melanocytic lesions which are not freckles, appear to lack metastatic potential and have been classified as naevi. (Confusingly a condition causing glaucoma and corneal decompensation is known as the iris naevus syndrome, but there is no evidence of abnormality within the melanocytic lineage, the condition being caused by corneal epithelial ectopia or metaplasia.)

A subpopulation of iris melanocytic tumours can grow rapidly, invading the drainage angle and causing blindness as a result of glaucoma. On cytological grounds these have been defined as aggressive iris naevi[8] but other authors dispute these tumours' supposed lack of malignant potential, suggesting that it is the small size of these lesions that explains their apparent inability to metastasise.[9]

METASTASIS

The concept of critical mass, determined by tumour dimension, plus the ability of tumour cells to penetrate vessel walls and survive within the bloodstream are part of the complex cascade of cellular events that result in successful establishment of metastases. Some cellular events resulting in increasing malignant potential are governed by genetic events, which may arise as mutations, other transcriptional changes may echo events that occur in normal embryogenesis. In ocular melanomas the phenotype of the tumour cell may correspond to the degree of malignancy. In uveal melanomas the number of epithelioid cells within the tumour is one of the major factors that have been shown to influence prognosis using multivariate analysis.[10]

UVEAL MELANOMA

Unequivocally malignant lesions occur in all three parts of the uvea, but lesions arising in the choroid are commoner than those arising in the ciliary body and the incidence of true iris melanomas is low. There are cytogenetic differences between ciliary body and choroidal melanomas but these may be dependent on size and age of the tumour, rather than location, since ciliary body tumours tend to present later and be larger at presentation than choroidal melanomas. Non random mutations of several chromosomes have been reported in uveal melanomas but monosomy of chromosomes 3, and 8 is reported as more likely to occur in ciliary body melanomas than choroidal melanomas.[11] Bilateral tumours are very rare.[12]

Size of the tumour is one of the most important factors to determine and following clinical observations and when appropriate histopathologic confirmation, uveal melanomas can be described as small, if they are less than 10 mm in diameter and 3 mm thick; medium if they are 10–15 mm in diameter and 3–5 mm thick and large if they exceed 15 mm diameter and 5 mm thick.[13]

Cells in malignant melanomas have been classified, initially by Callender in 1931 (in choroidal tumours) into spindle and epithelioid cells. Tumours can have admixtures of these elements and are then referred to as mixed. Spindle cells are further subdivided into spindle A cells which are long with grooved nuclei and inconspicuous nucleoli whilst spindle **B** cells are plumper, with prominent nucleoli. Epithelioid cells are large, with more cytoplasm, large rounded nuclei and prominent large nucleoli. They usually have fewer intermediate filaments in their cytoplasm than the spindle cells. They resemble the primitive cells at the neural crest, whilst the spindle cells resemble migrating neural crest cells. Balloon cells can also be seen within ocular melanomas. These are vaculolated lipid-filled cells with rather inconspicuous nuclei and are thought to metabolically less active and therefore less prone to enter mitosis and metastasise, although metastases with balloon cells have been reported.

Benign choroidal naevi are thought to occur in about 3–10% of the adult white population but malignant transformation has only been predicted to occur in 0.02% of these cases per annum. Transformed naevi show persistent radial growth and elevation, being greater than 3 mm in depth and are associated with disturbances of the retinal pigment epithelium (RPE) and subretinal exudates. Deeply pigmented jet black naevi (melanocytomas) usually occur in the optic nerve head but can be present in the choroid. Since they have a tendency to become necrotic [13] and liberate pigment; occasionally they are clinically thought to be melanomas. Other lesions that may mimic primary uveal malignant melanoma are choroidal haemangiomas and secondary tumours, including metastatic cutaneous melanoma.

In contrast to cutaneous melanoma, the peak incidence of uveal melanoma occurs between 50 and 70 years of age, although a congenital case has been reported, as have isolated cases in children. Less than 4% cases occur before the age of 30. Sunlight appears to be less unequivocally tumourigenic as there is no clear evidence of a current parallel increase in cases, although a predisposition to sunburn does increase risk. There is an increased incidence in non brown-eyed, particularly blue-eyed persons, especially if they live below latitude N°40. Hereditary factors are largely unimportant, familial uveal melanoma being very rare,[14] although an increased incidence has been suspected in patients with neurofibromatosis and both ocular and oculodermal melanocytosis have been suggested as risk factors as well as xeroderma pigmentosum and the atypical mole syndrome.[13] The clinical features of ocular melanoma are covered elsewhere in this issue (*see* Hungerford).

PATHOLOGY OF EYELID MELANOMAS

Despite the eyelids' extensive exposure to actinic irradiation malignant melanomas of the lids comprise less than 1% of all malignant neoplasms of the lid. In common with other skin melanomas, *in situ* and invasive forms occur so that the lesions may be classified into lentigo maligna, pagetoid malignant melanoma and nodular malignant melanoma.

Lentigo maligna

This lesion is identical to that seen elsewhere in the skin with rare progression to invasive lentigo malignant melanoma with slow peripheral extension and habit of becoming depigmented.[15] 5 year survival rate is 89% and metastasis is rare.

Pagetoid malignant melanoma

Invasive growth in an *in situ* pagetoid melanoma tends to be much more rapid than within lentigo maligna, often occurring within a year of presentation. Increasing pigmentation, induration and loss of surface epidermis and frank ulceration can all occur. 70% of eyelid melanomas fall into this category but cure rates of up to 78% have been reported in a follow-up period of 7.4 years.[4] These tumours may metastasise.

Nodular malignant melanoma

Nodular melanoma has a much worse prognosis, particularly if it involves the eyelid margin. The lesions appear as smooth grey or blue-black nodules usually in the fourth and fifth decades and are twice as common in men as in women. Growth is rapid and although spindle cells and pleomorphic cells can be seen, in practice most of the highly aggressive tumours contain large numbers of anaplastic or epithelioid cells which may be arranged in alveolar groups. Invasion is extensive and the death rate at 5 years is 60%. The Clark criteria and Breslow methodology widely applied to cutaneous melanomas elsewhere have been applied but in practice the most reliable diagnostic criterion has been found to be thickness of the primary lesion and sex, with improved survival in female patients.[16]

CONJUNCTIVAL MELANOMAS

Conjunctival melanoma is a rare unilateral disease, 2% of all ocular malignancies; predominantly confined to the elderly, although occasionally seen in young women, appearing to be associated with pregnancy or use of the contraceptive pill where some have been shown to have oestrogen receptor associated protein present [17]. In a recent, large series of 256 cases, 5 year survival was 82.9% and 10 year 69.3%. Multivariate analysis, coupled to Cox proportional hazard modelling showed that survival largely depended on location of the tumours. Tumours confined to the bulbar conjunctiva had a much better prognosis than those in unfavourable sites, often concealed from easy viewing, such as within the lid conjunctiva, tucked into the fornices, at sites of embryological or epithelial diversity such as the plica, or caruncle and lid margin where skin meets conjunctiva. These types of collision zones are known to be more unstable elsewhere in the body and melanomas developing at such sites, as for example, the anal verge, also have a tendency to do poorly. In the case of conjunctival melanomas developing at these unfavourable sites the mortality was 2.2 times higher than in those tumours confined to the limbal or epi-bulbar conjunctiva.[7] Multifocal epibulbar tumours were however associated with a five-fold increase in mortality. Other factors that influenced survival were whether the tumours had a mixed spindle and epithelioid cell population rather than being composed purely of spindle cells and whether the tumour had entered the extensive conjunctival lymphatic system. Tumour thickness did influence survival, with tumours greater than four millimetres increasing the death rate significantly, but this effect was confined to the tumours in unfavourable sites and not seen in epibulbar tumours.

Conjunctival melanomas arise in three clinical contexts. These are in association with pre-existing naevi, *de novo* and within the pigmentation of the conjunctiva that is called primary acquired melanosis (PAM).

Conjunctival naevi

These lesions which cause extensive, clinical and histopathologic diagnostic confusion with malignant melanoma, are amongst the commonest lesions to be referred for specialist opinion. Naevi commonly develop in the first two decades of life and can show rapid phases of apparent growth and change during adolescence or during pregnancy. This is often due to accumulation of mucins within the epithelial downgrowths containing goblet cells that are a feature of these lesions. Accumulation of inspissated mucins produces cystic areas which are nodular and can increase in size rapidly thus creating alarm that there is a malignant transformation within the lesion. However, if malignancy does occur, which is extremely rare, this is often within much younger patients [18] than melanoma developing *de novo* or within the context of PAM plus atypia. Naevus plus PAM with atypia (see below) was seen in 5 of 256 cases.[16]

Primary acquired melanosis

Acquired pigmentation of the conjunctiva can be idiopathic and primary or occur secondary to a variety of endogenous causes. Melanin deposition can be seen in Addison's disease, chronic conjunctival infections or inflammation such as trachoma or vernal conjunctivitis or after radiation or chemical insult.

Exogenous pigment resembling melanin can be seen after use of epinephrine, in argyrosis and as a result of foreign bodies including kohl and mascara.[15]

Primary (idiopathic) acquired melanosis has been recognised as occurring in two forms. The majority of cases (83%), remain benign, do not progress to melanoma and show no signs of atypia on histology (PAM minus atypia or PAM-). The other 17% a small but significant number of cases, exhibit atypia (PAM plus atypia, PAM+) and it is these lesions that have the capability to progress to conjunctival melanoma. These lesions can be multifocal, and probably represent a field change within the conjunctival melanocytes. They can be very difficult to monitor if they are unpigmented (PAM+ sine pigmento) and such pale lesions carry a worsened prognosis due to problems with clinical surveillance.[19]

PAM+ has been seen in patients with xeroderma pigmentosum[20] and the link between PAM+, the congenital dysplastic naevus syndrome and the incidence of ocular melanomas has been studied.[21,22]

PAM plus and minus atypia and the progression to melanoma has been extensively covered in a trio of papers by Folberg and associates.[23-25]

Primary acquired melanosis with atypia is characterised by increased numbers of irregular polyhedral, spindle or epithelioid melanocytes arranged in nests on the junction, extending up into the epithelium or spreading in a pagetoid fashion. Ninety percent of lesions with such pagetoid spread are associated with subsequent frank melanoma with invasion and 75% of those with epithelioid cells.[24] Histologically the use of S100 and HMB-45 immunohistochemical markers, with red chromogens, can be extremely helpful as there is also often substantial active chronic inflammation at the base of the lesions and degrees of invasiveness can be much more easily assessed. Invasive amelanotic melanoma cells not easily recognised amongst macrophages can be seen using these two techniques and melanophages differentiated from tumour cells. Clinically it is impossible to distinguish between PAM with and without atypia and frequent biopsy may be indicated. This can lead to scarring and symblepharon and monitoring can also be achieved with impression cytology.[26] Progression to melanoma can proceed at a variable pace and the lesions have been described as waxing and waning as cycles of inflammation occur. The influence of hormones is also recognised as these lesions may grow during pregnancy and the menopause.[17] The whole conjunctiva should be regarded as potentially unstable once atypia has developed. The unilaterality of the condition is puzzling and has led to the concept that the PAM is the conjunctival equivalent of an atypical mole or dysplastic naevus on the skin.

Conjunctival melanosis in association with melanosis oculi

There is some debate as to whether the increased pigmentation in the naevus of Ota, involving the skin in the area served by the trigeminal nerve and concomitant increased pigmentation of the coats of the eye, is associated with increased risk of malignancy,[13] and no excess of conjunctival melanomas is reported although multiple choroidal tumours is.

IRIS MELANOMAS

As stated in the introduction there are authors who believe that the vast majority of iris melanocytic lesions are essentially benign whilst admitting that there is a subset which are unequivocally malignant. The iris can also be involved as a secondary phenomenon by extension from a ciliary body tumour. There is also a form of ring melanoma and a more diffuse form that has been designated as a 'tapioca melanoma'.

A small increase in incidence of malignant melanomas of the iris has been reported from Denmark, a country with a high proportion of pale skinned blue eyed people, which it was considered could be due to increased actinic exposure.[27] The incidence was increased compared to choroidal melanoma and of the 80 cases recorded over a 25 year period 8 had died. Half of these patients had ring melanomas and the other half tumours that invaded the ciliary body. Jakobiec and Silbert's review[8] of a large number of cases of iris melanocytic tumours showed that up to nine grades of tumour could be recognised. The first three categories were melanocytosis, melanocytomas and epithelioid cell naevi; the second group, grades 4 to 6, were naevi of spindled type with a variable surface plaque which slid along the surface of the iris anterior border and obstructed the angle through arcs of up to 360 degrees and categories 7 to 9 were unequivocal melanomas of spindled, mixed or epithelioid type. These melanomas appear to be less able to metastasise, although long periods of apparent cure, can be followed by metastasis, 30 years being the longest interval reported. Dedifferentiation of tumours after surgical biopsy or resection can occur[28], with increase of numbers of epithelioid cells on the surface of the iris and infiltration through surgical resection lines or drainage channels such as trabeculectomy sites which adversely affects survival.

Markers of cell proliferation, including PCNA antibody and AgNORS, (silver staining of nucleolar regions) can help to define more aggressive tumours.[29] Familial aggressive naevi have been reported.[30]

PATHOLOGY OF CHOROIDAL AND CILIARY BODY UVEAL MELANOMAS

The decision to enucleate an eye as treatment for a malignant melanoma may occur after a period of surveillance, particularly if the lesion is flat and under 5 mm in diameter. Many of these flat lesions are naevi developing in adult life and can be safely left alone. There has been considerable controversy as to whether enucleation itself increases the risk of metastasis[31] or whether it is that tumours that are enucleated have already reached a size where metastasis is inevitable. Sub-clinical metastasis can occur before the primary tumour is removed when there is no overt disease,[3] and may account for many of the deaths within the first 2 years. Although manipulation of tumours during surgery has been shown experimentally to result in tumour cells within the circulation, but if those cells lack the capability to be able to leave the circulation and establish new colonies, then embolisation alone is unlikely to cause metastasis.

Eyes enucleated for uveal melanoma contain tumours ranging from 5 mm to 23 mm in diameter (when they fill the globe) composed of variably necrotic tumour which can be pure white to jet black or any intermediate shade of grey or brown colour. Pigmentation can vary from one part of the tumour to another; often extraocular extensions of tumour differ from the main tumour. Unsurprisingly albino patients, who cannot manufacture melanin, have snow white tumours[32]. Diffuse spread of a melanoma throughout the uvea carries a poor prognosis[33] but should not be confused with the paraneoplastic syndrome of bilateral diffuse uveal melanocytic proliferation (BDUMPF) that may accompany intra-abdominal malignancy[34], especially ovarian carcinoma.

Risk factors for the development of uveal melanoma include pale eye colour, exposure to actinic rays and atypical naevi in the skin [35] as well as the oculodermal melanocytosis discussed above.

Macroscopic appearance

Malignant melanomas of the choroid and ciliary body vary in shape and although mushroom shaped and collar stud lesions are most commonly illustrated, most choroidal tumours are oval and only achieve the 'waisted' appearance when they rupture through the constraints of Bruch's membrane and come to spread out beneath the retina. The fluid beneath the detached retina is usually serous: it is rare for tumour cells to rupture through or spread within the retina or along the vitreous interface although common for there to be retinal degeneration following the disruption of the choriocapillaris and thereby the homeostatic maintenance of the retinal outer segments by the retinal pigment epithelium (RPE). Spontaneous haemorrhagic necrosis may occur within the tumour and lymphocytic infiltrates in tumours have been shown to contain large numbers of T cells.[36]

Factors that determine survival

Multivariate analysis of variables and collaborative pooling of data has enabled researchers to define the most useful parameters to measure. These are related to tumour size, cell-type. invasiveness and aggressivity.

The maximum tumour dimension (MTD) has been shown by such analysis to be much the most important factor determining prognosis. Tumours less than 7 mm in any direction carry a much reduced risk of death. Although most tumours are widest across the base, occasionally the height of the tumour will be greater than its width. Patients with tumours less than 1 cm^3 in volume have good chances of survival although ciliary body tumours of equivalent size to choroidal tumours are said to have a poorer prognosis[37]. Cytologic factors include nucleolar size and pleomorphism[38] are discussed below but the degree of local aggressiveness which determines whether the tumour cells have access to vascular beds other than the specialised choroidal circulation may be important. If a tumour gains access to the conjunctival lymphatics or vessels or if it enters the orbital circulation there is a greater potential for metastasis.

It is, therefore, imperative to examine the enucleated globes for

evidence of extraocular spread along scleral channels in the advent-
itia of nerves or emissary vessels or entry into conjunctival lymphatics
and to establish whether the tumour has entered the large vortex
veins that drain the choroid. Occasionally tumours spread directly
up the optic nerve or within its sheaths. This is especially true of
peripapillary tumours, occurring in 80% of these cases.[13] Many of
these tumours are extensively necrotic and will have caused mel-
anolytic secondary glaucoma by accumulation of pigment within the
cells of the trabecular meshwork at the angle.

Rupture of Bruch's membrane, by itself is not a prognostic feature,
but does allow for seeding into the vitreous.

Some tumours develop collagenases that not only enable the first
steps of metastasis to proceed by lysis of the basement membranes
of vessels but also allow for dissolution of the sclera and spread into
the orbit. Orbital extension occurs in 10–23% of cases and is almost
always associated with other poor prognostic features such as the
presence of epithelioid cells or a large tumour.[13]

The presence of tumour within the eye may render it shrunken or
phthisical. This usually occurs in the context of a very necrotic
tumour or one that has induced glaucoma. Melanomas within
phthisical eyes can metastasize and kill the patient without adjuvant
surgical dissemination of tumour cells. (Self portraits of Sir Joshua
Reynolds document his phthsical eye and when John Hunter performed Reynolds' autopsy he was able to demonstrate a liver full of
metastatic melanoma).

Detection of circulating melanoma cells has been reported in patients with both cutaneous and ocular melanomas, but the presence
of cells in the circulation does not necessarily imply that metastasis
will occur. The polymerase chain reaction is a sensitive technique
capable of detecting 10 cells in 5 ml of blood[39] but tyrosinase RNA,
the marker used in these studies has been detected in other tumours
such as leiomyosarcomas[40] and is not absolutely specific for melanocytes.

The process of metastasis of any tumour is a series of sequential,
linked steps involving neovascularisation, invasion, embolism, arrest
in the capillary bed of the target organ, adherence, extravasation
and proliferation with further angiogenesis.[41] In other malignancies,
for example carcinoma of the breast, metastasis from metastases
occurs, so that cerebral secondary tumours and intraocular metastatic tumours are rare in the absence of pre-existing lung second-
aries[42]. Similarly it may be that in the case of malignant melanoma
of the uvea, that specific integrins[43] are developed that actively
promote metastasis to the liver, the preferred target organ, and this

may explain the late development of metastases elsewhere, which occur after the development of metastatic tumour in the liver.

The primary melanoma sits in one of the most richly vascularised areas of the body and choroidal vessels are copiously fenestrated. It could be thought paradoxical that metastasis does not occur early in the course of the disease. One of the most interesting recent discoveries is that vascular patterns develop within melanomas that are dissimilar from both normal choroidal circulation and those present within naevi.[44] These tumour vessels have abnormal basement membranes which are multilaminated, thick and fragmented. Normal eyes or those containing naevi have straight and parallel patterns but 'closed' vascular loops were seen twice as often after angiogenesis in eyes with melanoma which had metastasised. These features were associated with other independent predictors such as epithelioid cells and increased mitotic activity.[45,46]

The metastatic potential of uveal melanoma may be considerably less than that of cutaneous melanomas. In addition to integrin ligand interactions, cell adhesion is also determined by the lipophilic gangliosides that modulate adhesion to extracellular matrix proteins. In contrast to cutaneous melanomas, where upregulation of GD2 and GD3 gangliosides is seen at the expense of GM3, in vertical growth phase and metastases, uveal melanomas exhibit ganglioside profiles almost identical to normal resting melanocytes.[47]

Work on integrins has also shown interesting differences between primary ocular melanomas and cell lines derived from them, and cutaneous melanomas and secondary deposits. β subunits on the $\alpha\beta$ heterodimeric part of vitronectin receptor appear to have the greatest potential for variation. In cutaneous melanomas the acquisition of the β_3 subunit is associated with vertical growth phase and lymph node metastasis, but it is rare for ocular primary melanomas to have this subunit.[43,48]

Histological features

Callender's modified classification[49] divided tumours into spindled and epithelioid, with subsequent descriptions of spindle A tumours, which appear to have a very low potential for metastasis, and are regarded by some authors as naevoid cells and spindle B tumours. Cells at the edges of spindle B tumours are often compressed against the relatively rigid sclera and may appear more flattened and like spindle A cells. Mixtures of cells can occur so that the proportions of cells should be assessed. This classification, although broadly useful, is capable of great intra and inter observer variability but histopathologic misdiagnosis of melanoma is rare.[50]

In order to assess actuarial survival patterns, various other cellular parameters have been assessed. The proportion of epithelioid cells and their absolute numbers are important predictors of almost equal weight in determining outcome to MTD on multivariate analysis.

Since mitoses may be infrequent, methods of assessing nucleolar activity are often used. These include measuring the standard deviation of the nucleolar area (SDNA) by using automated image analysis, a method which is time consuming and expensive, although an accurate predictor. A variant which involves measuring the mean of the largest nucleoli (MTLN) at a magnification of 2000[51-53] is cheap and effective. Silver staining for nucleolar organiser regions[54] has also been used in choroidal and ciliary body tumours.

In 7–10% of uveal melanomas the tumour may be so necrotic, it is impossible to determine any of its cellular characteristics. Necrosis can arise as a result of T cell mediated immunity or following infarction and ischaemia. Although a small amount of necrosis, especially with a heavy T cell infiltrate might be thought advantageous, in practice, patients with necrotic tumours often do poorly, the necrosis indicating that the tumour may be swift growing. Electron microscopy may clinch the diagnosis as melanosomes may be demonstrable.

Since the differential diagnosis of an unpigmented intraocular mass in an adult should include metastatic tumours, immunohistochemistry may be of use. Over 60% of intraocular melanomas will stain with antibodies to S100 protein, the melanoma associated HMB-45 can be useful, vimentin will stain intermediate filaments in almost all tumours and 'neurone-specific' enolase is present in about 40% of tumours. Since this marker demonstrates use of the glyolytic pathway, it is often present in necrotic tumours. Widespread cytokeratin positivity may indicate a metastatic carcinoma, but cytokeratins involved in the mechanics of cell cycling[55] will also be shown in melanomas and should not be interpreted as indicating carcinoma, although they may be highlighted in epithelioid cells.

Spread into the orbit worsens the prognosis, but transecting the tumour extension does not necessarily lead to increased mortality, since adjuvant radiotherapy can eliminate small residual deposits. Most melanomas of the orbit are secondary, following local spread from within the globe, extension through the orbital septum of a conjunctival melanoma or extension up the nasolacrimal duct following incomplete clearance of a conjunctival or primary melanoma of the nasal passages or sinuses. Primary melanomas do occur, however, within the lacrimal sac[56] and metastatic lesions from cutaneous or ocular melanomas can occur. (In one such case seen recently the contralateral eye had been removed 16 years before the patient presented with proptosis due to metastatic melanoma behind the remaining eye).

Such bizarre behaviour and degree of latency underlines the difficulty in predicting outcomes on an individual basis for patients with this group of neoplasms but calculations based on some of the factors discussed above may enable the pathologist to give the referring clinician some useful information that may indicate further treatment and the likelihood of metastatic spread.

REFERENCES

1 Bowman CB, Guber D, Brown CH 3rd, Curtin VT. Cutaneous malignant melanoma with diffuse intraocular metastases. Arch Ophthamol 1994; 112: 1213–1216.

2 McCartney ACE 1994 Intraocular epithelial tumors and cysts. In: Pathobiology of ocular disease; a dynamic approach. Klintworth GK, Garner A, eds. New York: Marcel Dekker, 1994, Chap 47, 1405–1421.

3 Wang MX, Shields JA, Donoso LA. Subclinical metastasis of uveal melanoma. Int Ophthalmol Clin 1993; 33: 119–127.

4 Garner A, Koorneef L, Levene A, Collin JRO. Malignant melanoma of the eyelid skin; histopathology and behaviour. Br J Ophthalmol 1985; 69: 180–186.

5 Robertson DM, Hungerford JL, McCartney ACE. Pigmentation of the eyelid margin accompanying conjunctival melanoma. Am J Ophthalmol 1989; 108: 435–436.

6 Michelson JB, Shields JA. Relationship of iris nevi to malignant melanoma of the iris. Am J Ophthalmol 1977; 83: 694–696.

7 Paridaens ADA, Minassian D, McCartney ACE, Hungerford JL. Prognostic factors in malignant melanoma of the conjunctiva; a clinicopathological study of 256 cases. Br J Ophthalmol 1994; 78: 252–259.

8 Jakobiec FA, Silbert G 1981 Are most iris‡ melanomas‡ really nevi? A clinicopathologic study of 189 lesions. Arch Ophthalmol 1981; 99: 2117–2132.

9 Kersten RC, Tse DT, Anderson R. Iris melanoma. Nevus or malignancy? Surv Ophthalmol 1985; 29: 423–433.

10 Paul EV, Parnell BL,Fraker M. Prognosis of malignant melanomas of the choroid and ciliary body. Int Ophthalmol Clin 1962; 2: 387–402.

11 Sisley K, Cottam DW, Rennie IG et al. Non random abnormalities of chromosomes 3, 6, and 8 associated with posterior uveal melanoma. Genes Chromosom Cancer 1992; 5: 197–200.

12 Egan KM, Seddon JM, Glynn RJ, Gragoudas ES, Albert DM. Epidemiological aspects of uveal melanoma. Surv Ophthalmol 1988; 32: 239–251.

13 Grossniklaus HE, Green WR. Uveal tumors. In: Klintworth GK, Garner A, eds. Pathobiology of ocular disease : A dynamic approach. New York: Marcel Dekker. 1994; Ch 48: 1423–1477.

14 Jay M, McCartney ACE. Familial malignant melanoma of the uvea and p53: a Victorian detective story. Surv Ophthalmol 1993; 37: 457–462.

15 Campbell RJ Tumors of eyelid, conjunctiva, and cornea. In: Klintworth GK, Garner A, eds. Pathobiology of Ocular Disease: A dynamic approach. New York: Marcel Dekker. 1994, Ch 46: 1367–1396.

16 American Joint Committee on Cancer. Staging of cancer at specific anatomic sites: Ophthalmic tumours. In: Bearhs OH, Henson DE, Hutter RVP, Myers MH, eds. Manual for staging cancer, 3rd Edn. Philadelphia: Lippincott, 1988: 213–248.
17 Paridaens DA, Alexander RA, Hungerford JL, McCartney ACE. Oestrogen receptors in conjunctival melanoma: immunocytochemical study using formalin fixed paraffin wax sections. J Clin Pathol 1991; 44: 840–843.
18 McDonnell JM, Carpenter JD, Jacobs P, Wan WL, Gilmore JE. Conjunctival melanocytic lesions in children. Ophthalmology 1989; 96: 986–993.
19 Paridaens ADA, McCartney ACE, Hungerford JL. Multifocal amelanotic melanoma and acquired melanosis sine pigmento. Br J Ophthalmol 1992; 76: 163–165.
20 Paridaens ADA, McCartney ACE, Hungerford JL. Premalignant melanosis of the conjunctiva and the cornea in xeroderma pigmentosum. Br J Ophthalmol 1992; 76: 120–122.
21 McCarthy JM, Rootman J, Horsman D, White VA. Conjunctival and uveal melanoma in the dysplastic nevus syndrome. Surv Ophthalmol 1993; 37: 377–386.
22 Bataille V, Pinney E, Hungerford JL, Cuzick J, Bishop DT, Newton JA. Five cases of co-existent primary ocular and cutaneous melanoma. Arch Dermatol 1993; 129: 198–201.
23 Folberg R, McLean IW, Zimmerman LE. Conjunctival melanosis and melanoma. Ophthalmology 1984; 91: 673–678.
24 Folberg R, McLean IW, Zimmerman LE. Malignant melanoma of the conjunctiva. Hum Pathol 1985; 16: 136–143.
25 Folberg R, McLean IW, Zimmerman LE. Primary acquired melanosis of the conjunctiva. Hum Pathol 1985; 16: 129–135.
26 Paridaens ADA, McCartney ACE, Curling OM, Lyons CJ, Hungerford JL. Impression cytology of conjunctival melanosis and melanoma. Br J Ophthalmol 1992; 76: 198–201.
27 Jensen OA. Malignant melanoma of the iris. A 25-year analysis of Danish cases. Eur J Ophthalmol 1993; 3: 181–188.
28 Bechrakis N, Lee WR. Dedifferentiation potential of iris melanomas. Fortschr Ophthalmol 1991; 88: 651–656.
29 Deuble K, McCartney ACE. Nucleolar organiser regions in iris melanocytic tumours: an accurate predictor? Eye 1990; 4: 743–750.
30 Paridaens D, Lyons CJ, McCartney A, Hungerford JL. Familial iris aggressive naevi in childhood. Arch Ophthalmol 1991; 109: 1552–1554.
31 Zimmerman LE, McLean IW, Foster WD. Does enucleation of the eye containing a malignant melanoma prevent or accelerate dissemination of tumour cells? Br J Ophthalmol 1978; 62: 420–425.
32 Casswell AG, McCartney ACE, Hungerford JL. Choroidal malignant melanoma in an albino. Br J Ophthalmol 1989; 73: 840–847.
33 Font RL, Spaulding AG, Zimmerman LE. Diffuse malignant melanoma of the uveal tract. Trans Am Acad Ophthalmol Otolaryngol 1968; 72: 877–894.
34 Rohrbach JM, Roggendorf W, Thanos S, Steuhl KP, Theil HJ. Simultaneous bilateral diffuse melanocytic uveal hyperplasia. Am J Ophthalmol 1990; 110: 249–256.
35 Holly EA, Aston DA, Char DH, Kristiansen JJ, Ahn DK. Uveal melanoma in relation to ultraviolet light exposure and host factors. Cancer Res 1990; 50: 5773–5777.
36 Tobal K, Deuble K, McCartney A, Lightman S. Characterisation of cellular infiltration in choroidal melanoma Melanoma Res 1993; 3: 63–65.
37 Lee WR. Intraocular tumours. In: Ophthalmic Histopathology. London: Springer-Verlag 1993; Ch 5: 97–126.
38 Sorensen FB, Gamel JW, Jensen OA, Ladekarl M, McCurdy J. Prognostic value of nucleolar size and pleomorphism in choroidal melanomas. APMIS 1993; 101: 358–368.
39 Tobral K, Sherman LS, Foss AJ, Lightman SL. Detection of melanocytes from uveal melanoma in peripheral blood using the polymerase chain reaction. Invest Ophthalmol Vis Sci 1993; 34: 2622–2625.

40 Battyani Z, Xerri L, Hassoun J, Bonerandi JJ, Grob JJ. Tyrosinase gene expression in human tissues. Pigment Cell Res 1993; 6: 400–405.
41 Fidler I. Cancer metastasis. In: Sikora K, Evan G, Watson JV, eds. The cancer cell. Br Med Bull 1991; 47: 157–177.
42 McCartney ACE. Intraocular metastasis (Editorial) Br J Ophthalmol 1993; 77: 133.
43 Marshall JF, Rutherford DC, McCartney ACE, Mitjans F, Goodman S, Hart IR. $\alpha v \beta 1$ is a receptor for vitronectin and fibrinogen and acts with $\alpha 5 \beta 1$ to mediate spreading on fibronectin. J Cell Sci 1995 (In press).
44 Rummelt V, Folberg R, Rummelt C et al. Microcirculation architecture of melanocytic nevi and melanomas of the ciliary body and choroid. A comparative histopathologic and ultrastructural study. Ophthalmology 1994; 101: 718–727.
45 Folberg R, Rummelt V, Parys-Van Ginderdeuren R et al. The prognostic value of tumor vessel morphology in primary uveal melanoma. Ophthalmology 1993; 100: 1389–1398.
46 Folberg R, Pe'er J, Gruman LM et al. The morphololologic characteristics of tumor blood vessels as a marker of tumor progression in primary human uveal melanoma: a matched case-control study. Hum Pathol 1992; 23: 1298–1305.
47 Kanda S, Cochran AJ, Lee WR, Morton DL, Irie RF. Variations in the ganglioside profile of uveal melanoma correlate with cytologic heterogeneity. Int J Cancer 1992; 52: 682–687.
48 ten Berge PJM, Daren EHJ, van Muijen GNP, Jager MJ, Ruiter DJ. Integrin expression i-unveal melanoma differs from cutaneous melanoma. Invest Ophthalmol Vis Sci 1993; 34: 3635–3640.
49 Callender GR. Malignant melanotic tumors of the eye. A study of histologic types in 111 cases. Trans Am Acad Ophthalmol 1964; 1667: 225–-238.
50 Anonymous. Accuracy of diagnosis of choroidal melanoma in the Collaborative Ocular Melanoma Study. COMS report no. Arch Ophthalmol 1990; 108: 1268–1273.
51 McCurdy J, Gamel J, McLean I. A simple, efficient, and reproducible method for estimating the malignant potential of uveal melanoma from routine H & E slides. Pathol Res Pract 1991; 187: 1025–1027.
52 Gamel JW, McCurdy JB, McLean IW. A comparison of prognostic covariates for uveal melanoma. Invest Ophthalmol Vis Sci 1992; 33: 1919–1922.
53 Gamel JW, McLean IW, McCurdy JB. Biologic distinctions between cure and time to death in 2892 patients with intraocular melanoma. Cancer 1993; 71: 2299–2305.
54 Marcus DM, Minkovitz JB, Wardwell SD, Albert DM. The value of nucleolar organiser regions in uveal melanoma. The Collaborative Ocular Melanoma Study Group. Am J Ophthalmol 1990; 110: 527–534.
55 Fuchs U, Kivela T, Summanen P, Immonen I, Tarkkanen A. An immunohistochemical and prognostic analysis of cytokeratin expression in malignant uveal melanoma. Am J Pathol 1992; 141: 169–-181.
56 Harry JH, Ashton N. The pathology of tumours of the lacrimal sac. Trans Ophthalmol Soc UK 1968; 88: 19–35.

British Medical Bulletin 1995, Vol 51, No. 3 pp. 694–716
©The British Council 1995

Management of ocular melanoma

J L Hungerford

Department of Ophthalmology, aint Bartholomew's Hospital and Moorfields Eye Hospital, London, UK

Most melanomas in the orbital region are primary tumours. The uveal tract is the commonest site though the skin of the eyelids, the conjunctiva and, very occasionally, the orbit itself may be involved. Direct spread may cause the tumour to present in an adjacent structure so that a uveal tract melanoma with an extrascleral nodule may appear to arise in the conjunctiva or in the orbit whilst a conjunctival melanoma may first be apparent in the adjacent eyelid skin. Metastatic deposits from cutaneous melanoma may occasionally present in the eye or ocular adnexa.[1]

MELANOMA OF THE UVEAL TRACT

The iris, ciliary body and choroid comprise the uveal tract which is the most frequent site of origin of primary melanoma in the orbital region. Uveal melanoma is the commonest primary intraocular tumour. Any age or racial group may be affected but the tumour occurs predominantly in white Caucasian adults with a peak incidence in late middle age. There are approximately 7 new cases per million each year.[2] Environmental factors have not been shown to play a part in the aetiology of uveal melanoma. In particular, sunlight exposure does not seem to predispose to the development of this tumour.[3] A Danish study demonstrated no overall increase in the incidence of uveal melanoma during a period in which cutaneous melanoma became 5 or 6 times commoner.[4] Host factors, however, play an important part in the development of this tumour in the uveal tract. Most uveal melanomas are thought to arise in pre-existing naevi which have been reported in up to 2% of eyes on clinical examination and 6.5% at autopsy, though the chance of malignant change has been estimated to be less than 1 in 500 during a 10-year period.[5] Uveal melanoma is strongly associated with oculodermal melanocytosis (naevus of Ota) and ocular melanocytosis[6]: annual ophthalmoscopic review under full mydriasis is recommended for individuals with either condition. Familial uveal melanomas have been reported.[7,8] Some of these and cases of bilateral uveal melanoma have been linked to the atypical mole syndrome (AMS)[8] in which there is an increased incidence of uveal naevi[9] as well as of dysplastic cutaneous moles. Ocular melanoma patients with a family history of ocular or cutaneous melanoma, with an excessive number of choroidal naevi or with bilateral uveal melanoma should be screened for the AMS.

The diagnosis of uveal melanoma is largely based on clinical criteria aided by non-invasive ancillary tests. Using this approach, specialists in ocular oncology can distinguish melanoma from simulating lesions with an accuracy approaching 98%.[10,11] Cases of doubt may be resolved by biopsy. Fine needle aspiration has become popular though the cytological results are much harder to interpret than those of a formal incisional biopsy. In general, the latter technique is preferred for accessible anterior tumours and the former for more posteriorly located lesions. There is a small risk of local extraocular extension and orbital recurrence after biopsy and, bearing in mind the accuracy of clinical diagnosis, a tissue diagnosis is sought in less than 5% of cases.

There is no evidence that survival rates are better following radical treatment by enucleation of the affected eye than after treatments which aim to conserve the eye and, pending the results of the formal prospective randomised Collaborative Ocular Melanoma ('COMS') Study underway in the United States, most uveal melanomas are now treated conservatively where possible. Good visual function may be retained after such treatments, especially of small melanomas. The technology of treating ocular melanoma is now such that most tumours are managed in specialist centres. Several treatment modalities are available, some more expensive than others. Although some centres tend to favour one treatment method over another, there is no single tecnhnique which is ideal for all tumours. In London, all treatment methods are available and efforts are made to tailor therapy to the clinical features of individual tumours. With experience of treating several thousand melanomas the selection criteria for one treatment method or another have been refined progressively, whilst at the same time bearing in mind considerations of cost-effectiveness and quality of life. Many small melanomas can be treated effectively by simple treatments using radioactive scleral plaques and do not require expensive treatments using charged particles which may have the additional disadvantage of severe side effects. Although charged particle therapy may have the capability of bringing about regression of very large uveal melanomas, useful vision is rarely retained in such cases and severe late effects may substantially impair quality of life. In London we have learned that it is rarely justified to treat very large and extensive melanomas conservatively and that there is still a role for primary enucleation. Many of the side effects of treating melanomas by radiation take several years to develop and we have reached this view point by a rigid policy of long-term follow-up. Nevertheless ours is a view which is not universally held and many very large melanomas are still treated conservatively, committing the patient to a high likelihood of disfiguring side effects and the disappointment of the ultimate loss of the eye. This point will have been reached after a long period of follow up during which doubts about tumour control makes many patients anxious and which would have been avoided had enucleation been chosen in the first place.

The treatment of choice for any particular melanoma depends mainly on the size of the tumour at presentation and on its site of origin within the eye. The precise watershed between tumours which can be managed conservatively and those which should be treated by enucleation is not well defined. Eyes which have a poor chance of being saved by conservative therapy are still treated and this is often justified by there being defective vision in the other eye. It should be borne in mind that the fact that the other eye has poor vision makes such an eye no more likely to be retained and that, most importantly, vision is rarely preserved even when conservative treatment allows an eye with a very large tumour to be retained. The visual status of the other eye should therefore be taken into account only when the affected eye is otherwise suitable for the conservative approach.

Uveal melanoma is life-threatening and carries a high mortality rate. Prognosis, too, depends substantially on whether or not a uveal melanoma is detected early and this in turn is dependent on location. Large tumour size is the most important clinical indicator of a poor life prognosis.[12] The tumour cell type is also highly predictive of outcome and the mortality rate is worse following treatment of tumours containing epithelioid cells than it is after that of spindle cell melanomas.[13,14] Clinical and histopathological features of uveal melanomas may not be independent predictors of outlook because large tumour volume is closely associated with epithelioid cell histology.[15] Moreover, although local extrascleral extension has an adverse influence on outcome, this feature too is closely associated with epithelioid cell histology[16] and multivariate analysis has not demonstrated that extrascleral spread has an independent adverse influence on survival rate.[17] In some series location within the uveal tract has a prognostic significance which appears to be independent of tumour size whereas in others correcting for size eliminates such differences. Small tumours in some locations appear to have a very good prognosis.and this is particularly so for melanomas of the iris. The low overall mortality rate of around 5% for iris melanomas may depend on the fact that they are clearly visible to the patient when very small and so are detected early in their evolution. Additionally or alternatively the good reputation of some iris melanomas may have been gained under false pretences because they are, in reality, not malignant. tumours. Iris melanomas, unlike their choroidal and ciliary body counterparts, are notable for containing few epithelioid cells and a preponderance of naevoid or spindle A cells of questionable malignancy.[18] In the iris the dividing line between benign and malignant is less distinct than elsewhere in the uveal tract[19] and this led one author to reclassify 87% of a group of iris melanocytic tumours, previously considered malignant, as benign tumours.[20] Recently, a group of spindle-cell iris tumours originally categorised as leiomyomas has been reclassified as melanocytic, further swelling the numbers of relatively benign iris lesions[21] though we know some 10% of iris melanomas which do contain epithelioid cells will metastasise even though they may be very small.[22]

Iris melanoma

Melanomas of the iris comprise 8% of malignant melanocytic tumours of the uveal tract. They are commoner in light-coloured than in dark irides.[23] Iris melanomas seem to be commoner in the inferior portion of the iris which is not covered by the upper eyelid suggesting that, in this location unlike others in the uveal tract, melanoma may be related to exposure to sunlight. Ultraviolet rays do not penetrate deeply into the eye but it is conceivable that they reach the exposed inferior iris. Being easily visible to the patient, iris melanomas tend to be detected at an earler age[24] and when smaller[25] than ciliary body and choroidal tumours. They may adopt a nodular or superficial spreading growth pattern so that they may be circumscibed or diffuse. They may be variably pigmented but tend to be relatively pale in colour. An iris melanoma is often very difficult to distinguish clinally from an iris naevus and ancillary tests, such as ultrasound and fluorescein angiography, are much less helpful in the categorisation of iris tumours than of those arising elsewhere in the uveal tract.[18] Malignant iris tumours tend to contain prominent and abnormal blood vessels. In pale melanomas these can be seen without the aid of fluorescein angiography and in darker tumours they are masked by pigment so that the test is helpful in only 50% of cases.[26] Large size, documented enlargement, nodular shape and distortion of the pupil have come to be regarded traditionally as indicators of malignancy in a pigmented iris tumour but may all be seen in benign naevi. Excision of an iris tumour produces a noticeable cosmetic defect as well as significant photophobia. Because of the good overall outlook, most small iris melanocytic tumours are managed by observation and only about 5% will be seen to grow in a 5-year period.[27] Tumours which grow are best excised if it is technically possible though many will be reported as benign naevi despite enlargement. Large, nodular tumours are best excised without waiting for evidence of growth. Tumours not involving the root of the iris may be removed by simple sector iridectomy but those extending to the drainage angle will require irido-trabeculectomy. Significant ciliary body involvement demands irido-cyclectomy. Diffuse melanomas involving more than one quadrant of the iris cannot be excised and should be managed by incisional biopsy followed promptly by enucleation if there is unequivocal evidence of malignancy.[28]

Ciliary body melanoma

Approximately 12% of uveal melanomas arise in the ciliary body. This structure is the most difficult part of the uveal tract to visualise ophthalmoscopically and melanomas in this location tend to remain occult until they disturb vision by growing across the visual axis or by invading the choroid to produce a retinal detachment. Alternatively they may become noticeable to the patient because of iris root involvement, sentinel blood vessels in the episclera, an extra-scleral nodule or pain from glaucoma. Because of their tendency towards late presentation, most ciliary body melanomas are large at diagnosis. Although large size at diagnosis undoubtedly contributes to the poor prognosis of ciliary body melanomas, anterior location has been reported to have an adverse effect on the survival rate which is independent of size.[14]

Ciliary body melanomas may be nodular or diffuse. Diffuse melanomas of the ciliary body are extremely difficult to diagnose until late in their evolution. These tumours tend to grow circumferentially around the eye, invading the trabecular meshwork and ultimately presenting with glaucoma. Even at this stage the diagnosis may be delayed for months because of difficulty establishing the cause of the glaucoma. This entity is described as ring melanoma. Ciliary body melanomas may be variably pigmented. The origin of ciliary body melanomas is interesting because naevi are said to be rare in this location. Perhaps they are commoner than we suppose but difficult to see.

Just as they are in the iris, ancillary diagnostic tests are relatively unhelpful in the ciliary body. Standard ophthalmic B-scan ultrasound machines resolve anterior tumours poorly and generally only larger tumours can be seen. New higher frequency ultrasound machines can detect small tumours but have a limited range in tissue. The microanatomical features which make ultrasound such an effective tool for distinguishing choroidal melanomas from other simulating lesions are not present in the ciliary body and this limits the capability of the test in elucidating the differential diagnosis. This is particularly important because there is a wider range of lesions simulating melanoma in the ciliary body than elsewhere in the uveal tract. The difficulties of establishing the diagnosis of melanoma in the ciliary body have an important bearing on management and in doubtful cases biopsy should be considered. If the lesion occupies less than one quadrant and does not extend behind the ora serrata, an excisional biopsy should be performed by cyclectomy or iridocyclectomy and may also serve as the definitive treatment. Larger lesions for which the diagnosis is in doubt should undergo incisional biopsy followed by active treatment if the tumour is a melanoma.

Cyclectomy

Cyclectomy is performed under a partial thickness scleral flap. It is technically straightforward but is commonly complicated by late retinal detachment. For this reason small, typical melanomas which do not require biopsy are best treated by radiation brachytherapy using a radioactive scleral applicator and the same technique more commonly applied to choroidal melanomas. Modern plaques are shielded on their outer suface and the eyelids and lacrimal apparatus are protected. A radiation cataract may supervene but may be removed and an intraocular lens prosthesis inserted with a good visual outcome. Proton beam radiotherapy results in unacceptable damage to the eyelids when used to treat anteriorly located melanomas. When the upper eyelid is in the full dose volume of proton treatment, in addition to poor cosmesis from lash loss and skin pallor, keratinisation of the lid margin ensues and leads to a painful keratitis. Proton therapy should not be used to treat ciliary body melanomas too large to manage by cyclectomy or plaque radiotherapy, particularly when they are located superiorly under the upper eyelid. Such tumours should be managed by enucleation. The same applies to any ciliary body melanoma which has produced a secondary glaucoma, even though it may appear to be localised, and to ring melanomas. Localised ciliary body melanomas with extrasceral extension are best managed by plaque therapy. Cyclectomy can be considered but the full thickness of involved sclera will need to be removed and replaced, preferably with a half thickness autograft from the same eye. It should be stressed that both plaque therapy and cyclectomy are contraindicated when a tumour with extrasceral extension is associated with glaucoma. If plaque therapy is attempted in the presence of raised pressure, the weakened sclera will bulge and the result will be a massive staphyloma. If cyclectomy is performed, the graft will dehisce.

Choroidal melanoma

Approximately 80% of melanomas in the uveal tract arise in the choroid. Small, asymptomatic tumours may be detected during routine sight testing whereas larger lesions may present with a disturbance of visual acuity or of the field of vision caused by the tumour itself or by an associated retinal detachment or vitreous haemorrhage. Most choroidal melanomas adopt a nodular growth pattern and the characteristic collar stud contour they develop as they rupture the Bruch's inner limiting membrane of the choroid, is an important feature assisting in the clinical diagnosis. Other types of tumour rarely have a collar stud contour. Melanomas tend to bleed into the vitreous as they breach Bruch's membrane. Occasionally, a choroidal melanoma will exhibit a diffuse pattern of growth with a pronounced tendency to extend extrasclerally.[29] Diffuse melanomas may involve a substantial part of the choroid. Choroidal melanomas of either growth pattern may be pigmented or amelanotic and some show variations of pigmentation within the same tumour. The shallow contour of some small melanomas and particularly that of diffuse melanomas can be difficult to distinguish from that of a solitary metastasis from an unsuspected primary cancer elsewhere. In this case the primary will most commonly be in the lung. Metastatic deposits from breast cancer can usually be distinguished from melanoma by the fact that they are frequently multiple and bilateral. The most helpful ancillary test is B-scan ultrasound which, as well as demonstrating the contour of the tumour better than ophthalmoscopy, may show low internal reflectivity and choroidal excavation characteristic of melanoma and not seen in other simulating lesions. If ultrasound, a search for a distant primary, or radioim-munoscintigraphy[30] are unhelpful, biopsy may be considered.

The maximum size of choroidal melanoma which is cureable is not known. Large tumours have a very poor outlook and many are probably incurable at diagnosis. On the other hand, small mela-nomas have a good life prognosis and, although lead time bias may contribute to this, there is a need to recognise them as soon as possible. Early detection of small melanomas is difficult because they are hard to distinguish clinically from choroidal naevi. Choroidal naevi are common and small, flat or nearly flat lesions can be ignored. Large and thick lesions are characterised as suspicious naevi and warrant follow up. They are generally too thin to be amenable to biopsy and the finding of intrinsic vasculature on fundus fluorescein angiography correctly predicts malignancy in less than 50% of cases.[31] Although radioimmunoscintigraphy can distinguish between melanocytic and non-melanocytic tumours, it cannot differentiate between a melanoma and a naevus.[32] One approach commonly adopted is to follow such tumours with serial fundus photographs and ultrasound measurements of size, looking for evidence of growth. Although some naevi may be seen to grow for a period, sustained growth is suggestive of malignancy. Tumour thickness of greater than 1.5 mm, presence of orange lipofuscin pigment on the surface of the tumour, and leakage of fluid under to retina to produce a serous retinal detachment are all predictive of malignancy[33] and small peripheral lesions demonstrating all three of these features are best treated urgently as small melanomas without waiting for documentary evidence of growth. Treatment of melanomas near the macula or optic disc may be associated with significant loss of vision and it may be better to document growth before treating suspicious lesions in these locations.

Enucleation still plays an important role in the management of eyes with large choroidal melanomas having a volume greater than 1.5 cubic centimetres, in eyes with glaucoma or extensive local extra-scleral extension, and in eyes in which conservative treatment has failed or has produced severe side effects. Unless there is pain or extrascleral spread, patients planned for enucleation should first undergo a metastatic evaluation including a chest X-ray and abdomi-nal ultrasound. Postoperative radiotherapy to the orbit is rec-ommended to reduce the incidence of local orbital recurrence when an eye with a nodular extrascleral exension has been removed.[34] Rarely, orbital exenteration may be needed for a neglected melanoma with massive extrascleral spread.

Conservative treatment may be considered for all other choroidal melanomas. A small posterior melanoma up to 3 mm thick, located outside the vascular arcades of the macula, not touching the edge of the optic disc, and without an overlying retinal detachment may be treated by direct xenon arc photocoagulation[35] when it is considered to be too close to the disc to avoid radiation optic neuropathy from plaque or proton therapy. Most choroidal melanomas, however, are treated by radiotherapy.

The relatively unusual approaches chosen for radiotherapy to ocular melanomas depend on the need to deliver a high dose of between 60 and 100 Gy to this relatively radioresistant tumour whilst at the same time, and if possible, keeping the dose to the adjacent retina, choroid and optic nerve below the 50 Gy tolerated by these structures. Radioactive plaques achieve these aims because their radiation is attenuated rapidly with increasing distance from the source. Their advantages in this respect are progressively lost with increasing tumour thickness. The size of melanoma which can be treated by plaque without serious side effects depends on the energy of the radiation source and the thickness of the tumour.[36] In the choroid, melanomas up to 5 mm thick can be treated by ruthenium-106/rhodium-106 plaques emitting beta rays[37] and tumours up to 8 mm thick by iodine-125 plaques emitting X-rays[38] (Fig. 1), in both instances employing a dose of 100 Gy to the apex of the tumour at

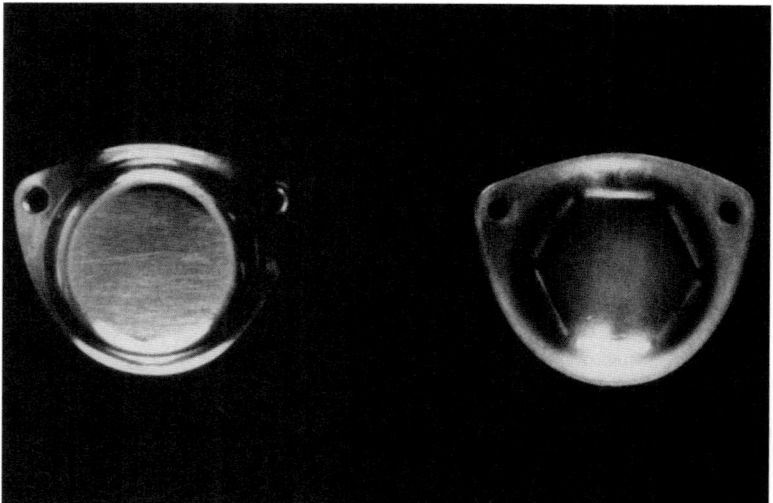

Fig. 1 Obverse and reverse views of 10 millimetre diameter circular iodine-125 scleral applicator in use at Saint Bartholomew's Hospital, London. Six radioactive iodine seeds are embedded in epoxy resin in a gold carrier.

a minimum dose rate of 45 cGy per h. Unlike the older cobalt-60 applicators which they have largely replaced, these modern applicators are shielded on their external surface and produce little in the way of side effects on the ocular adnexa.

Plaques do not produce reliable local tumour control when used to treat melanomas adjacent to the optic disc. These tumours and melanomas over 8 mm thick may benefit from radiotherapy techniques which utilise the dose distribution advantages of positively charged particles, usually protons[39] (Fig. 2). The finely collimated beam is directed towards the tumour with the aid of surgically applied tantalum marker clips and a uniform dose of 60 Gy is given to the whole melanoma in 4 or 5 daily fractions The Bragg peak of protons means that the entry dose is reduced and that the exit dose is zero for posterior tumours but the superficial radiation sparing effect is progressively lost with increasing modulation of the beam to treat larger and more anteriorly located melanomas. Eyelid damage is greater following proton therapy of more anteriorly located choroidal melanomas than it is after plaque therapy which should be used in preference to proton treatment whenever possible. With careful case selection, more than 90% of eyes can be retained after

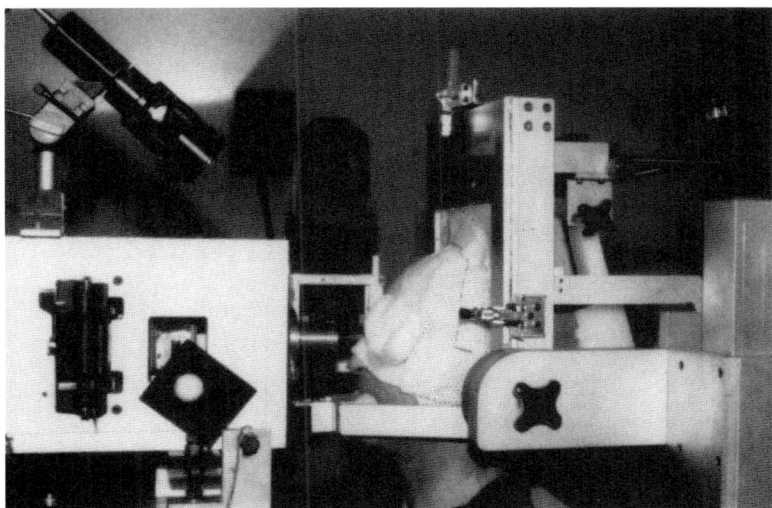

Fig. 2 Proton beam radiotherapy set up for treatment of ocular melanoma. The patient is seated with his head fixed rigidly by a bite block and a face mask. His eye position is maintained by viewing a target and can be monitored during treatment by closed circuit television. The position of his marker clips can be checked by X-rays using polaroid cameras.

plaque or proton radiotherapy, most with useful acuity or field of vision.

Regression of choroidal melanomas does not usually begin until at least 4 months after radiotherapy and may continue for 2 or more years (Figs 4 & 5). When the retina is detached, reattachment may take place within 4 months but extensive detachments may not resolve quickly enough to prevent ischaemic changes which lead to

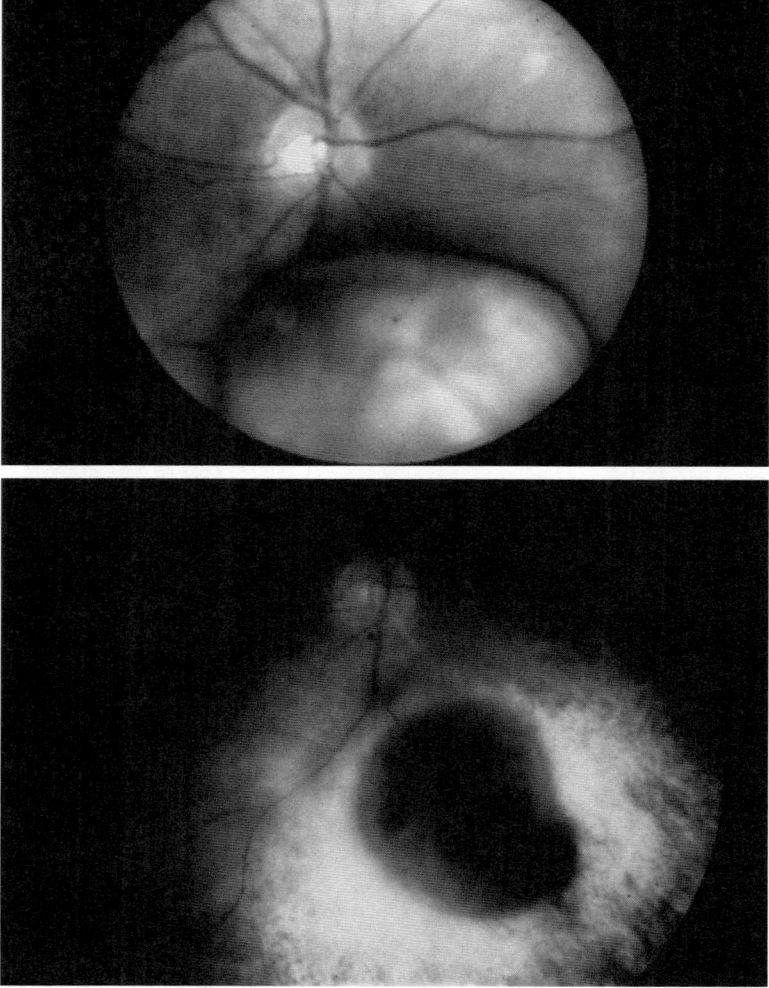

Fig. 3 Choroidal melanoma a) before and b) 15 months after iodin125 plaque therapy.

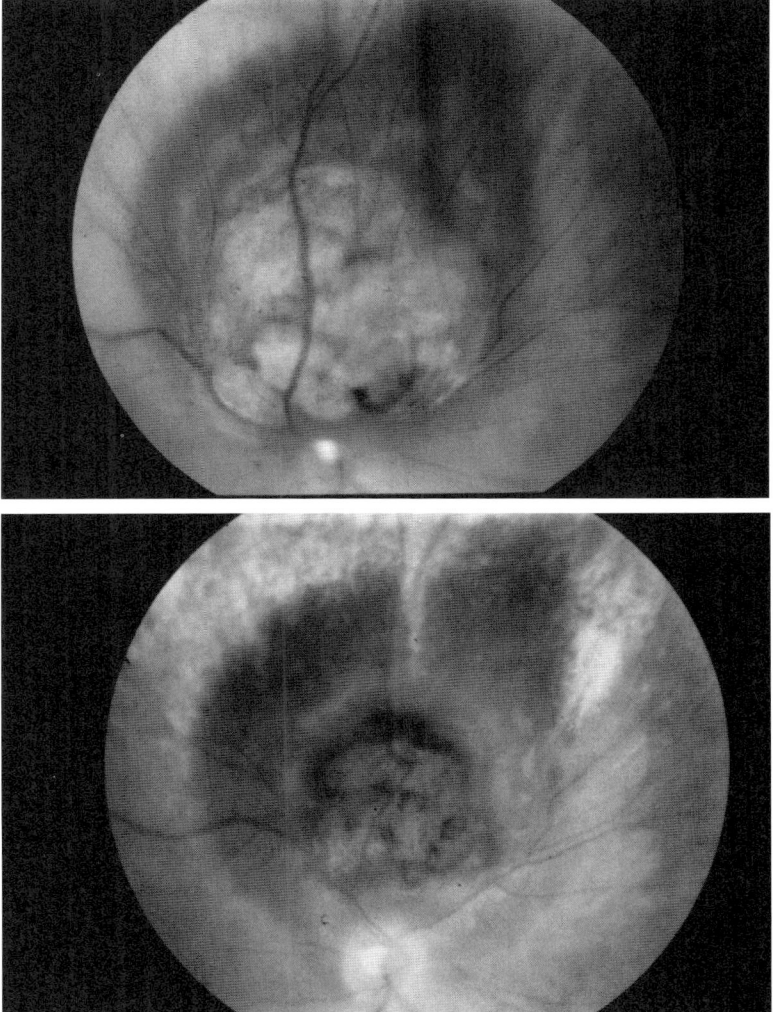

Fig. 4 Juxtapapillary choroidal melanoma a) before and b) 2 years after proton beam radiotherapy.

neovascular glaucoma. This type of glaucoma is a common late event in the natural history of untreated melanoma and is not strictly a side effect of radiotherapy. Nevertheless, it is one of the main factors limiting the success of radiation treatments. Modern microsurgery allows choroidal melanomas which do not extend to the optic disc to be resected.[40] Retinal reattachment occurs more rapidly after resection though two operations may be required to achieve it.

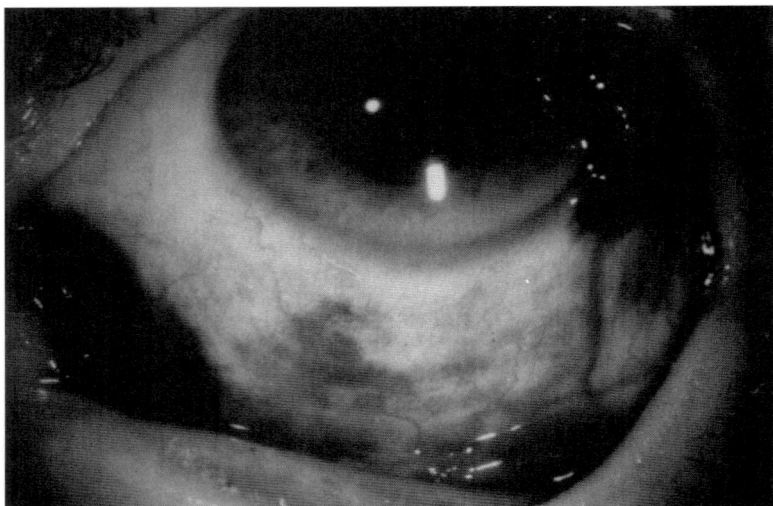

Fig. 5 Multifocal malignant melanoma of the conjunctiva arising in primary acquired melanosis. Two tumours have arisen simultaneously, a nodular melanoma at the temporal limbus.and a diffuse melanoma in the plica. The limbal melanoma is heralded by a feeder vessel.

Larger tumours with extensive retinal detachment are better managed by resection though the operation requires profound hypotensive anaesthesia and is only applicable to younger patients with no history of cardiovascular disease.

MELANOMA OF THE SKIN OF THE EYELID

Primary eyelid skin melanomas are rare and account for only 1% of lid tumours.[41] They may arise *de novo*, in a pre-existing naevus, or in an area of lentigo maligna. They are frequently associated with primary acquired melanosis (PAM)[42] and occasionally with oculodermal melanocytosis. Eyelid skin melanoma associated with PAM usually develops as a late manifestation long after conjunctival pigmentation is first noted but, rarely, the lid tumour may present first.[43] About half exhibit a superficial spreading and half a nodular growth pattern and they are often amelanotic.[42] Occasional metastases in the eyelids from distant cutaneous melanoma may be distinguished from primaries by their characteristic subepithelial location.

Treatment of small, cicumscribed tumours is by wide excision followed by plastic repair of the eyelid. A careful search should be made for any evidence of associated melanosis or melanocytosis. Large and diffuse melanomas are best managed by orbital exenteration after diagnostic biopsy and the same radical approach will be required for local recurrence. Eyelid melanomas frequently spread to preauricular or submandibular lymph nodes. Thick and nodular tumours and those with spread to regional nodes have a poor prognosis though the outlook is better than for cutaneous melanoma.[41]

MELANOMA OF THE CONJUNCTIVA

Primary conjunctival melanoma is uncommon and comprises 2% of ocular malignancies.[44] It may arise in the bulbar or palpebral conjunctiva or in that of the conjunctival fornices or plica semilunaris. Rare examples develop in the caruncle which, with its epidermal tissue and hair follicles, has more histological similarities with skin than with conjunctiva. Conjunctival melanomas may also be of superficial spreading or nodular growth pattern and variably pigmented. There is no known association with solar exposure but host risk factors are prominent in its aetiology. The majority of conjunctival melanomas develop in a pre-exsting pigmented conjunctival lesion.[45] Approximately 18% arise in a conjunctival naevus and these tumours, like occasional melanomas arising *de novo*, tend to be solitary and circumscribed. About 57% of tumours arise in primary acquired melanosis and are usually multifocal and often diffuse (Fig. 5). Some tumours, apparently arising *de novo* or in a naevus, eventually show signs of PAM, suggesting that naevus formation may be a step in the development of malignant melanocytic tumours of the conjunctiva in some individuals with acquired melanosis.

Primary acquired melanosis usually presents in middle age with flat, granular, intraepithelial reddish-brown pigmentary change which is clinically similar to racial pigmentation. Typically, it is first noticed in the bulbar conjunctiva. A benign variant has been described which is said not to progress to the precancerous form to which the term PAM is now usually applied. The version with atypia is commoner and in it the atypical melanocytes then spread contiguously or non-contiguously and over a period of years to involve the palpebral conjunctiva and that of the fornices and plica, the skin of the eyelids[42] and even the corneal epithelium.[46] Ultimately, multifocal melanoma develops sequentially in most cases in which atypia are found. The degree of pigmentation found in PAM may vary with time and the waxing and waning characteristic of the disorder may be so extreme that it may seem to disappear. Apparent spontaneous resolution of this type is rarely sustained. This feature of PAM and the fact that multifocal melanomas have been reported to arise in amelanotic PAM[47] suggests that what is changing is pigment production. Pigmentation may also vary in the same individual with pregnancy and in this respect it may be significant that approximately 40% of conjunctival melanomas have been found to contain oestrogen receptors.[48] There is recent evidence to suggest that PAM may be a manifestation of the atypical mole syndrome.[49]

The incidence and time scale of malignant change in PAM is difficult to estimate, not least because most patients with acquired melanosis do not present until they have developed their first melanoma. The number of individuals with as yet undiagnosed PAM is unknown so that the denominator of the fraction who develop malignancy is uncertain. Moreover, many patients with conjunctival melanoma describe ipsilateral reddish discolouration of the bulbar conjunctiva, suggestive of PAM, for decades. This is often mistaken for inflammation and not infrequently treated as such for long periods, making it difficult to ascertain how long acquired melanosis has been present. Nevertheless malignancy has been reported to supervene in between 17% of PAM patients in a 5-year period[50] and 50% overall.[51]

It is as important to be alert to the possibility of malignant change in any pigmented conjunctival lesion as it is in the skin. Clinical features suggestive of malignant transformation are increased thickness, a change in pigmentation, the appearance of prominent blood vessels feeding a tumour, and tethering of the conjunctiva to the underlying sclera in areas where it is usually mobile. In adolescence, a short period of benign enlargement due to epithelial downgrowth with cyst formation is almost the rule in bulbar conunctival naevi but increase in size later in life and particularly sustained growth should be regarded with suspicion. Melanomas arising *de novo* or in a naevus tend to present in the bulbar conjunctiva exposed within the interpalpebral fissure where they are soon noticed by the patient. By contrast, melanomas arising in PAM may develop anywhere within the conjunctiva and frequently in areas hidden from view. Such tumours may become very large before they are first noticed because of a lump in the eyelid or because of bleeding or a mass protruding under the lid. When a melanoma arises at a site other than in the interpalpebral bulbar conjunctiva, it almost always does so in PAM. A careful clinical or histopathological search should always be made for PAM in such tumours.

The treatment of conjunctival malignant melanoma is essentially surgical. The life prognosis is much better for solitary, thin melanomas arising in the bulbar conjunctiva and not associated with PAM than it is for multiple and thick tumours developing in unfavourable locations including the palpebral conjunctiva, the fornices, the plica and the caruncle and associated with acquired melanosis.[45] Melanomas arising in high risk locations have twice the mortality of epibulbar tumours and mixed cell lesions have 3 times the mortality of spindle cell melanomas.[45] Differences in access to lymphatics may be the underlying reason why some locations are less favourable than others and histological evidence of lymphatic invasion carries a 4-fold increase in the mortality rate.[45] Development of new tumours in PAM may contribute to the higher mortality rates that are seen the longer patients are followed.[42,51,52] These various risk factors conspire to make conjunctival melanoma arising in PAM a much more serious disease than melanoma arising *de novo* or in a naevus. Because of these differences, solitary bulbar conjunctival tumours have tended to be managed by conservative local excision whereas multiple melanomas elsewhere in the conjunctiva have been treated mainly by orbital exenteration.

Any new, raised pigmented patch appearing in the conjunctiva of an adult and any area of increased thickness or vascularity within a pre-existing naevus or area of PAM should be excised, if possible with a 3 mm margin. Frequently, excision biopsy of this type will also serve as the definitive treatment of a conjunctival melanoma. Bulbar conjunctival melanomas not involving the corneoscleral limbus are amenable to simple excision with a low recurrence rate. Most recurrences arising after excision of such a tumour are, in reality, new foci of melanoma arising in PAM: the development of multiple local recurrences in a patient not diagnosed to have PAM should always raise suspicion of this disorder. The interpalpebral limbus is a frequent site for conjunctival melanoma. At the limbus, the conjunctiva is adherent to the underlying sclera and melanomas arising in this location tend to recur if not properly excised. Melanomas tend not to invade the corneal and scleral lamellae and the incidence of this type of recurrence may be greatly reduced by performing a block excision of the tumour with the underlying superficial one third of the adjacent cornea and sclera. Separation of the corneal epithelium at the tumour margin is facilitated by application of absolute alcohol. In the unlikely event that corneal invasion occurs significantly beyond the limbus, transparency may be maintained by replacing lost corneal tissue with a lamellar graft.[46] After incomplete excision the recurrence rate may be reduced by adjunctive treatment either by radiotherapy[53] or cryotherapy.[54] Beta radiotherapy using a strontium-90 surface applicator is preferred and the surface dose should be at least 50 Gray (Gy) given in 5 daily fractions. Strenuous efforts should be made to avoid irradiating the whole limbus to this dose or serious corneal toxicity may ensue. Survival rates are excellent following excision of solitary circumscribed bulbar conjunctival melanomas not associated with PAM.

Melanomas arising in the palpebral conjunctiva, the fornices, the plica, and the caruncle are more difficult to eradicate, partly because adjunctive treatments are more difficult to apply in these locations. For this reason standard treatment has tended towards orbital exenteration for such lesions, and particlarly for large, extensive or multiple tumours. A recent study, however, suggests that an attempt at conservative excision is legitimate before resorting to exenteration if this approach fails.[55] Two groups of exenterated patients have been compared retrospectively. The indications for orbital exenteration were similar in both, namely conjunctival melanoma in an unfavourable location for conservative excison. One group of patients underwent orbital exenteration as the primary treatment of conjunctival melanoma whilst the other group were exenterated only when conservative excision failed. Survival rates were similar in both groups and the key to survival appeared to be the thickness of the largest tumour rather than the treatment method. The melanoma-related mortality rate in this series of poor prognosis patients ranged between zero in tumours with a maximum thickness of 1 mm and 50% in those in excess of 2 mm thick. A particularly poor outcome was recorded for melanoma of the caruncle with 6 out of 7 patients dying despite primary exenteration. Orbital exenteration, frequently advocated for caruncular melanoma, is an illogical operation for tumours in this location because it can achieve a clearance margin of only a millimetre or two without a good survival prospect and with a severe cosmetic deficit. Caruncular melanomas may be better managed by local excision followed by local radiotherapy to the tumour bed with protons and to the nasal passages with photons. This approach achieves a local control rate as good as exenteration and, although insufficient patients have as yet been treated in this way to determine whether survival rates are as good, they could hardly be much worse.

In conservatively treated patients who survive their initial tumours, the natural history of melanoma arising in PAM tends towards an aggressive phase in which the interval between the development of new malignancies shortens and new lesions form simultaneously throughout the conjunctival sac. Exenteration continues to play an important part in palliating such patients in whom conservative therapy has failed and others who present with massive neglected melanomas. There is no need to exenterate the posterior orbit and the procedure can almost always be achieved through a lid-splitting approach with primary closure of skin and orbicularis muscle salvaged from the eyelid. Following exenteration the patient may be fitted with a specacle-mounted prosthesis. Advanced melanomas ultimately invade lymphatics and spread to preauricular, submandibular and cervical nodes before disseminating locally to the parotid gland or widely, usually to liver, subcutaneous tissues or brain. Although patients about to undergo exenteration should undergo a metastatic evaluation including chest X-ray, liver function tests and abdominal ultrasound, prior to surgery many will require the operation for local tumour control even in the presence of asymptomatic metastases. Patients who develop spread to regional glands or the parotid are best managed by excision of all visible local disease followed by radiotherapy to the neck. In this way unpleasant local recurrence may be avoided but this treatment is unlikely to prevent widespread dissemination.

Following exenteration, recurrence in the orbit, nasal passages and paranasal sinsus has been noted in some patients.[56,57] Orbital recurrence tends to occur following treatment of large, neglected lesions and nasal recurrence after that of inner canthal tumours, presumeably because of implantation of tumour cells shed down the nasolacrimal duct. At Saint Bartholomew's Hospital, patients exenterated for large melanomas are now offered postoperative adjunctive orbital radiotherapy and those who have undergone exenteration for inner canthal melanomas radiotherapy to the ipsilateral nasal passages in the hope of eliminating local recurrence.

Conjunctival melanomas may respond to radiotherapy[58] but high doses in the region of 100 Gy are required to achieve tumour regression. As with uveal tumours, shrinkage may take several years[59] and, since these tumours are very visible, most prefer to excise them and to employ radiotherapy where appropriate in an adjuvant setting. Just as they would be in uveal melanoma, doses of this order are far too toxic to apply to a large volume including the whole conjunctiva and the adjacent eye. Radiotherapy therefore has limited value in the treatment of diffuse and superficial spreading melanomas associated with PAM but beta-irradiation of small, circumscribed melanomas of the bulbar conjunctiva using strontium-90 surface applicators has been found to be effective.[59] Practical considerations make it difficult to apply surface brachytherapy using low penetrance beta rays to melanomas of the palpebral conjunctiva, the fornix, the plica and the caruncle. Proton beam radiotherapy may be effective for inner canthal melanomas and combinations of charged particle therapy and brachytherapy using gamma emissions from cobalt-60 plaques have been tried for the treatment of extensive melanomas elsewhere in the bulbar and palpebral conjunctiva. Cobalt plaques have the advantage of practically equal emissions from both their inner and outer surfaces and this property is useful when treating juxtaposed areas of involved bulbar and palpebral conjunctiva. The plaque is positioned in the conjunctival fornix between the adjacent layers of affected conjunctiva and secured with sutures through the conjunctival tissue and into the underlying sclera. Unfortunately, the dose distribution of protons is not favourable in such locations because there is no superficial sparing effect for lesions close to the surface. This, together with the high penetrance of gamma emissions from cobalt-60 and the high doses required means that these treatments result in considerable damage to the eye, to normal eyelid structures and to the lacrimal apparatus, though the full effect of such changes may not be apparent for several years. Radiation may induce uveitis and painful neovascular glaucoma which demands enucleation. Such eyes as are retained are dry and uncomfortable. Radiation-induced telangiectasia make these eyes chronically red and unsightly. Permanent loss of eyelashes occurs and depigmentation is noticeable in dark skinned patients. When the upper eyelid is irradiated, keratinisation leads to abrasion of the cornea and subsequently to corneal vascularisation and opacification which is not amenable to treatment. In general, therefore, radiotherapy is not a satisfactory substitute for orbital exenteration in advanced conjunctival melanoma because it rarely results in a seeing eye, the cosmetic appearance is often worse than that achieved with a prosthesis and, perhaps most important of all, the irradiated eye is chronically painful.

The particular risk factors associated with PAM contribute significantly to the high mortality rate of conjunctival melanoma. All patients with PAM should undergo twice yearly re-evaluation looking for evidence of malignant change and they should be encouraged to report any changes between visits. Although PAM with atypia is commoner than that without, it is difficult to differentiate clinically between the two and the diagnosis should be confirmed histologically to justify time-consuming follow-up. Impression cytology may be helpful if it gives a positive result[60] but a possibility of false negatives exists and cytological absence of melanocytic atypia requires confirmation by incisional biopsy. Cryotherapy may be able to kill conjunctival melanoma cells selectively and has been recommended for melanosis in which atypia have been demonstrated in the hope of preventing malignant change.[61] Cryotherapy certainly reduces pigmentation but some of this effect may result from alterations of pigment production and there is insufficient experience of this approach at present to determine how effective it will be. Present evidence suggests that it cannot prevent all new melanomas and that the best we can hope for is that it may be able to postpone malignant change and reduce the number of new tumours. Moreover, there are no means of detecting areas of amelanotic PAM and this entity defies any form of prophylactic treatment at present.

MELANOMA OF THE ORBIT

Primary melanomas of the orbit are very rare and melanoma in this location usually represents an extension from an intraocular or conjunctival source.[62] The aetiology and management differ according to the age of the patient. In younger individuals primary orbital melanoma tends to arise in a cellular blue naevus.[62,63] Tumours with this type of origin tend to be relatively benign and circumscribed lesions may be managed by local excision. In older patients the tumours usually arise in ocular or oculodermal melanocytosis.[64-66] Melanomas originating in this way may be seen in black patients.[67] They are more malignant and are best treated by orbital exenteration.

REFERENCES

1 Stephens RF, Shields JA. Diagnosis and management of cancer metastatic to the eye: a study of 70 cases. Ophthalmology 1979; 86: 1336–1349.
2 Egan KM, Seddon JM, Glynn R, Gragoudas ES, Albert DM. Epidemiologic aspects of uveal melanoma. Survey Ophthalmol 1988; 32: 239–251.
3 Dolin PJ, Foss AJE. Hungerford JL. Uveal melanoma: is solar ultraviolet radiation a risk factor? Ophthalmic Epidemiol 1994; 1: 27–30.
4 Østerlind A. Trends in incidence of ocular malignant melanoma in Denmark 1943–1982. Int J Cancer 1987; 40: 161–164.
5 Ganley JP, Comstock GW. Benign nevi and malignant melanomas of the choroid. Am J Ophthalmol 1973; 76: 19–25.
6 Gonder JR, Shields JA, Albert DM, Augsburger JJ, Lavin PT. Uvealmalignant melanoma associated with ocular and oculodermal melanocytosis. Ophthalmology 1982; 89: 953–960.
7 Canning CR, Hungerford JL. Familial uveal melanoma. Am J Ophthalmol 1988; 72: 241–243.
8 Oosterhuis JA, Wenrt LN, Lynch HT. Primary choroidal and cutaneous melanomas, and familial occurrence of melanomas. Br J Ophthalmol 1982; 66: 230–233.
9 Rodriguez-Sains RS. Ocular findings in patients with dysplastic nevus syndrome. Ophthalmology 1986; 93: 661–665.
10 Robertson DM, Campbell RJ. Errors in the diagnosis of malignant melanoma of the choroid. Am J Ophthalmol 1979; 87: 269–275.
11 Char DH, Stone RD. Irvine AR et al. Diagnostic modalities in choroidal melanoma. Am J Ophthalmol 1980; 89: 223–230.
12 Flocks M, Gerende JH, Zimmerman LE. The size and shape of malignant melanomas of the choroid and ciliary body in relation to prognosis and histlogical

characteristics: a statisticial study of 210 tumors. Trans Am Acad Ophthalmol Otolaryngol 1955; 59: 740–758.

13 McLean IW, Foster WD, Zimmerman LE. Prognostic factors in small malignant melanomas of the choroid and ciliary body. Arch Ophthalmol 1977; 95: 48–58.

14 Shammas HF, Blodi FC. Prognostic factors in choroidal and ciliary body melanomas. Arch Ophthalmol 1977, 95: 63–69.

15 Davidorf FH, Lang JR. The natural history of melanoma of the choroid: small versus large tumors. Ophthalmology 1975; 79: 310–320.

16 Starr HJ, Zimmerman LE. Extrascleral extension and orbital recurrence of malignant melanoma of the choroid and ciliary body. Int Ophthalmol Clin 1962; 2: 369–384.

17 Kidd MN, Lyness RW, Patterson CC, Johnston PB, Archer DB. Prognostic factors in malignant melanoma of the choroid: a retrospective survey of cases occurring in Northern Ireland between 1965 and 1980. Trans Ophthalmol Soc UK 1986; 105: 114–121.

18 Hungerford J. Prognosis in ocular melanoma. Br J Ophthalmol 1989; 73: 689–690.

19 Rones B, Zimmerman LE. The prognosis of primary tumors of the iris treated by iridectomy. Arch Ophthalmol 1958; 60: 193–205.

20 Jakobiec FA. Are most iris 'melanomas' really nevi? Arch Ophthalmol 1981; 99: 2117–2132.

21 Foss AJE, Pecorella I, Alexander RA et al. Are most intraocular 'leiomyomas' really melanocytic lesions? Ophthalmology 1994; 101: 919–924.

22 Geisse LJ, Robertson DM. Iris melanomas. Am J Ophthalmol 1985; 60: 193–205.

23 Shields JA, Annesly WH, Spaeth GL. Necrotic melanocytoma of iris with secondary glaucoma. Am J Ophthalmol 1977; 84: 826–829.

24 Ashton N. Primary tumours of the iris. Br J Ophthalmol 1964; 48: 650–668.

25 Geisse LJ, Robertson DM. The prognosis of primary tumors of the iris treated by iridectomy. Arch Ophthalmol 1985; 99: 638–648.

26 Dart JK, Marsh RJ, Garner A, Cooling RJ. Fluorescein angiography of anterior uveal melanocytic tumours. Br J Ophthalmol 1988; 72: 326–337.

27 Territo C, Shields CL, Shields JA, Augsburger JJ, Schroeder RP. Natural course of melanocytic tumors of the iris. Ophthalmology 1988; 95: 1251–1255.

28 Kersten RC, Tse DT, Anderson R. Iris melanoma: nevus or malignancy? Surv Ophthalmol 1985; 29: 423–433.

29 Font RL, Spaulding AG, Zimmerman LE. Diffuse malignant melanoma of the uveal tract: a clinicopathologic report of 54 cases. Trans Am Acad Ophthalmol Otolaryngol 1968; 72: 877–895.

30 Bomanji J, Hungerford JL, Granowska M, Britton KE. Radioimmunoscintigraphy of ocular melanoma with ^{99m}Tc labelled cutaneous melanoma antibody fragments. Br J Ophthalmol 1987; 71: 651–658.

31 Char DH, Stone RD, Irvine AR, et al. Diagnostic modalities in choroidal melanoma. Am J Ophthalmol 1980; 89: 223–230.

32 Bomanji J, Hungerford JL, Granowska M, Britton KE. Uptake of ^{99m}Tc labelled (Fab')$_2$ fragments of monoclonal antibody 225.28S by a benign ocular naevus. Eur J Nuclear Med 1988; 14: 165–166.

33 Augsburger JJ, Schroeder RP, Territo C et al. Clinical parameters predictive of enlargement of melanocytic choroidal lesions. Br J Ophthalmol 1989; 73: 911–917.

34 Hykin PG, McCartney ACE, Plowman PN, Hungerford JL. Postenucleation radiotherapy for the treatment of malignant melanoma of the choroid with extrascleral extension. Br J Ophthalmol 1990; 74: 36–39.

35 Vogel MH. Treatment of malignant melanomas with photocoagulation: evaluation of 10-year follow-up data. Am J Ophthalmol 1982; 74: 1–11.

36 Hungerford J. Treatment of uveal melanoma by radioactive scleral plaque. In Easty DL, ed Current Ophthalmic Surgery. London: Baillière Tindall, 1990, 459–472.

37 Lommatzsch P. β-Irradiation of choroidal melanoma with ^{106}Ru/^{106}Rh applicators: 16 years' experience. Arch Ophthalmol 1983; 101: 713–717.
38 Packer S. Iodine-125 radiation of posterior uveal melanoma. Ophthalmology 1987; 94: 1621–1625.
39 Munzenrider JE, Gragoudas ES, Seddon JM, et al. Conservative treatment of uveal melanoma: probability of eye retention after proton treatment. Int J Radiat Oncol Biol Physics 1988; 15: 553–558.
40 Foulds WS. Experience with local resection of uveal melanomas. Trans Ophthalmol Soc UK 1977; 97: 412–415.
41 Garner A, Koornneef L, Levane A, Collin JR. Malignant melanoma of the eyelid skin: histopathology and behaviour. Br J Ophthalmol 1985; 69: 180–186.
42 Robertson DM, Hungerford JL, McCartney ACE. Pigmentation of the eyelid margin accompanying conjunctival melanoma. Am J Ophthalmol 1989; 108: 435–439.
43 Hicks C, Liu C, Hiranandani M, Garner A, Hungerford J. Conjunctival melanoma after excision of a lentigo maligna melanoma in the ipsilateral eyelid skin. Br J Ophthalmol 1994; 78: 317–318.
44 Scotto J, Fraumeni JF Jr., Lee JA. Melanomas of the eye and other non-cutaneous sites: epidemiological aspects. J Natl Cancer Inst 1976; 56: 489–491.
45 Paridaens ADA, Minassian DC, McCartney ACE, Hungerford JL. Prognostic factors in primary malignant melanoma of the conjunctiva: a clinicopathological study of 256 cases. Br J Ophthalmol 1994; 78: 252–259.
46 Paridaens ADA, Kirkness CM, Garner A, Hungerford, JL. Recurrent malignant melanoma of the corneal stroma: a case of 'black cornea'. Br J Ophthalmol 1992; 76: 444–446.
47 Paridaens ADA, McCartney ACE, Hungerford JL. Multifocal amelanotic conjunctival melanoma and acquired melanosis sine pigmento. Br J Ophthalmol 1992; 76: 163–165.
48 Paridaens ADA, Alexander RA, Hungerford JL, McCartney ACE. Oestrogen receptors in conjunctival malignant melanoma: immunocytochemical study using formalin fixed paraffin wax sections. J Clin Path 1991; 44: 840–843.
49 Bataille V, Boyle J, Hungerford JL, Newton, JA. Three cases of primary acquired melanosis of the conjunctiva as a manifesation of the atypical mole syndrome. Br J Dermatol 1993; 128: 86–90.
50 Reese AB. Precancerous and cancerous melanosis. Am J Ophthalmol 1966, 61: 1272–1277.
51 Folberg R, McLean IW, Zimmerman LE. Malignant melanoma of the conjunctiva. Hum Pathol 1985; 16: 136–143.
52 Jay B. Naevi and melanomata of the conjunctiva. Br J Ophthalmol 1965; 49, 169–204.
53 Lederman M, Wybar K, Busby E. Malignant epibulbar melanoma: natural history and treatment by radiotherapy. Br J Ophthalmol 1984; 68: 605–617.
54 Collin JRO, Allen LH, Garner A, Hungerford JL. Malignant melanoma of the eyelid and conjunctiva. Australian N Z J of Ophthalmol 1986; 14: 29–34.
55 Paridaens ADA, McCartney ACE, Minassian DC, Hungerford JL. Orbital exenteration in 95 cases of conjunctival malignant melanoma. Br J Ophthalmol 1994; 78: 520–528.
56 Robertson DM, Hungerford JL, McCartney ACE. Malignant melanomas of the conjunctiva, nasal cavity, and paranasal sinuses. Am J Ophthalmol 1989; 108: 440–442.
57 Paridaens ADA, McCartney ACE, Lavelle RJ, Hungerford JL. Nasal and orbital recurrence of conjunctival melanoma 21 years after exenteration. Br J Ophthalmol 1992; 76: 369–371.
58 Lederman M. Radiotherapy of epibulbar malignant melanomata. Trans Ophthalmol Soc UK 1953; 73: 399–413.
59 Lommatzsch PK. Beta-ray treatment of malignant epibulbar melanoma. Albrecht von Graefes Arch Klin Exp Ophthalmol 1978; 209: 111–124.

60 Paridaens ADA, McCartney ACE, Curling OM, Lyons CJ, Hungerford JL. Impression cytology of conjunctival melanosis and melanoma. Br J Ophthalmol 1992; 76, 198–201.

61 Jakobiec FA, Rini FJ, Fraunfelder FT, Brownstein S. Cryotherapy for conjunctival primary acquired melanosis and malignant melanoma. Ophthalmology 1988; 95: 1058–1070.

62 Rottino A, Kelly AS. Primary orbital melanoma. Case report with review of the literature. Arch Ophthalmol 1942; 27: 934–949.

63 Wolter JR, Bryson JM, Blackhurst RT. Primary orbital melanoma. Ear Nose Throat Mon 1966; 76: 307–308.

64 Jay B. Malignant melanoma of the orbit in a case of oculodermal melanocytosis (Naevus of Ota). Br J Ophthalmol 1965; 49: 359–363.

65 Hagler WS, Brown CC. Malignant melanoma of the orbit arising in a nevus of Ota. Trans Am Acad Ophthalmol Otolaryngol 1966; 78: 817–822.

66 Haim T, Meyer E, Kerner H, Zonis S. Oculodermal melanocytosis (nevus of Ota) and orbital malignant melanoma. Ann Ophthalmol 1982; 14: 1132–1136.

67 Wilkes SR, Uthman BO, Thornton CN, Randall EC. Malignant melanoma of the orbit in a black patient with ocular melanocytosis. Arch Ophthalmol 1984; 102: 904–906.

British Medical Bulletin 1995, Vol 51, No. 3 pp. 717–746
©The British Council 1995

Prospectives for cutaneous malignant melanoma
Considerations of the precursor state and heritability

W H Clark

Department of Pathology, Harvard Medical School, The Beth Israel Hospital, Boston, MA, USA; Pathology Services Inc., Cambridge, MA, USA: The Pigmented Lesion Group, University of Pennsylvania, School of Medicine, Philadelphia, PA, USA.

A M Goldstein and M A Tucker

Genetic Epidemiology Branch, National Cancer Institute USA, Bethesda, MD, USA

Each of the discoveries through the years has begotten a series of Gordian knots. We must patiently inspect our new collection of mysteries and focus on those where our efforts may well change the course of the disease to the benefit of affected patients. The proper management of the precursor state, the beginning of the disease, and the patient exploration of the complexities of heritability would seem to be appropriate beginnings.

Neoplastic systems come into being and are manifest through induction, development, and progression. These phenomena of tumor biology are characteristic of neoplasia and may be classified into six categories. The generic categories applicable to all neoplastic systems are indicated by bold face type in the following list.[1-3] In melanocytic neoplasia, the specific terminology for some of the categories follows the generic category term.

1. Events at the beginning (inductive events)

2. The precursor state

Melanoma development may not be limited to origin from evident lesions. The entire organ, the skin, is in an altered state and melanomas may from specific kinds of precursor lesions or may arise from altered melanocytes that are not a part of evident precursor lesions.

3. Primary cancer without competence for metastasis (intermediate lesions): Malignant melanoma *in situ* and radial growth phase primary melanoma.

This class of lesions in tumor progression has acquired the property of continuous growth, but has not acquired capacity for metastasis. Melanoma *in situ* shows all tumor cells to be in the epidermal compartment, separated from the dermis by the basement membrane. Radial growth phase melanoma is characterized by tumor cells in the epidermis and papillary dermis similar in appearance to the cells of melanoma *in situ*. Although tumor cells extend into the papillary dermis in the radial growth phase there is no evident capacity for growth there and competence for metastasis is not manifest by this stage of tumor development.[4] We have termed these lesions intermediate for their behavior is intermediate between the distal end of precursor state lesions and primary cancer with competence for metastasis. They differ from late precursor lesions in several respects; the most important of which is continuous growth, albeit quite slow, of intermediate lesions when compared with late precursor state lesions. Intermediate lesions lack the manifest competence for metastasis frequently expressed in primary cancers with competence for metastasis.

4. Primary cancer with competence for metastasis: Primary melanoma that has progressed to the vertical growth phase.

Vertical growth phase melanoma refers to a stage in melanoma progression that is characterized by dermal invasion; the ability to grow in the dermis; and some metastatic capacity. Vertical growth phase is not a synonym for invasion. Vertical growth phase melanomas not only extend into the dermis, they **grow** there. The phrase does imply acquisition of metastatic competence, which may or may not be expressed. Invasion and metastasis are separable properties; clearly attested to by the differences between radial growth phase (invasive capacity, but no metastatic capacity) and the vertical growth phase (invasive capacity, competence for growth in a second tissue compartment, the dermis, and capacity for metastasis).[2,5]

5. Metastasis

6. Metastasis from metastasis

Under some of the foregoing categories we will discuss current problems in the study of melanoma and delineate reasonable directions for future study.

EVENTS AT THE BEGINNING

The events at the beginning are the interactions between agents or mechanisms (endogenous or exogenous) and the target organ. The result of such interactions is an altered target organ. The alterations constitute a predisposition to the development of malignant melanoma and may or may not be manifested by demonstrable or recognizable lesions or other tissue changes. Recent epidemiologic studies of melanoma have delineated some of the *manifest* changes in the skin, the target organ for human cutaneous melanomas. The manifest changes constitute most of the known risk factors for melanoma development. The risk factors, with few variations, have been similar in different studies.[6–10] The risk factors usually include the following attributes.

- An increased number of melanocytic nevi (nevi in this paper are melanocytic nevi) 2–4 mm in width[11]
- An increased number of clinically atypical nevi and dysplastic nevi[12–17]
- A family history of melanoma[18–22]
- Freckling[6]
- Fair complexion[7]
- Excessive exposure to sunlight and severe sunburns[23–27]
- A cutaneous phenotype that burns rather than tans[10,26,27]

A review of melanoma epidemiology and risk factors is not one of the objectives of this article. Studies of such factors, however, clearly delineate major problems related to melanoma induction and progression. Several of these problems are fascinating and these will be discussed.

THE PRECURSOR STATE

One of the most intriguing, and largely unappreciated, aspects of tumor biology is the manifestation of the very beginnings of neoplasia: the initial response to inductive agents and mechanisms is not cancer. Rather, the agents induce the precursor state. As a generality, the development of cancer, itself, is rare when compared with the evident lesions of the precursor state. Thus, the precursor state and its lesions are most often end stage phenomena; they are not 'pre-anything'.[28] 'Premalignant lesion', with its obvious semantic infer-ence, is the usual term for some lesions of the precursor state and the term is an egregious misnomer. The precursor state is an organ-wide alteration which predisposes the organ to the development of cancer; in the context of this paper a predisposition to the devel-opment of primary cutaneous malignant melanoma. The precursor state may not be apparent or it may be manifested by the various proliferative lesions and atypical cells of the melanocytic system that are confined to a single tissue compartment and only grow for a limited time (growth is temporally restricted or constrained). When growth ceases the precursor lesions become indolent or quiescent.

[A tissue compartment is composed of one or more cellular pheno-types in organized array separated from an adjacent tissue com-partment by a basement membrane. When one states that a proliferative lesion of the precursor state is confined to a single tissue compartment, the foregoing definition of a tissue compartment is usually satisfactory. For example, the parenchymal cells of a tubular adenoma of the colon are all separated from the lamina propria by a basement membrane. However, on causal inspection, the definition is not applicable to a compound nevus or a dermal nevus (nevus refers to a melanocytic nevus in this paper. Studies have shown, however, that dermal nevic cells are surrounded by a basement membrane; in this sense they are still within the epidermal tissue compartment.[29]]

The atypical cells of the precursor state, when present, may be within clinically manifest (macroscopic) lesions or they may be scat-tered throughout an organ in individual cell array (microscopic lesions). A cutaneous phenotype manifested by freckles, sun sen-sitivity and solar degeneration of the dermis is also a predisposition to melanoma development; a precursor state without nevi. Pro-gression to cancer from a given precursor lesion or from a precursor state without melanocytic nevi is optional, not obligatory.[2]

Organ-wide alteration

Organ-wide, in the present context, refers to alteration of all epi-dermal and dermal structures, epithelial and mesenchymal. Thus, the alteration characterized by increased melanoma susceptibility may not be confined to a demonstrable lesion, such as some form of a melanocytic nevus. The evidence supporting the concept of organ-wide is as follows. Even though there is wide variation in the reported number of melanomas associated with nevi, all studies concerned with the association of nevi and melanoma have some subset of cases wherein the melanoma develops without an associated nevus.[30-32] Further, some white children and teenagers (and *many* black children and teenagers) have no melanocytic nevi on examination by trained observers.[33,34] It follows that some melanomas develop in skin without a demonstrable precursor lesion at the site of the melanoma or elsewhere on the skin. In addition, we have personally observed and photographically documented patients with many clinically atypical nevi who, in follow-up, developed a melanoma at a site where there was no previously visible precursor lesion. In fact, it has been stated that all of the known risk factors account for only about one half of melanoma cases.[9,35] We regard this figure as low, but are fully aware that a significant number of melanomas arise in patients that lack most of the *known* risk factors for the disease. Studies of induced neoplasia in experimental animals and studies of in vitro transformation also indicate that a precursor state (incipient neoplasia) is induced in that portion of an organ exposed to a carcinogen. Foulds defined incipient neoplasia (the precursor state) as a region coextensive with the area of exposure to carcinogenic treatment that has a permanent replicable new reactivity or increased capacity for neoplastic development.[36] In vitro, increased saturation density and growth constraint, X-ray treatment, and chemical carcinogens induce a state of incipient neoplasia in *all* treated cells not just the cells of transformed foci.[37-40]

Clinical and histologic definitions of melanocytic precursor state lesions

In the previous section there was evidence presented suggesting that the entire organ, coextensive with exposure to the inductive mechanism, is altered. However, in practice, the existence of the precursor state and its potential for progression to melanoma is based upon recognizable lesions. The most important of these lesions are common nevi, clinically atypical nevi, and dysplastic nevi. Other melanocytic lesions, such as small and large congenital nevi *may* be precursor lesions and may indicate a precursor state, but will not be considered here. There are problems with terminology applied to the cells composing melanocytic nevi and with definitions of common nevi, clinically atypical nevi, and dysplastic nevi. Our usage of terms and our definitions follow.

The terminology of cells composing nevi

A chronic problem with the terminology of the cells in nevi exists. The intraepidermal melanocytes arrayed as single cells in nevi are difficult to distinguish from some melanocytes in the epidermis adjacent to the nevus. Consequently, many observers simply call this intraepidermal population of nevic cells, melanocytes. The superficial cells in the dermal component of a nevus synthesize pigment, but do not have the form of melanocytes with dendrites. Further into the dermis, the nevus cells are rounded, lack pigment, or tyrosinase, and differentiate into elongate cells that are Schwannian in character. Some authors call the cells in the dermis (and epidermis) nevomelanocytes, even though most of the cells have few properties that may be rightfully regarded as those of dendritic intraepidermal melanocytes. One could designate all of the cells as nevic cells of melanocytic origin and designate their location. Such a descriptive designation is semantically cumbersome. We refer to the intraepidermal cells of nevi as melanocytes, either in single cell array or in nests. The cells in the dermis are termed dermal nevic cells. We are not satisfied with any terminology, including our own, and lean toward descriptive designations for accuracy in transmission of concepts.

Definitions of lesions and disorders manifested by the lesions

Common nevi – clinical definitions. The following definition of a nevus is acceptably vague and comprehensive, but it lacks precision. A melanocytic nevus is a sharply circumscribed area where there is a great increase in the number of melanocytes and nevic cells in the surface epithelium, or in the dermis, or in both epidermis and dermis, when compared with the surrounding, unaffected skin. Melanocytic nevi may be found in the skin, in the mucosae, and rarely in other tissues and organs.

- Lentigo and junctional nevus
  The lesions are sharply delineated, oval or circular in outline, dark tan or brown. Angulation is rare. They are flat or barely palpable. By definition, for this report, the lesions are $\leqslant 4$ mm in width. Lesions $\geqslant 4$ mm in width, along with other characteristics given later, are, again by definition, clinically atypical nevi. Different observers use a different size for the designation of a lesion as clinically atypical; $\geqslant 5$ mm in width seems to be the most common size in use as one of the criteria for clinical atypia.

- Compound nevus and dermal nevus
  The lesions are also sharply delineated, usually circular in outline, brown, dark brown, or flesh colored. They are elevated and may

be polypoidal, but, if the latter, have a stalk virtually the same width as the lesion.

Common nevi – histologic definitions. The descriptions in standard texts of cutaneous pathology usually give 4 histologic kinds of nevi. This statement does not include congenital melanocytic nevi, blue nevi and several other diverse and uncommon nevi. Some texts separate the simple lentigo from the other histologic appearances of nevi. We regard the lentigoes and junctional, compound, and dermal nevi as **one** distinctive category of melanocytic proliferation presenting in different stages of evolution. Circumscribed melanocytic proliferations begin with an increase in the number of basilar melanocytes associated with elongation of rete (in other words, as a lentigo) and may progress to junctional, compound and dermal nevi. The incidence of such progression is totally unknown and available evidence suggests that this process of evolution may become arrested at any stage. Thus, one may have a lentigo or compound nevus, for example, that is stable for years. All nevi in the group we are discussing here are common, appear in the first three decades of life, and may or may not be related to the cutaneous effects of light.

- Lentigo
  The hallmarks of a lentigo are an increased number of melanocytes along regularly elongated rete and increased basilar pigmentation.

- Junctional nevus
  A junctional nevus shows an increased number of intraepidermal melanocytes disposed in nests. The cells in the nests are lymphocyte-like, being small, with a scanty amount of cytoplasm. Dendrites are not observed. The individual cells of the nests are no larger than the usual, inactive basilar melanocytes of the epidermis. The nests tend to be equally spaced and at the tips of rete. As will be discussed, lesions fulfilling the foregoing histologic criteria are rare and the entity still exists more through custom than evidence or even conventional wisdom.

- Compound nevus
  The intraepidermal melanocytic component is similar to that just described for an idealized junctional nevus. The cells of the dermal component, just below the epidermis, are round, delimited by a basement membrane and variably pigmented. Deeper in the dermis, the pigment is absent and, still deeper, some of the cells are elongated and show various neuroidal forms. Such a deep component is usually interpreted as showing Schwannian differentiation.

- Dermal nevus

  There is no epidermal melanocytic component, but the epidermis may be hyperpigmented. The lesion is similar to the dermal component of a compound nevus, but neurotization tends to be more prominent.

  The weakest link in the evolutionary chain of nevi is the junctional nevus.[41] Meticulous search of a large histologic collection of cutaneous pigmented lesions by one of us has shown but the rarest example of a junctional nevus with the histologic criteria given above (WHC). Further, a careful histologic systematist (Aldo Gonzales-Serva, personal communication, 1994) has told us that he has difficulty with the histologic diagnosis of a junctional nevus and rarely makes such a diagnosis, without qualification.

Clinically atypical nevus. The clinically atypical nevus is ≥ 4 mm (others use ≥ 5 mm) in diameter and has a macular component and two or more of the following characteristics: an irregular border, an indistinct or hazy margin, two or more tan-brown colors, and erythema.

Dysplastic nevus. A dysplastic nevus shows an array of intra-epidermal melanocytes that is different from that seen in a lentigo or compound nevus. The different array may be seen as irregular nests of melanocytes along the margins of rete or over dermal papillae or as a bridge of melanocytes extending from one rete to the next. In addition, readily discernible atypical melanocytes must be seen in those areas showing the different disposition of intraepidermal melanocytes. The subjacent dermis is altered. The fibroblasts, both bipolar and dendritic, are increased in number. The collagen may appear as an intensely eosinophilic band parallel with the epidermal basal layer, or as parallel layers of collagen and bipolar fibroblasts (lamellar fibroplasia). Scattered patches of lymphocytes and macrophages are also seen in the dermis.

  Controversies concerning the term dysplastic nevus are discussed with the related controversies concerning the dysplastic nevus syndrome.

Familial melanoma. When a family has two or more first degree relatives with melanoma it is affected by familial melanoma. The existence of familial melanoma does not imply heredity, but does identify kindreds that may be studied for hereditary mechanisms.

- The dysplastic nevus syndrome

  Dysplastic nevus syndrome was used to designate a familial melanoma family member who had clinically atypical nevi and dysplastic nevi. A member of a familial melanoma family who has clinically atypical nevi or dysplastic nevi or both is stated to be affected by the dysplastic nevus syndrome. The term, dysplastic nevus, has been lifted from its histologic context (it is a histologic term) when used to designate the syndrome.[42] Controversies concerning the term dysplastic nevus syndrome, clinically atypical nevus and familial melanoma have been so vigorous that they form a small industry characterized by divisiveness, a profusion of papers, a plethora of terms for the same entity, seminars and large conferences.[43-48] It would seem unwise to us to continue to use dysplastic nevus syndrome for the following reasons. First, the term implies a common pathway for cutaneous malignant melanoma and dysplastic nevi. This may or may not be true. Both cutaneous malignant melanoma and dysplastic nevi in an individual and in a family are remarkably complex in presentation, histology, and heritable mechanisms. Given such complexity, it is likely that the developmental and even the causal paths of cutaneous malignant melanoma and dysplastic nevi may be intersecting, independent, or overlapping. Secondly, some formal definitions of syndrome state that multiple tissue-organ systems must be involved. Thirdly, familial melanoma may occur without dysplastic nevi, and in this context there can be no relationship between the two lesions.[22] For these reasons, we do not use the term dysplastic nevus syndrome.

In contrast, the histologic term, dysplastic nevus is satisfactory and should be retained for it designates a pivotal lesion of biologic significance, when dysplasia is used as it is in other neoplastic systems. In other neoplastic systems dysplasia designates a class of lesions having considerable propensity for progression to overt cancer. However, even this common usage is associated with controversy that may be quite acrimonious.[49] The controversies are readily understood for dysplasia occurs in the lesions of a grey area in neoplastic development: a vast collection of diverse proliferative lesions that span the broad developmental time zone between induction and cancer. The distal end of the grey area, has lesions that show readily recognizable cytologic atypia, harbors dysplastic lesions. The pathology of the lesions of the distal precursor state is not easy in most neoplastic systems but of great importance, for it informs tumor biology and arguably identifies, with some precision, the lesions and sites most likely to progress to overt cancer.[50,51] In this regard, Antonioli has stated that many conditions such as atrophy and intestinal metaplasia are associated with gastric carcinoma, '... but only epithelial *dysplasia* has a positive predictive value for malignancy.[52] Prominent melanocytic atypia in dysplastic nevi may prove to be as important in melanocytic neoplastic biology and progression as it is in gastric tumor progression and tumor progression in other neoplastic systems. Augustsson et al. found that a single lesion with histologic dysplasia was second only in relative risk for melanoma to ⩾3 clinically dysplastic nevi (clinically atypical nevi).[55] In spite of contrary recommendations, the terms dysplastic nevus and dysplasia should be used, for only such use affords some uniformity in terminology and biologic significance from one neoplastic system to another neoplastic system.

Light in relationship to nevi and melanoma

Many epidemiologic studies of melanoma, addressing inductive factors, have been reported, but, thus far, light is the only exogenous inductive agent consistently identified as of significance.[10,53-56] The role of light in the induction of melanoma is, to say the least, complex. The following categories include only some of the divergent roles light may play as an exogenous factor in the interactive complexities of melanoma causation.[57]

The induction of common nevi by light

Evidence for induction of common nevi by light. As far as we are able to determine, the foregoing clinical and histologic definitions constitute the lesions ⩽4 mm (or ⩽5 mm) in width counted and evaluated histologically in most epidemiologic studies of melanoma. There is an abundance of evidence that light plays a significant role in the induction of such nevi (the common nevi). Clinically atypical nevi and dysplastic nevi will be discussed in a subsequent section. Trained observers studying the skin surface routinely and easily note the presence of nevi in areas exposed to the sun and the virtual absence of nevi in areas usually covered by clothing and rarely exposed to light. Methods used in nevic counts vary widely and comparisons of the counts of nevi in various studies are, consequently, of little value. Until methods and ability of observers are standardized, reliable and consistent counts of nevi will be unusual. Augustsson and her associates, however, have done careful studies on a random sample of Swedish people 30–50 years of age and compared the sample with melanoma cases also 30–50 years of age. Their studies afford quantitation of nevic numbers in relationship to exposure to sunlight. Therefore, we will present the results of their studies in some detail.[53-56,58] We emphasize that the results of other studies are similar but not so readily quantifiable.[59-61]

The Swedish workers (Augustsson, Stierner, Rosdahl, Suurkla) compared a population sample and melanoma cases. The random sample from the census file in Göteborg resulted in 379 subjects (183 men and 196 women) that could be analyzed. 121 melanoma cases (of 197 original cases from the Regional Cancer Register), who were also between 30 and 50 years of age could be analyzed. The main reasons for exclusion of cases from analysis were death and inability to histologically review or confirm the original diagnosis of melanoma. One specific objective of their studies was to investigate the possible role of UV-irradiation in the development of melanocytic nevi. Another objective of their studies was to evaluate both common nevi and dysplastic nevi as risk markers for melanoma. All subjects were evaluated by a single trained dermatologist and a random sample of 20 subjects was assessed by another dermatologist to assure uniformity in diagnosis and counting. The pathology of all cases was reviewed. The evaluation and counting of nevi was done in two parts.

• All subjects had the macular and raised nevi $\geqslant 2$ mm in width, of the entire body surface, counted. If there was difficulty in distinguishing between nevi, lentigines, and freckles, the questionable lesion was not counted.

• A different method was used to carefully distinguish between protected and exposed areas. A protected area 14×28 cm over the buttocks was compared with an exposed area of the same size on the back, 14 cm above the buttock area. The differences between the exposed and protected areas were expressed as the *Ex-Pr* difference.

The major clinical criterion used to define dysplastic nevi was a diameter $\geqslant 5$ mm. (These workers use dysplastic nevus as a clinical as well as a histologic term. They give precise definitions for both the clinical and histologic usage.) In addition to size, at least two of the following criteria were required before a lesion was classified as dysplastic on clinical grounds: an ill-defined or an irregular border, speckled pigmentation, erythema or a pebbled surface. The histological criteria required for classification of a lesion as a dysplastic nevus included:

(a) irregular melanocytic hyperplasia in the basal epidermal layer;

(b) minimal nesting of the increased number of basilar melanocytes;

(c) lentiginous elongation of the rete;

(d) stromal changes including fibrosis and a lymphocytic infiltrate;

(e) a thin dermal nevic component that was not as wide as the epidermal component;

(f) cytologic atypia that was not more prominent than that seen in lentigo maligna.

The criteria are similar to those of Elder and Sagebiel et al. and are not as fully described here as in the original papers.[62-64]

Augustsson and her coworkers have shown a quantitative relationship between light exposure and the number of common nevi. The number of nevi on exposed areas of the body surface was significantly higher than in areas rarely exposed to light. Cutaneous surfaces categorized as having intermittent light exposure (back above the waist, for example) had larger numbers of nevi than chronically exposed areas (face and backs of the hands). Subjects reporting > 3 sunburns had higher total nevus counts than patients with < 3 sunburns. Somewhat surprisingly, chronically exposed areas had about the same number of nevi as areas rarely exposed to light (bathing trunk area and inner aspects of the upper extremity). The 14×28 cm defined area on the back, the exposed area, had more nevi than the protected area of the same size on the buttocks. The total number of nevi and the difference in number of nevi between the two areas was greater in melanoma cases than in controls. Also, the number of nevi in both areas was higher in patients with dysplastic nevi when compared with individuals without dysplastic nevi. Dysplastic nevi did not have the same regional distribution as common nevi, none being recorded on the face and they were uncommon on the extremities. While it is hard to disagree with the compelling evidence relating sun exposure to nevi, there has been a study that denies such a relationship.[65] In that work, however, comparative nevic counts on exposed and protected areas were not done; only nevi on the chest, back and legs were counted and the results were related to anamnestic information concerning sun exposure and exposure to artificial sources of UV-light.

The development of melanocytic nevi without the direct effect of light

There is no question, however that nevi develop without any relationship to the **direct** effects of light. Melanocytic nevi occur in sites with little or no exposure to the direct effects of light. They are relatively common subungually and on the plantar surfaces of blacks and whites, and they are observed in the oral cavity, the vagina, the perineum and in the capsule of lymph nodes.[66-68] The origin of nevi without a discernible relationship to UV-light exposure suggests several areas for future study. Such sites are referred to herein as unusual sites.

- What are the inductive mechanisms for nevi in these sites?
- Are nevi in the unusual sites formal histogenetic precursors of melanoma?
- Do they indicate a precursor state for the unusual site?
- One of the more intriguing thoughts concerning nevi in unusual sites is generated by reflecting on nevi in the capsule of lymph nodes. These nevi are composed of small round, pigment-free nevic cells of the kind seen in the mid-portion of dermal nevi. Standard histogenetic thinking concerning the development of the dermal nevus tells us that its component cells arise from the melanocytes of the epidermis, which then migrate into the dermis and form the various structures that constitute a dermal nevus. Such a mechanism could hardly apply to the nevi in the lymph node capsule. What are its origins? Could true dermal nevi in the skin have histogenetic pathways that are different from our maxims?

Experimentally, melanocytic nevi can be induced by chemical carcinogens.[69,70] Lesions so induced are remarkably similar to common junctional and compound nevi of human skin, and this again attests to the repeated observation that the early manifest lesions of neoplastic systems are similar regardless of the nature of the inductive mechanism.[2,3] Accordingly, nevi in unusual sites could be related to inductive agents and mechanisms other than light. A search for these disparate agents could be fruitful. It would seem especially important to inquire into the nature of pigmented lesions on the plantar surfaces, and to determine whether or not such lesions are a part of a distinctive precursor state of a melanocytic neoplastic system on the sole of the foot. Mishima and Nakanishi have reported a plantar precursor lesion under the term plantar premalignant melanosis, but a systematic epidemiologic and histologic study of the problem of a precursor state or precursor lesions of plantar melanomas has not been done, to our knowledge.[71,72] Plantar malignant melanoma seems to be a different form of the disease than that which occurs over the other cutaneous surfaces and for this reason alone the disease on the sole of the foot warrants careful scrutiny.[73] The paper of Lewis' on melanoma in Uganda specifically addressed the problem of precursor lesions of plantar melanoma. He did not use terms commonly applied to nevi, but adopted a grading system for pigmentation of the sole of the foot.

- Grade I   No pigment seen.
- Grade II   Areas of light brown to dark brown pigment of various sizes, often with irregular outlines.
- Grade III   Discrete, small black areas of pigment with clear-cut margins.

The pigmentation varied with age and from *tribe to tribe*. The feet of children were more or less pigment free. Grade II pigmentation appeared about the time of puberty and became more prominent and common during adolescence. Grade III pigmentation was not commonly observed until the affected individuals were about 20 years of age. Lewis regarded Grade II pigmentation as 'simple melanosis' not related to Grade III pigmentation nor to melanoma. On the other hand he correlated Grade III pigmentation with 'clear cell' hyperplasia and junctional activity. Further, he correlated the site of Grade III pigmentation with sites of plantar melanoma and concluded that Grade III pigmentation was a precursor lesion to plantar melanoma. The observations of Gordon and Henry corroborated Lewis' work.[74] Nevi and melanomas on the sole of the foot have frequently been attributed to trauma to the sole of the foot in the African, but there is little evidence to support this. For one thing plantar melanomas are about as common in whites as in blacks. Even though the vast majority of melanomas in blacks are on the sole of the foot, the incidence of the plantar disease in the two races is probably about the same, at least in North America.[75] If there are differences in incidence of plantar melanoma in different countries and tribes in Africa and if any such differences distinguish the disease from that seen in North American blacks, there would be urgent reasons for appropriate case control studies to tease out suggestions as to causation. In fact, one would hope that future studies of melanoma would focus on disease in unusual sites as being informative of mechanisms important in nevus/melanoma induction other than light and complex heritable factors.

What is a melanocytic nevus?

It is remarkably difficult to answer this question with any confidence that answer is anything but a parroting of conventional wisdom gleaned from any standard text on cutaneous pathology. One problem is the frequently glib assignment by pathologists of pigmented lesions to the categories of lentigo, junctional nevus, compound nevus, and dermal nevus. There are few critical studies of biology, histogenesis, and histology of common nevi. For example, comparative histologic studies of nevi, matched by site, age and sex, in different cutaneous phenotypes could be quite informative. What *are* the differences between nevi located in the scapular area of 16 year old female individuals, one group being black and the other red-haired frecklers? More directly, are there different kinds of common nevi, dependent upon race, inductive mechanisms, or other factors, as yet unknown?

Is a melanocytic nevus a manifestation of 'spottiness'? Exposure to sunlight – depending on such factors as dosage, skin color and the like – will evoke melanocytic and keratinocytic mitogenesis as well as pigment synthesis. The tanning response to light occurs more or less uniformly in an area coextensive with the area of light exposure. In addition, exposure of a large area of the skin surface to light will evoke a mild tanning response in a protected area.[76] By inference, systemic factors may be evoked by cutaneous light exposure, including some that are mitogenic. If light is important in nevogenesis and if the responses to light are more or less uniform in the area exposed to light, why is a nevus a *sharply circumscribed* area having a great increase in melanocytic density? Obviously, a similar question may be asked about the initial manifest lesions of any neoplastic system and answers to the question would cover many topics related to cellular injury and necrosis, and to the nature and quantity of carcinogenic stimuli. Here, we would like to focus speculations on focality to the phenomenon of cutaneous spottiness. The late Ian Whimster wrote with remarkable imagination on this topic.[77,78] Briefly, Whimster showed that many cutaneous diseases, (such as neurofibromas, xanthomas, and the Köbner phenomena) show a 'spotty' quality. When the inductive mechanism is continuous over a given area, say a scratch mark in a patient with psoriasis, the resultant lesions are initially focal (spotty) and not coextensive with the scratch mark. Later the lesions induced by the trauma may or may not become confluent. Whimster posited that spottiness was the result of a response of mosaics forming the skin. He further suggested that there were differential responses between different mosaics, possibly dependent upon neural control. The term mosaicism is most commonly used in a genetic sense today. 'Mosaicism in an individual or in one or more tissues is a condition in which there are two or more cell lines, derived from a single zygote but differing genetically because of post zygotic mutation or nondisjunction.'[78a] Whimster viewed the entire human skin as organ having '...a planned and organized composition built up of initially separate pieces with differing qualities, purposefully chosen and individually placed together so that together they form a picture or pattern, designed to fulfill an intention.' He showed that reptilian skin was clearly so formed and a spot of a given color was fixed at a site. If the spot was excised the healing skin initially showed no spot, but in time the spot returned exactly as it was before surgery. Spots could either be fixed (the red and green scales of the lizard *Phelsuma laticauda*) or they could come and go (the chameleon, *Chamelo dilepsis*), but the coming and going was always in the same spot. He suggested that human skin was a mosaic and that there could be a differential response of its mosaic tiles (if you will) based upon internal factors controlling the mosaic, factors possibly related to the autonomic nervous system. There are studies of genetic mosaicism in relationship to cutaneous and other diseases and these genetic factors may play a role from time to time in unusual patterns of melanocytic nevi, but Whimster was referring to a mosaicism present in the skin of all individuals having a role in disease manifestation. (*See* Happle for a discussion of genetic mosaicism and cutaneous disease.[79]) Jean Bolognia and her associates have given us an excellent discussion of Blaschko's lines and these intriguing structures may have some relationship to the mosaicism discussed by Whimster. In fact, Crelin suggested to Bolognia that the lines could represent the distribution of autonomic motor innervation.[80]

Light and the induction of clinically atypical nevi and dysplastic nevi

Clinically atypical nevi have a body site distribution that differs from common nevi. They are uncommon on the arms when compared with common nevi, while clinically atypical nevi are more frequent on the buttocks than common nevi.[81] We have also noted clinically atypical nevi and dysplastic nevi (histologic dysplasia) commonly on the covered area of the female breast and in the scalp. It is of considerable interest that melanoma is rare on the covered area of the breast of females in the United States and the buttocks of both sexes. The various discrepancies between the site distribution between common nevi, clinically atypical nevi, and melanoma pose several questions.

What is the relationship between common nevi and dysplastic nevi? Dysplasia may develop in a common nevus that has been present for some years. There is no question that classical dysplasia occurs in association with a classical histologic pattern of a common nevus. It is difficult to *prove*, however, that the common nevus preceded the dysplasia. If one assumes the common nevus → dysplastic nevus path to occur in temporal sequence, with a period of quiescence between the two lesions, it follows that the dysplasia is the result of causative mechanisms in addition to those responsible for the common nevus. Consider two different cutaneous phenotypes in support of the foregoing statement. One phenotype is represented by an individual who tans with ease and forms nevi. Many such individuals expose themselves extensively to sunlight and may well have over 100 common nevi, but some individuals with this phenotype, perhaps the majority, do *not* develop dysplasia. Thus, one important nevogenic agent, light, *may* not induce a dysplastic nevus even when the dosage is quite high. In contrast, the second phenotype, frequently burns and tans poorly *and* forms nevi and such nevi may well develop dysplasia. One infers, if not concludes, that the dysplasia developed in this second cutaneous phenotype because of an inherent difference in the skin; a different biological skin from the first phenotype. The difference could well act conjointly with light to induce dysplasia. A further point illuminating differences between ordinary nevi and dysplastic nevi is the natural history of the two lesions. Common nevi do not, as a rule, form after 30 years of age. Dysplastic nevi continue to form in more than 20% of patients > 50 years of age.[82] The foregoing discussion considered light as a force driving nevi to dysplasia. However, 'spontaneous' progression from a common nevus to a dysplastic nevus is a significant possibility, at least on theoretical grounds. Compound nevi have spherical nests of melanocytes at the tips of epidermal rete and nevic cells in the dermis. If one conflates such a histologic picture with the life history of some nevi, one may state that the intraepidermal nests of a compound nevus have a great increase in melanocytic density when compared with the adjacent uninvolved epidermis and such a lesion may have ceased growing. A repetitive theme in neoplastic development is growth, cessation of growth, growth, cessation of growth, growth, cessation of growth....[3,83,84] Foulds' has shown that tumor progression occurs in neoplastic systems during periods of growth cessation. **Foulds' Rule III. Progression is independent of growth.** Progression occurs in latent tumor cells and in tumors whose growth is arrested. Progression without manifest growth may account for long delayed recurrences and metastases. Progression that is independent of growth may also account for the development of cancer in a precursor lesion that had been stable for years. Foulds also states, in discussing the significance of time in neoplastic development, that neoplastic capacity may increase autonomously with time without repeated carcinogenic stimuli.[84] Strauss has presented evidence that mutation may be time dependent rather than replication dependent.[85]

In an elegant series of in vitro experiments using a subline of NIH3T3 cells, Rubin has shown that increased saturation density and growth constraint will induce transformation with tumorigenic foci similar to the effects of ionizing irradiation or chemical carcinogens.[37,86,87] One may suggest that events similar to those observed by Foulds in studying experimental rodent mammary carcinogenesis and events observed by Rubin in his in vitro experiments with fibroblasts, occur, from time to time, during nevic growth and cessation of growth. In such instances, one sees a nest of intraepidermal melanocytes. These nests of a compound nevus show small melanocytes crowded into a compact sphere. When compared with the distribution of melanocytes in the adjacent skin, the lesion manifests increased saturation density and may well have ceased growth (growth constraint). With regrowth, the intraepidermal pattern of melanocytes is entirely different and some of the cells are atypical: dysplasia has followed increased saturation density and one or more periods of growth constraint. If such a mechanism is one of the pathways to the development of dysplasia, it would exemplify progression from a compound nevus to a dysplastic nevus without the necessity of further action of additional exogenous agents. The diverse paths of progression to a dysplastic nevus just discussed, further emphasize the complex and heterogeneous nature of nevi, dysplastic nevi, and melanoma. It is likely that **all** of the paths are operative in the development and progression of the melanocytic neoplastic system.

Dysplasia may arise concomitantly with the development of a common nevus. This histogenetic proposal suggests that a common nevus develops and concomitantly shows dysplasia somewhere within the lesion. Direct observations suggest that this may be a common mechanism of histogenesis of dysplasia. The difficulty with such evidence is that most patients subjected to extensive sequential photography are patients from families with heritable melanoma. Nevertheless, we have photographically documented the development of a nevus that was both common and dysplastic. The site of the lesion was the posterior shoulder of an 8 year old girl. The site was photographed showing no manifest lesion. Sequential photographs showed a continually evolving lesion: initially macular; then elevated centrally with a macular periphery; and, finally, irregularity of the border. When excised the central elevated portion of the lesion was a compound nevus and the periphery of the lesion dysplastic. One cannot **prove** that the common nevus and the dysplastic nevus arose simultaneously, but, in this instance, the two certainly formed a continuum. Such histogenesis implies that the combination of common nevus and dysplastic nevus may develop simultaneously and, in all likelihood, the inductive mechanisms for both forms of nevi were present at the same time. Such mechanisms could be both endogenous and exogenous. In the instance just referred to, the individual was a member of a melanoma family most of whom had a cutaneous phenotype characterized by: numerous clinically atypical nevi and dysplastic nevi, freckles, difficulty in tanning, and ease of sunburn. Common nevi and dysplastic nevi may develop separately from each other, both spatially and temporally. When this occurs, and it would seem to be the most frequent presentation of common and clinically atypical nevi, one may observe a separate population of common nevi, dysplastic nevi, and lesions that are a combination of the two.

What is the relationship between light and dysplastic nevi? In this paper we have reviewed evidence that intermittent light exposure is nevogenic (for common nevi). Is light also an inductive factor for dysplastic nevi? It would seem that both 'Yes' and 'No' are correct answers to the question.

Yes. Weinstock and his associates, as a result of a case control study, stated than sun sensitivity was associated with dysplastic nevus (clinically atypical nevi and dysplastic nevi – 54% showed histologic dysplasia) risk, (clinically atypical nevi and dysplastic nevi – 54% showed histologic dysplasia).[88] Clinical observations showing dysplastic nevi in sites of intermittent sun-exposure provide impressive evidence of a relationship between light and dysplastic nevi.

No. We have previously discussed, in this paper, dysplastic nevi occurring on the buttocks, on the scalp and on the covered area of the breasts (of US women). Dysplastic nevi also occur on the vulva. One may conclude that dysplastic nevi do appear where direct light exposure is minimal or absent.

Is the continuing action of light required as an engine driving common nevi to dysplastic nevi, and, in turn, driving dysplastic nevi to melanoma? The precursor state of many neoplastic systems seems to be driven forward by the continuing action of its initial inductive mechanisms. The best example of this is the effect of tobacco smoke. Cessation of smoking greatly decreases the subsequent incidence of bronchogenic carcinoma. In this regard, the reader should study the experimental work of Iverson. He has shown that very small doses of DMBA stated to have no promoting potency act synergistically as a strong promoter of DMBA-initiated mouse skin.[89] Thus, the continuing action of the inductive agent drove the system down the pathroad of tumor progression.

A critical study has not been done wherein patients with clinically atypical nevi and proven dysplastic nevi are protected from light; and patients, so protected, are subsequently shown to have a decreased incidence of melanoma and changing dysplastic nevi. Tucker and her associates have suggested that additional sun exposure is important in the progression from clinically atypical nevi and dysplastic nevi to melanoma. Family members followed prospectively after the family had been shown to be affected by melanoma had a lower incidence of melanoma after 5 years than during the first 5 years of follow up when compared with the incidence of melanoma in family members prior to knowledge of the family being affected. In addition, those followed prospectively had fewer changing moles and fewer biopsies in the later time periods. Upon questioning, it was discovered that the prospective follow-up group had significantly changed their sun exposure habits early in the follow up; their insolation was definitely decreased.[90]

Light and a cutaneous phenotype incapable of forming nevi

The sun-reactive skin types in common usage are:
  I.   Always burn, never tan
  II. Usually burn, tans with difficulty
  III. Sometimes burns, tans about average
  IV. Rarely burns, tans with ease to deep brown.

There are individuals of types I and II who do not form any nevi. We do not know of any extensive discussion of this phenotype. It is known, however, that such individuals not only develop melanoma, but are at high risk for its development when they have a history of many damaging sunburns. Thus, we have opposed phenotypes: the mucosae and dark brown to black skin form nevi without the direct effects of light and some sun-reactive skin types with significant light exposure cannot form nevi. One may suggest that the latter group has epidermal melanocytes that produce a high level of pheomelanin (aminohydroxyphenylalanine – AHP), as do dysplastic melanocytic nevi.[91] However, work by Salopek et al. indicates that the normal skin of patients with dysplastic nevi had a lower content of pheomelanin than did dysplastic nevi. There are, however, individual cases whose pheomelanin content in their *normal* skin was as high as the median of the dysplastic nevus cases in the Salopek study.[92] In addition, one cannot tell from their data whether or not they studied individuals with a cutaneous phenotype that cannot form nevi. Therefore, there is still a possibility that the 'no-mole' phenotype has a distinctive melanocyte, characterized by pheomelanin synthesis.

FATAL MALIGNANT MELANOMA: PRIMARY MELANOMA AND DISSEMINATED METASTATIC DISEASE

Most studies of prognostic factors indicating a high risk of dissemination and death use attributes of the primary melanoma and attributes of the host bearing that melanoma. These factors are now well known and include such features as mitotic count, thickness, sex of the patient, site of the melanoma and other useful attributes. There are not, however, detailed studies of patients and their primaries when the outcome was death due to disease. If such cases be studied in comparison with nonfatal cases (say matched by thickness, mitotic count, host lymphocytic response, site and sex) will a distinctive group of fatal melanomas emerge? Heenan (unpublished observations and personal communication, 1994) has suggested that there may be a core of 'fatal melanoma' in the cases in Western Australia. In that province both the public and the profession are knowledgeable concerning the early stages of the disease, but the mortality rate has flattened in recent years. It has not declined in spite of identification and treatment of the early, 'thin' melanomas.

PROSPECTIVES FOR THE STUDY OF THE MELANOCYTIC PRECURSOR STATE, PRIMARY MELANOMAS, AND METASTATIC MELANOMA

- What are the inductive mechanisms when light apparently has no direct effect?
  - (a) Do nevi have a different histogenesis and histology in light skin when compared with dark skin?
  - (b) What is the histogenesis of nevi of the mucosae and other uncommon sites, such as the capsules of lymph nodes, when the epithelium has few or no melanocytes or there is no epithelium?
- What alteration of the skin marks the precursor state in interlesional skin?
- What alteration of the skin marks the precursor state when the cutaneous phenotype cannot form common or dysplastic nevi?

- What is the nature of the precursor state when progression to melanoma has been documented?
    - (a) Will this nature, if it can be defined, be unique and partially explain the remarkable rarity of progression from the precursor state to overt melanoma?
- What is an atypical cell in a precursor lesion?
    - (a) Does such an atypical cell differ from the cells of an overt melanoma?
    - (b) Are atypical cells required for melanoma to develop?
- What are the defining characteristics of acral lentiginous and mucosal melanoma?
    - (a) What is the precursor state for these distinctive forms of melanoma?
- What is the nature of primary melanomas that lead to disseminated disease?
    - (a) Is this a subset of melanomas awaiting delineation?
- Should we all revisit Whimster and the lizard's tail?

HERITABILITY. WHAT IS INHERITED IN FAMILIAL SYSTEMS?

Consider the following aspects of malignant melanoma.
- The interaction of light with white skin of an individual for the first 30 years of life may result in the following different manifestations in the epidermal melanocytic system. The list is partial and does not include tanning or changes in the dermal connective tissue.

> No clinically manifest lesions.
> Freckles, no moles.
> Freckles and moles.
> Common nevi.
> Common nevi and clinically atypical nevi.
> Common nevi, clinically atypical nevi, and dysplastic nevi.

*Malignant melanoma.

> *Lentigo maligna type*
> *Superficial spreading type*
> *Nodular type.*

- Malignant melanoma and nevi occur in sites without a direct effect of light: oral mucous membrane, vaginal mucous membrane, the capsule of lymph nodes, leptomeninges, urinary bladder, gall bladder, hepatic and common bile ducts, esophagus, anus, and other sites.

- Nevi and melanomas occur on the plantar surfaces of blacks, as do nevi. Nevi and melanomas may or may not be related in these sites. The incidence of plantar nevi in Uganda varies from tribe to tribe.

- The incidence of melanoma is exquisitely rare when compared with the number of nevi.

If one merges the preceding lists with the fact that no 2 melanomas are alike (as no 2 multicellular organisms are alike[93]) and the fact that only some 8–12% of melanomas are familial, what, from the infinite (the term is used literally) maze of phenomena, is inherited?[94] Even if one adds reasonable constraints to both the speculations and the questions, and addresses only familial melanoma (two or more first degree relatives affected), the problem of heritability in melanocytic neoplasia (and any form of cancer) is still incomprehensibly complex. A common history of melanocytic neoplastic evolution may be seen in children whose families are affected by familial melanoma. The initial manifestation is the appearance of nevi, which arise, enlarge and may merge imperceptibly into clinically atypical nevi and dysplastic nevi (when examined microscopically). Such individuals may not progress to melanoma. Did these children only inherit a predisposition to the development of nevi, clinically atypical nevi, and dysplastic nevi? If so what kind of gene product could be responsible for such a predisposition? Other children, siblings indeed, may have a similar history of nevic emergence and evolution *and* develop melanoma? Did such children have a different genetic heritability or did environmental factors drive their nevi into melanoma? Then, there are familial melanoma families without clinically atypical nevi or dysplastic nevi.[22] Did they inherit a predisposition to melanoma only? The complexities do not end and cannot be explained by the product of a single susceptibility gene. If such genes are shown to actually exist they are can be but *markers* of a disorder. Their products are not autonomous forces driving the system. From the foregoing description of the different presentations of familial melanoma, one would assume that the disease is heterogeneous. In fact, a variety of genetic studies confirm this.

Familial melanoma

Two of the authors (AMG, MAT) have recently reviewed the genetic epidemiology of familial melanoma.[95] Different methods are used to demonstrate genetic factors, including the study of tumor tissue for changes in chromosomes, oncogenes, tumor suppressor genes, DNA repair genes, genes controlling the cell cycle (molecular check point genes), and linkages studies. Herlyn has recently reviewed abnormalities in chromosomes, oncogenes, and tumor suppressor genes.[96] Here, we shall discuss linkage studies. In 1989, Bale and her associates demonstrated linkage of a combined cmm/dn (cutaneous malignant melanoma/dysplastic nevus) trait to chromosome 1p markers d1s47 and pnd. One important criticism of Bale's work was that the objective phenotype of cutaneous malignant melanoma, alone, was not linked to 1p. Although controversy about the matter still exists, linkage of cutaneous malignant melanoma without dysplastic nevi, as a phenotype, has been linked to 1p.[97] Subsequent studies by Cannon-Albright et al and Nancarrow, et al showed linkage of a familial melanoma locus (mlm) to chromosome region 9p13–9p22 near interferon-α (INFA) and d9si26.[98,99] Quite recent studies by Cannon-Albright and her associates have placed the mlm locus to a 2-cM region between D9S736 and D9S171.[100] A study of the estimated power to detect linkage in different data sets indicated that the discrepant findings in the data sets were likely to be due to genetic heterogeneity rather than spurious results.[101] The p16 CDKN2 gene, a strong candidate for a melanoma tumor suppressor gene, has been localized to 9p21 in the region implicated in melanoma in linkage, cytogenetic and heterozygosity studies.[102] The candidate gene binds to cyclin dependent kinase 4 and, thus, inhibits the activity of certain cell cycle enzymes. In this capacity it may affect the balance between functional p16 and cyclin D and alter growth control. However, the demonstration of involvement of the p16 gene (CDKN2) has been shown in only a fraction of cases.[103] If the p16 gene should actually be shown to be a melanoma tumor suppressor gene in the fraction of cases, its action(s) would fail to explain but the smallest portion of the manifest and manifold phenomena of the disease. Many studies of oncogenes and tumor suppressor genes have only addressed *growth* in neoplastic systems. However, neoplastic systems are characterized by growth and cessation of growth in repetitive cycles covering years of neoplastic development and progression. Further, the appearance of strikingly atypical cells, some indistinguishable from many cells in fully evolved cancers, apparently occurs in the precursor state during periods of growth cessation. The emergence of such atypical cells precedes fully evolved cancer by years (in human systems).

Presently, it must be concluded that linkage studies show significant evidence of heterogeneity, with some showing linkage to 1p, others to 9p and others without demonstrable linkage. Explanations for genetic heterogeneity include the strong possibility that the disease is actually heterogeneous. We would be surprised if a disorder as complex as melanocytic neoplasia (or any neoplastic system, for that matter) would or could have a monogenic explanation. Monogenic explanations (or searches for *a* cause or *an* etiology) for neoplastic disease seem to reflect the human mind entrapped in a theoretical and historical prison of reductionism, and also entrapped in the contemporary fashion for molecular explanations, rather than a human mind curiously probing the natural history of a disease as it actually occurs.[3,104]

ACKNOWLEDGEMENT

This work was supported by grants from the National Cancer Institute, USA: CA-58845 and CA-25298.

REFERENCES

1 Clark WH. Tumour progression and the nature of cancer. Brit J Cancer 1991; 64: 631–644.
2 Clark WH, Jr. The role of tumor progression in prevention of cancer and reduction of cancer mortality. In: Greenwald P, Kramer BS, Weed DL, eds. Cancer prevention and control. New York: Marcel-Dekker, Inc., 1994: 135–160.
3 Clark WH, Jr. The nature of cancer: Morphogenesis and progressive (self)-disorganization in neoplastic development and progression. Acta Oncol 1994 (In press).
4 Guerry D, Synnestvedt M, Elder DE, Schultz D. Lessons from tumor progression – the invasive radial growth phase of melanoma is common, incapable of metastasis, and indolent. J Invest Dermatol 1993; 100: S342–S345.
5 Clark WH, Jr., Elder DE, Guerry DI et al. Model predicting survival in stage I melanoma based on tumor progression. J Natl Cancer Inst. 1989; 81: 1893–1904.
6 MacKie RM, Freudenberger T, Aitchison TC. Personal risk-factor chart for cutaneous melanoma. Lancet 1989; 2: 487–490.
7 Østerlind A, Tucker MA, Hou-Jensen K, Stone BJ, Engholm G, Jensen OM. The Danish case-control study of cutaneous malignant melanoma. I. Importance of host factors. Int J Cancer 1988; 42: 200–206.
8 Østerlind A. Epidemiology on malignant melanoma in Europe. Acta Oncol 1992; 31: 903–908.
9 Lee JAH. The melanoma epidemic thus far. Mayo Clinic Proc 1990; 65: 1368–1371.
10 Armstrong BK, Kricker A. Cutaneous melanoma. Cancer Surveys 1994; 20: 219–240.
11 Holly EA, Kelly JW, Shpall SN, Chiu S-H. Number of melanocytic nevi as a major risk factor for malignant melanoma. J Am Acad Dermatol 1987; 17: 459–468.
12 Clark WH, Reimer RR, Greene M, Ainsworth AM, Mastrangelo MJ. Origin of familial malignant melanomas from heritable melanocytic lesions. The B-K mole syndrome. Arch Dermatol 1978; 114: 732–738.
13 Elder DE, Clark WH,, Elenitsas R, Guerry DI, Halpern AC. The early and

intermediate precursor lesions of tumor progression in the melanocytic system: Common acquired nevi and atypical (dysplastic) nevi. In: Cochran A, ed. Seminars in Diagnostic Pathology 1993: 18–35.

14 Grob JJ, Gouvernet J, Aymar D et al. Count of benign melanocytic nevi as a major indicator of risk for nonfamilial nodular and superficial spreading melanoma. Cancer 1990; 66: 387–395.

15 Rigel DS, Rivers JK, Kopf AK et al. Dysplastic nevi. Markers for increased risk for melanoma. Cancer 1989; 63: 386–389.

16 Halpern AC, Guerry D, Elder DE et al. Dysplastic nevi as risk markers of sporadic (nonfamilial) melanoma – a case-control study. Arch Dermatol 1991; 127: 995–999.

17 Halpern AC, Guerry D, Elder DE, Trock B, Synnestvedt M. A cohort study of melanoma in patients with dysplastic nevi. J Invest Dermatol 1993; 100: S346–S349.

18 Bale SJ, Goldstein AM, Tucker MA. Description of the National Cancer Institute Melanoma Families. Cytogenet Cell Genet 1992; 59: 159–160.

19 Bergman W, Gruis NA, Frants RR. The Dutch FAMMM Family Material – Clinical and Genetic Data. Cytogenet Cell Genet 1992; 59: 161–164.

20 Dracopoli NC, Bale SJ, Fountain JW. Genetic analysis of familial melanoma. In: Brandi ML, White R, eds. Hereditary Tumors. New York: Raven Press, 19??; 39–45.

21 Goldstein AM, Fraser MC, Clark WH, Tucker MA. Age at diagnosis and transmission of invasive melanoma in 23 families with cutaneous malignant melanoma dysplastic nevi. J Nat Cancer Inst 1994; 86: 1385–1390.

22 Salmon JA, Rivers JK, Donald JA, Shaw HM, Mccarthy WH, Kefford RF. Clinical Aspects of Hereditary Melanoma in Australia. Cytogenet Cell Genet 1992; 59: 170–172.

23 Weinstock MA, Colditz GA, Willett WC et al. Melanoma and the sun – The effect of swimsuits and a healthy tan on the risk of nonfamilial malignant melanoma in women. Am J Epidemiol 19??; 134: 462–470.

24 Westerdahl J, Olsson H, Ingvar C, Brandt L, Jonsson PE, Moller T. Southern travelling habits with special reference to tumour site in Swedish melanoma patients. Anticancer Res 1992; 12: 1539–1542.

25 White E, Kirkpatrick CS, Lee JAH. Case-control of malignant melanoma in Washington State .1 Constitutional factors and sun exposure. Am J Epidemiol 19??; 139: 857–868.

26 Koh HK, Kligler BE, Lew RA. Sunlight and cutaneous melanoma: Evidence for and against causation. Photochem Photobiol 1990; 51: 765–779.

27 Gallagher RP, McLean DI, Yang P et al. Suntan, sunburn, pigmentation factors and the frequency of acquired melanocytic nevi in children. Similarities to melanoma: The Vancouver mole study. Arch Dermatol 1990; 126: 770–776.

28 Foulds L. Neoplastic Development. New York: Academic Press, 1969: 81.

29 Yaar M, Woodley DT, Gilchrist BA. Human nevocellular nevus cells are surrounded by basement membrane components. Immunohistologic studies of human nevus cells and melanocytes in vivo and in vitro. Lab Invest 1988; 58: 157–162.

30 Stolz W, Schmoeckel C, Landthaler M, Braun-Falco O. Association of early malignant melanoma with nevocytic nevi. Cancer 1989; 63: 550–555.

31 . Sagebiel RW. Melanocytic nevi in histologic association with primary cutaneous melanoma of superficial spreading and nodular types – effect of tumor thickness. J Invest Dermatol 1993; 100: S322–S325.

32 Weinstock MA, Colditz GA, Willett WC et al. Moles and site-specific risk of nonfamilial cutaneous malignant melanoma in women. J Natl Cancer Inst 1989; 81: 948–952.

33 Gallagher RP, Rivers JK, Yang CP, Mclean DI, Coldman AJ, Silver HKB. Melanocytic nevus density in Asian, Indo-Pakistani, and white children – The Vancouver mole study. J Am Acad Dermatol 1991; 25: 507–512.

34 Pope DJ, Sorahan T, Marsden JR, Ball PM, Grimley RP, Peck IM. Benign pigmented nevi in children – prevalence and associated factors – the West Midlands, United Kingdom mole study. Arch Dermatol 1992; 128: 1201–1206.

35 English DR, Armstrong B. Identifying people at high risk of cutaneous malignant melanoma: results from a case-control study in Western Australia. BMJ 1988; 296: 1285–1288.

36 Foulds L. Neoplastic Development. London and New York: Academic Press, 1969: p 44.

37 Rubin H. Incipient and overt stages of neoplastic transformation. Proc Natl Acad Sci USA 1994 (In press).

38 Kennedy AR, Fox M, Murphy G, Little JB. Relationship between X-ray exposure and malignant transformation in C3H 10T1/2 cells. Proc Natl Acad Sci USA 1980; 77: 7262–7266.

39 Kennedy AR, Cairns J, Little JB. Timing in the steps in transformation of C3H 10T1/2 cells by X-irradiation. Nature 1984; 307: 85–86.

40 Mondal S, Heidelberger C. In vitro malignant transformation by methylcholanthrene of the progeny of single cells derived from the C3H mouse prostate. Proc Natl Acad Sci USA 1970; 65: 219–229.

41 Clark WH Jr., Elder DE, Guerry D. IV. Dysplastic nevi and malignant melanoma. In: Farmer ER, Hood AF, editors. Pathology of the skin. Norwalk, Connecticut: Appleton & Lange, 1990: 684–756.

42 Greene MH. Dysplastic nevus syndrome. Hospital Practice January,1984: 91–108 43 Consensus Statement. National Institutes of Health. Diagnosis and treatment of early melanoma. NIH Consensus development conference 1992; 10: 1–26.

44 Greene MH, Fraser MC, Clark WH Jr, Elder DE, Guerry D IV, Kraemer KH. For the record: The history of precursors to malignant melanoma. Arch Dermatol 1984; 120: 18–19.

45 Greene MH. Rashomon and the Procrustean bed - A tale of dysplastic nevi. J Natl Cancer Inst 1991; 83: 1720–1724.

46 Frichot BCIII, Lynch HT, Guirgis HA, Harris RE, Lynch JF. A new cutaneous phenotype in familial melanoma. Lancet 1977; 1: 864–865.

47 Lynch HT, Frichot BCIII, Lynch JF. Familial atypical multiple mole-melanoma syndrome. J Med Genetics 1978; 15: 352–356.

48 de Wit PEJ, Vanthofgrootenboer B, Ruiter DJ et al. Validity of the histopathological criteria used for diagnosing dysplastic naevi – an interobserver study by the pathology subgroup of the EORTC malignant melanoma cooperative group. Eur J Cancer 1993; 29A: 831–839.

49 Pascal RR. Consistency in the terminology of colorectal dysplasia. Human Pathol 1988; 19: 1240–1250.

50 You WC, Blot WJ, Chang YS et al. Comparison of the anatomic distribution of stomach cancer and precancerous gastric lesions. Jpn J Cancer Res 1992; 83: 1150–1153.

51 Farinati F, Rugge M, Dimario F, Valiante F, Baffa R. Early and advanced gastric cancer in the follow-up of moderate and severe gastric dysplasia patients – a prospective study. Endoscopy 1993; 25: 261–264.

52 Antonioli DA. Precursors of gastric carcinoma: A critical review with a brief description of early (curable) gastric carcinoma. Human Pathol 1994; 25: 994–1005.

53 Augustsson A. Melanocytic nevi, melanoma and sun exposure [dissertation]. Göteborg, Sweden: Department of Dermatology, University of Göteborg, Göteborg, Sweden; Graphic Systems AB, Göteborg 1991.

54 Augustsson A. Melanocytic naevi, melanoma and sun exposure. Acta Derm Venereol (Stockh) 1991; S166: 2–34.

55 Augustsson A, Stierner U, Rosdahl I, Suurkula M. Common and dysplastic naevi as risk factors for cutaneous malignant melanoma in a Swedish population. Acta Derm Venereol (Stockh) 1991; 71: 518–524.

56 Augustsson A, Stierner U, Rosdahl I, Suurkula M. Melanocytic naevi in sun-exposed and protected skin in melanoma patients and controls. Acta Derm Venereol (Stockh) 1991; 71: 512–517.
57 Stierner U. Melanocytes, moles, and melanoma [dissertation]. Göteborg, Sweden: University of Göteborg; 1991.
58 Augustsson A, Stierner U, Rosdahl I, Suurkula M. Regional distribution of melanocytic nevi in relation to sun exposure, and site-specific counts predicting total number of naevi. Acta Derm Venereol (Stockh) 1992; 72: 123–127.
59 Green A, Swerdlow AJ. Epidemiology of melanocytic nevi. Epidemiologic Rev 1989; 11: 204–221.
60 English DR, Armstrong BK. Melanocytic nevi in children .1 Anatomic sites and demographic and host factors. Am J Epidemiol 1994; 139: 390–401.
61 Coombs BD, Sharples KJ, Cooke KR, Skegg DCG, Elwood JM. Variation and covariates of the number of benign nevi in adolescents. Am J Epidemiol 1992; 136: 344–355.
62 Elder D. The dysplastic nevus. Pathol 1985; 17: 291–297.
63 Sagebiel RW, Banda PW, Schneider JS, Crutcher WA. Age distribution and histologic patterns of dysplastic nevi. J Am Acad Dermatol 1985; 13: 975–982.
64 Augustsson A, Stierner U, Suurkula M, Rosdahl I. Prevalence of common and dysplastic naevi in a Swedish population. Br J Dermatol 1991; 124: 152–156.
65 Rampen FHJ, Fleuren BAM, de Boo TM, Lemmens WAJ. Prevalence of common 'acquired' nevocytic nevi and dysplastic nevi is not related to ultraviolet exposure. J Am Acad Dermatol 1988; 18: 679–683.
66 Buchner A, Leider AS, Merrill PW, Carpenter WM. Melanocytic nevi of the oral mucosa: a clinicopathologic study of 130 cases from northern California. J Oral Pathol Med 1990; 19: 197–201.
67 Johnson WT, Helwig EG. Benign nevus cells in the capsule of lymph nodes. Cancer 1969; 23: 747–753.
68 Hruban RH, Eckert F, Baricevic B. Melanocytes of a melanocytic nevus in a lymph node from a patient with a primary cutaneous melanoma associated with a small congenital nevus. Am J Dermatopathol 1990; 12: 402–407.
69 Pawlowski A, Lea PJ. Nevi and melanoma induced by chemical carcinogens in laboratory animals: similarities and differences with human lesions. J Cutaneous Pathol 1983; 10: 81–110.
70 Pawlowski A, Haberman HF, Menon A. Junctional and compound pigmented nevi induced by 9, 10–dimethyl-1,2–benzanthracene in skin of albino guinea pigs. Cancer Res 1976; 36: 2813–2821.
71 Mishima Y, Nakanishi T. Acral lentiginous melanoma and its precursor – Heterogeneity of palmo-plantar melanomas. Pathol 1985; 17: 258–265.
72 Umeda M, Mishima Y, Teranobu O, Nakanishi K, Shimada K. Heterogeneity of primary malignant melanomas in oral mucosa: An analysis of 43 cases in Japan. Pathology 1988; 20: 234–241.
73 Dwyer PK, Mackie RM, Watt DC, Aitchison TC. Plantar malignant melanoma in a white Caucasian population. Br J Dermatol 1993; 128: 115–120.
74 Gordon JA, Henry SA. Pigmentation of the sole of the foot in Rhodesian Africans. S A Med J 1971; 45: 88–91.
75 Stevens NG, Liff JM, Weiss NS. Plantar melanoma: Is the incidence of melanoma of the sole of the foot really higher in blacks than whites? Int J Cancer 1990; 45: 691–693.
76 Stierner U, Rosdahl I, Augustsson A, KŒgedal B. UVB irradiation induces melanocyte increase in both exposed and shielded human skin. J Invest Dermatol 1989; 92: 561–564.
77 Whimster IW. The mosaic nature of pigmentary change in diseased skin. Ann Ital Dermatol Clin Sperimentali 1960; 16: 357–384.
78 Whimster IW. An experimental approach to the problem of spottiness. Brit J Dermatol 1965; 77: 397–420.
78a Thompson MW, McInnes RR, Willard HF. Thompson & Thompson Genetics in Medicine. Philadelphia: Saunder. Harcourt Brace Jonavich Inc. 1991: p 436.

79 Happle R. Mosaicism in human skin – understanding the patterns and mech-
    anisms. Arch Dermatol 1993 Nov; 129: 1460–1470.
80 Bolognia JL, Orlow SJ, Glick SA. Lines of Blaschko. J Am Acad Dermatol 1994;
    31: 157–190.
81 Stierner U, Augustsson A, Rosdahl I, Suurküla. Regional distribution of com-
    mon and dysplastic naevi in relation to melanoma site and sun exposure. A case-
    control study. Melanoma Research 1991; 1: 367–375.
82 Halpern AC, Guerry D, Elder DE, Trock B, Synnestvedt M, Humphreys T.
    Natural history of dysplastic nevi. J Am Acad Dermatol 1993; 29: 51–57.
83 Rubin H. Experimental control of neoplastic progression in cell populations:
    Foulds' rules revisited. Proc Natl Acad Sci USA 1994; 91: 6619–6623.
84 Foulds L. Neoplastic Development. New York: Academic Press, 1969: pp. 69–
    75.
85 Strauss BS. The origin of point mutations in human tumor cells. Cancer Res
    1992; 52: 249–253.
86 Rubin H. Experimental control of neoplastic progression in cell populations:
    Foulds' rules revisited. Proc Natl Acad Sci USA 1994; 91: 6619–6623.
87 Rubin H. Cellular epigenetics: Effect of passage history on competence of cells
    for 'spontaneous' transformation. Proc Natl Acad Sci USA 1993; 90: 10715–
    10719.
88 Weinstock MA, Stryker WS, Stampfer MJ, Lew RA, Willett WC, Sober AJ.
    Sunlight and dysplastic nevus risk. Results of a clinic-based case-control study.
    Cancer 1991; 67: 1701–1706.
89 Iversen OH. A course of very small doses of DMBA, each of them with allegedly
    no promoting potency, acts with clear synergistic effect as a strong promoter of
    DMBA-initiated mouse skin carcinogenesis. APMIS 1994; 102, Supplementum
    No. 41: 1–38.
90 Tucker MA, Fraser MC, Goldstein AM, Elder DE, Guerry D, Organic SM. Risk
    of melanoma and other cancers in melanoma-prone families. J Invest Dermatol
    1993; 100: S350–S355.
91 Jimbow K, Lee SK, King MG, Hara H, Chen H, Dakour J, Marusyk H. Melanin
    pigments and melanosomal proteins as differentiation markers unique to normal
    and neoplastic melanocytes. J Invest Dermatol 1993; 100: S259–S268.
92 Salopek TG, Yamada K, Ito S, Jimbow K. Dysplastic melanocytic nevi contain
    high levels of pheomelanin: Quantitative comparison of pheomelanin/eumelanin
    levels between normal skin, common nevi, and dysplastic nevi. Pigment Cell Res
    1991; 4: 172–179. (See Fig. 1).
93 Elsasser WM. Reflections on a theory of organisms. Quebec, Canada: Editions
    Orbis, 1987:
94 Clark WH Jr. What is inherited in neoplastic systems? Animal models of
    cutaneous malignant melanoma. Lab Invest 1994; 71: 1–4.
95 Goldstein AM, Tucker MA. Genetic epidemiology of familial melanoma. Derm-
    atol Clin 1994 (In press).
96 Herlyn M. Molecular and cellular biology of melanoma. Austin, Texas: R.G.
    Landis Co., 1993.
97 Goldstein AM, Dracopoli NC, Ho EC et al. Further evidence for a locus for
    cutaneous malignant melanoma-dysplastic nevus (CMM/DN) on chromosome
    1p and evidence for genetic heterogeneity. Am J Hum Genet 1993; 52: 537–550.
98 Cannon-Albright LA, Goldgar DE, Meyer LJ. Science 1992; 258: 1148–1152.
99 Nancarrow DJ, Mann GJ, Holland EA et al. Confirmation of chromosome-9P
    linkage in familial melanoma. Am J Hum Genet 1993; 53: 936–942.
100 Cannon-Albright LA, Goldgar DE, Neuhausen S et al. Localization of the 9p
    melanoma susceptibility locus (MLM) to a 2–cM region between D9S736 and
    D9S171 Genomics 1994; 23: 265–268.
101 Prenger VL, Colyer CR, Mellen BG, Harris EL, Beaty TH, Meyers DA. Esti-
    mated power to detect linkage in three CM/DN data sets. Cytogenet Cell Genet
    1992; 59: 220–222.

102 Serrano M, Hannon GJ, Beach D. A new regulatory motif in cell-cycle control causing specific inhibition of cyclin D/CDK4 Nature 1993; 366: 704–707.

103 Ohta M, Nagai H, Shimizu M et al. Rarity of somatic and germline mutations of the cyclin-dependent kinase 4 inhibitor gene, CDK4I, in melanoma. Cancer Res 19??; 54: 5269–5272.

104 Strohman R. Epigenesis: The missing beat in technology. Bio/Technology 1994; 12: 156–164.

British Medical Bulletin (1995) Vol. 51, No. 3, pp. 747–753
© The British Council 1995

Key references

I R Hart, S B Kaye, R M Mackie and D S Soutar

Autier P, Dore JF, Schifflers E, *et al.* **Melanoma and use of sunscreens: an EORTC case control study in Germany, Belgium and France.** Int J Cancer 1995; 61: 1–7.
An important case, control study which suggests that use of sunscreens does not protect against melanoma, but is indeed a risk factor for the development of melanoma. Furthermore the use of psoralen containing sunscreens (now banned) appears to be associated with greater risk than with other types of sunscreens. This is an important paper in terms of the public health message which must be delivered regarding sensible and safe sun exposure.

Bajetta E, Dileo A, Zampino M, *et al.* **Multicentre randomized trial of dacarbazine alone or in combination with 2 different doses and schedules of interferon alpha-2a in treatment of advanced melanoma.** J Clin Oncol 1994; 12: 806–811.

Balch CM, Urist MM, Karakousis CP, Smith TJ, Temple WJ, Drwewiecki K, *et al.* **Efficacy of 2 cm surgical margins for intermediate thickness melanoma (1 to 4 mm). Results of a multi-institutional randomised surgical trial. Narrow excision (1 cm).** Ann Surg 1993; 218: 262–267.
This prospective multi-institutional randomised trial is based on 486 patients with intermediate thickness (1–4 mm thick) primary cutaneous malignant melanoma. Controversy surrounding this paper concerns the relatively short follow up (median 72 months) and the additional randomization regarding treatment of regional lymph nodes.

Binder M, Scharz M, Winkler A *et al.* **Epiluminescence microscopy.** Arch Dermatol 1995; 131: 286–291.
A useful review of this technique which in the hands of the expert is probably of value in differentiating melanocytic from non-melanocytic lesions. However, recent studies have suggested that in the hands of the non-expert it can actually decrease rather than increase pre-operative accuracy.

Brichard V, Van Pel A, Wolfel T, et al. **The tyrosinase gene codes for an antigen recognised by autologous cytolytic T lymphocytes on HLA-A2 melanomas.** J Exp Med 1993; 178: 489–495.
Reports on the cloning of a cDNA encoding an antigen recognised by cytolytic T lymphocytes, stimulated with autologous tumour cells, isolated from melanoma patients. The cDNA was shown to code for tyrosinase suggesting that this enzyme, which directs melanin biosynthesis and whose expression is limited to melanocytes, may constitute a selective target for anti-melanoma immunotherapy.

Burden AD, Vestey JP, Sirel JM *et al.* **Multiple primary malignant melanoma risk factors and prognostic implications.** BMJ 1994; 309: 375–376.
A useful study of 45 patients who developed multiple primary melanomas from a population of 38,018. Readers should be aware that patients with thin melanomas are at greater risk of a second primary than of developing recurrence from a thin melanoma.

Burton RC, Armstrong BK. **Recent incidents trends imply a non-metastatizing form of invasive melanoma.** Melanoma Res 1994; 4: 107–113.
*An intriguing and well argued paper which suggests that in the Hunter Valley of New South Wales the recent very steep increase in the incidence of thinner melanomas may include a **proportion** of tumours which do not have the capacity to metastasize. It is difficult to prove this hypothesis but, if true, it is important in terms of generating unnecessary work with early detection campaigns which result only in the removal of thin tumours and not in a reduction in the numbers of thick tumours removed.*

Cascinelli N, Krutmann J, MacKie R, *et al.* **Sun lamps UVA and risk of skin cancer.** Eur J Cancer 1994; 30A: 548–560.
A useful account reporting on the importance of sun exposure UVA lamps and the risk of skin cancer.

Cox AL, Skipper J, Chen Y, et al. **Identification of a peptide recognised by five melanoma-specific human cytotoxic T cell lines.** Science 1994; 264: 716–719.
The extraction and fractionation of peptides from HLA-A2.1 molecules was followed by screening with melanoma-specific cytotoxic T lymphocytes to identify particular peptide epitopes. Tandem mass spectrometry was then used to sequence this nine-residue peptide which could constitute a promising candidate for use in peptide-based vaccination protocols.

Franceschi S, Vecchia CL, Lucchini F. Cristofolini M. **The epidemiology of cutaneous malignant melanoma: aetiology and European data.** Eur J Cancer Prevention 1991; 1: 9–22.
A useful review by the Italian group of the steadily increasing incidence of malignant melanoma in European countries.

Fritschi L. McHenry P, Green A *et al.* **Naevi in school children in Scotland and Australia.** Br J Dermatol 1994; 130: 599–603.
This useful study of III Australian children and 222 Scottish children clearly demonstrate that by the early teenage years the Australian children have larger numbers of naevi than their Scottish counterparts. As naevi are the most important known risk factor for malignant melanoma, this observation has implications with regard to primary prevention of melanoma and education of young children and their parents.

Karakonsis C, Blumenson L *et al.* **Adjuvant chemotherapy with a nitrosourea based protocol in advanced malignant melanoma.** Eur J Cancer 1993; 29A: 1831–1835.
*Total of 173 patients with completely resected regional or distant metastases randomized to observation or adjuvant chemotherapy with BCNU actinomycin D and vincristine. A significant (P = 0.03) difference in progression-free survival, but **not** overall survival was seen. The authors postulate that additional immunotherapy might be the next step.*

Kawakami Y, Eliyahu, Delgado CH, et al. **Cloning of the gene coding for a shared human melanoma antigen recognised by autologous T cells infiltrating into tumor.** Proc Natl Acad Sci USA 1994; 91: 3515–3519.
Using similar approaches to those outlined in the paper by Brichard et al. (1993) these authors have isolated a gene encoding a melanocyte lineage-specific protein (MART-1; melanoma antigen recognised by T cells 1) which they also suggest could be useful for establishing immunotherapeutic protocols.

Khayat D, Borel C. Towani J *et al.* **Sequential chemoimmunotherapy with cisplatin, interleukin-2 and interferon alpha-2a for metastatic melanoma.** J Clin Oncol 1993; 11: 2173–2180.
Total of 39 patients with metastatic melanoma, 79% previously treated with chemotherapy. The response rate was a remarkable 54% (including 5 complete responses) and the toxicity was `manageable'.

Krementz ET, Carter DL, Sutherland CM, Muchmore JH, Ryan CF, Creech O. **Regional chemotherapy for melanomas. A 35-year experience.** Ann Surg 1994; 220: 520-538.
This paper reports an extensive study of 1139 patients with malignant melanoma treated between 1957 and 1992. Cumulative 10 year survival figures are given together with indications for isolated limb perfusion based on their extensive experience.

Lee SM, Margison G, Woodcock A and Thatcher N. **Sequential administration of varying doses of dacarbazine and fotemustine in advanced malignant melanoma.** Br J Cancer 1993; 67: 1356–1360.
Total of 60 patients treated with escalating doses of DTIC followed by fotemustine, aimed at synergism based on ATase depletion. Overall 30% response rate, and increasing toxicity seen with increasing DTIC doses.

Lejeune F, Bauer J. Leyvraz S, *et al.* **Disseminated melanoma, preclinical therapeutic studies, clinical trials and patient treatment.** Curr Opin Oncol 1993; 5: 390–396.
A useful overview of a number of areas with recommended references including 1992.

MacKie RM, Aitchison T, Sirel JM et al. **Prognostic models for subgroups of melanoma patients from the Scottish Melanoma Group Database 1979-86, and their subsequent validation.** Br J Cancer 1995; 71: 173–176.
A study based on 1978 patients which uses prognostic data to develop charts to enable the working physician to more accurately compute prognosis for individual patients once the age, sex, site and tumour thickness of the melanoma is made available.

MacKie RM, McHenry P, Hole D. **Accelerated detection with prospective surveillance for cutaneous malignant melanoma in high-risk groups.** Lancet 1993; 341: 1618–1620.
A useful surveillance study of 116 patients at increased risk of developing malignant melanoma. The important point here is that 3 or more atypical naevi increased the relative risk on a factor of times 90, and that a family history of melanoma in association with such naevi increases the relative risk by times 400. Useful information for follow-up and possibly for screening strategies.

McCarthy WH, Shaw HM, Cascinelli N, Santinami M, Belli F. **Elective lymph node dissection for melanoma: Two perspectives.** World J Surg 1992; 10: 203–213.
This paper highlights the differences in opinion between surgeons in Europe and those in the United States and Australia surrounding the efficacy of elective regional lymph node dissection.

Meisenberg B, Ross M. Voedenburgh T *et al.* **Randomized trial of high dose chemotherapy with autologous bone marrow support as adjuvant therapy for high-risk multi-node positive malignant melanoma.** J Nat Cancer Inst 1993; 85: 1080–1085.
Total of 39(!) patients randomized to observation or immediate high dose chemotherapy with cisplatin, BCNU and cyclophosphamide. The trial was terminated much too early; a non-significant doubling of median time to progression (16 weeks versus 35 weeks) was seen, and the danger of extrapolating from this very small study is the main message.

Moriwaki S, Nishigori C, Takebe H and Imamura S. **O^6-alkylguanine-DNA alkyltransferase activity in human malignant melanoma.** J Dermat Science 1992; 4: 610.
Levels of O^6-Agt documented in 13 patients with melanoma. These varied widely, but were generally higher than normal tissue, indicating potential for clinical modulation.

Morton DL, Wen DR, Wong JH, Economou JS, Cagle LA, Storm FK, Foshal LJ, Cochran AJ. **Technical details of intraoperative lymphatic mapping for early stage melanoma.** Arch Surg 1992; 127: 392–399.
This paper discusses the pros and cons of elective lymph node dissection and points the way to an alternative method of determining lymph node involvement based on the experience of 237 lymphadenectomy specimens.

Nabel GJ, Nabel EJ, Yang Z-Y, et al. **Direct gene transfer with DNA-liposome complexes in melanoma: Expression, biologic activity and lack of toxicity in humans.** Proc Natl Acad Sci USA 1993; 90: 11307-11311.
Five HLA-B7-negative patients with stage IV melanoma received direct injections of DNA-liposome complexes into cutaneous tumour nodules on more than one occasion. Plasmid DNA was detected in biopsied material from treated tumours but not in the serum of these patients. Expression of HLA-B7, encoded for by the injected cDNA, was found by immunohistochemistry and one patient demonstrated regression of an injected nodule associated with a response at distant sites. These results showed that not only was the direct injection of DNA into tumour tissue a safe procedure but also that it was followed by expression of the encoded protein which could lead to a potentially therapeutic response.

Pardoll DM. **Tumour antigens: a new look for the 1990s. News and Views.** Nature 1994; 369: 357–358.
Succinct review of the relevance of recent identifications of tumour-specific antigens, particularly from malignant melanomas, and their potential for immunotherapy.

Park KGM, Blessing K, McLaren KM, Watson ACH. **A study of thin (<1.5 mm) malignant melanomas with poor prognosis.** Br J Plast Surg 1993; 46: 607–610.
This study, using the Scottish Melanoma Group (SMG) database, identified 555 cases of which 30 recurred locally or metastasized during follow up. No local recurrence was found in completely excised tumours less than 1 mm thickness irrespective of the width of excision.

Richards JM, Mehta N, Ramming K, et al. **Sequential chemoimmunotherapy in the treatment of metastatic melanoma.** J Clin Oncol 1992; 10: 1338–1343.
Total of 74 cases treated with DTIC, BCNU, cisplatin and tamoxifen, IL-2 and IFN-α(!). Overall response rate of 55% including 15% CR), with a median time to progression if 9 months. Interestingly, 50% of cases developed vitiligo, presumably an autoimmune phenomenon.

Rosenberg S, Yang JC, Topalian S, et al. **Treatment of 283 consecutive patients with metastatic melanoma or renal cell cancer using high dose bolus IL-2.** J Am Med Assoc 1994; 271: 907–913.
Large review of 7 years experience at NCI, with IL-2, including 135 patients with melanoma. Of these 9 (7%) achieved CR and 14 (10%) achieved PR. Those achieving CR have had remarkably long remissions, free of disease.

Rosenberg S. **The immunotherapy and gene therapy of cancer.** J Clin Oncol 1992; 10: 180–199.

Soong S-J, Shaw HM, Balch CM, McCarthy WH, Urist MM, Lee JY. **Predicting survival and recurrence in localised melanoma: a multivariate approach.** World J Surg 1992; 16: 191–195.
An analysis on extensive data base (4568 patients) combining the series of University of Alabama (UAB) and the Sydney Melanoma Unit (SMU) which identified tumour thickness at diagnosis as the single most important prognostic indicator for all outcomes.

Timmons MJ, Merion Thomas J. **The width of excision of cutaneous melanoma.** Eur J Surg Oncol 1993; 19: 313–315.
This concise paper is an excellent up date with regards to attitudes surrounding width of excision of cutaneous malignant melanoma. It highlights the need for further research which has led to the prospective study undertaken by the Melanoma Group and the British Association of Plastic Surgeons currently in progress.

Timmons MJ. **Malignant melanoma excision margins: Plastic Surgery audit in Britain and Ireland, 1991, and review.** Br J Plast Surg 1993; 46: 525–531.
This paper identifies the discrepancy in treatment amongst British plastic surgeons and provides an excellent review of surgical practices.

Topalian S, Rivoltini L, Mancini M, et al. **Human CD4+ T cells specifically recognise a shared melanoma-associated antigen encoded by the tyrosinase gene.** Proc Natl Acad Sci USA 1994; 91: 9461–9465.
Based upon the specific release of cytokines from melanoma-specific CD4+ T cell lines in response to tumour antigens presented by Epstein-Barr virus-transformed B cells it proved possible to identify an immunodominant epitope from melanoma cells. This epitope was characterised as a product of the tyrosinase gene (see Brichard et al. 1993) indicating that it is presented by both class I and class II major histocompatibility molecules.

Veronesi U, Cascinelli N. **Narrow excision (1 cm margin): a safe procedure for thin cutaneous melanoma.** Arch Surg 1991; 126: 438–441.
This paper was instrumental in opening up the debate surrounding the width of excision for primary cutaneous melanoma. It reports on a WHO randomised prospective study of 612 patients with primary cutaneous malignant melanoma 1 mm. 84 patients (13.7%) have relapsed with disease within the eight year follow up but width of excision – 1 cm versus 3 cm did not affect overall survival.

Westerdahl J, Olsson H, Masback A, et al. **Use of sunbeds or sunlamps and malignant melanoma in southern Sweden.** Am J Epidemiol 1994; 140: 691–699.
This well conducted large case controlled study shows that the use of artificial sources of UV, including sunbeds, add to the risk of melanoma, particularly in younger people. A worrying fact in this paper is the observation that relatively small numbers of exposures to sunbeds are associated with statistically significant increase in melanoma risk in young people.

Whiteman D, Green A. **Melanoma and sunburn.** Cancer Causes Control 1994; 5: 564–572.
A useful review of 16 case control studies assessing sunburn as a risk factor for malignant melanoma. These well respected authors conclude, that only 4 studies have data which is of value, but do show that in all but one study sunburn is a risk factor for melanoma. This meta analysis does not however confirm that childhood sunburn is more dangerous than adult sunburn.

Wong JH, Skinner KA, Kim KA, Foshag LJ, Morton DL. **The role of surgery in the treatment of non regionally recurrent melanoma.** Surgery 1993; 113: 389–394.
This paper is based on 144 patients and using Cox regression analysis identifies anatomic site and number of metastases as important prognostic indicators for survival.

Index